Econometric Analysis of Health Data

Econometric Analysis of Health Data

Edited by

Andrew M. Jones

Department of Economics and Related Studies, University of York, UK

and

Owen O'Donnell

Department of Balkan, Slavic and Oriental Studies, University of Macdeonia, Greece

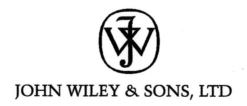

JOHN WILEY & SONS, LTD

Other Wiley Editorial Offices

John Wiley & Sons, Inc., 605 Third Avenue,
New York, NY 10158-0012, USA

Wiley-VCH Verlag GmbH, Pappelallee 3,
D-69469 Weinheim, Germany

John Wiley & Sons (Australia) Ltd, 33 Park Road, Milton,
Queensland 4064, Australia

John Wiley & Sons (Asia) Pte Ltd, 2 Clementi Loop #02-01,
Jin Xing Distripark, Singapore 129809

John Wiley & Sons (Canada) Ltd, 22 Worcester Road,
Rexdale, Ontario M9W 1L1, Canada

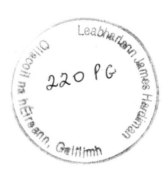

British Library Cataloguing in Publication Data

A catalogue record for this book is available from the British Library

ISBN 0-470-84145-1

Typeset in 9/11pt Times by Vision Typesetting, Manchester

Printed and Bound by Antony Rowe Ltd

Dedication

As secretary for the European Workshop series, Barbara Olive has been largely responsible for the smooth running of the preparations for the meetings. This dedication is a token of our gratitude. We wish her great happiness in her retirement.

Contents

Contributors

Richard Blundell *University College London, Department of Economics, Gower Street, London, WC1E 6BT, UK*

Partha Deb *Department of Economics, Indiana University Purdue University, Indianapolis, 425 University Boulevard, Indianapolis IN 46202, USA*

Dorly Deeg *Free University of Amsterdam, DeBoelelaan 1105, 1081 HV Amsterdam, The Netherlands*

Manfred Erbsland *Fachhochscule Neubrandenburg, Studiengang Pflege U Gesundh, 17041 Neubrandenburg, Germany*

Paul V. Grootendorst *Centre for Evaluation of Medicines, St Joseph's Hospital, Martha Wing Room H-3 19, 50 Charlton Ave East, Hamilton Ontario, Canada L8N 4A6*

Barton H. Hamilton *John M. Olin School of Business, Washington University in St Louis, Campus Box 1133, One Brookings Drive, St Louis MO 63130, USA*

Vivian H. Ho *Health Care Organization and Policy, Department of General Practice, University of Alabama Birmingham, RPHB 330, 1530 3rd Ave. South, Birmingham, AL 35294-0022, USA*

Ann M. Holmes *801 W. Michigan St., Room 4070, Spea-IUOUI, Indianapolis, IN 46202 5199, USA*

Sergi Jiménez-Martín *Department of Economics, Universidad Carlos III de Madrid, c/Madrid, 126E-28903 Getafe, Madrid, Spain*

Andrew M. Jones *Department of Economics and Related Studies, University of York, Heslington York YO10 5DD, UK*

Marcel Kerkhofs *Organisation of Labour Market Research, Tilburg University, PO Box 90153 5000 LE Tilberg, The Netherlands*

Jose M. Labeaga *Universidad Nacional De Educacion A Distancia, Facultad De CC. Economicas Y Empresariales, Departamento De Analisis Economico, Senda Del Rey, 11, 28040 Madrid, Spain*

Saturo Kobayashi *Institute of Policy and Planning Sciences, University of Tsukuba, Tsukuba, Ibaraki 305-8573, Japan*

Kajal Lahiri *Department of Economics, University of Albany: SUNY, 1400 Washington Avenue, Albany NY 12222, USA*

Myoung-jae Lee *Department of Economics, Sungkyunkwan University, 3–53 Myongryun-dony, Seoul 110-745, South Korea*

Maarten Lindeboom *Department of Economics, Vrije Universiteit, De Boelelaan 1105 1081 HV Amsterdam, The Netherlands*

Angel López-Nicolás *Universitat Pompen Fabra, Departmento de Economia Y Epresa CIRamon Trias Fargas 25-27, 08005-Barcelona, Spain*

Maite Martínez-Granado *Department of Economics, Department of Psychiatry, Universidad Carlos III de Madrid, c/Madrid, 126.E-28903 Getafe, Madrid, Spain*

Owen O'Donnell *Department of Balkan, Slavic and Oriental Studies, University of Macedonia, 156 Egnatia Street, Thessaloniki, 54006, Greece*

David Parkin *Department of Economics, City University, Northampton Square, London, EC1V 0HB, UK*

France Portrait *Faculty of Econometrics, Vrije Universiteit, De Boelelaan 1105 1081 HV Amsterdam, The Netherlands*

Nigel Rice *Centre for Health Economics, University of York, Heslington York YO1 5DD, UK*

Walter Ried   *Department of Economics, University of Mannheim, Seminargbaude AS, B247, 68131 Mannheim, Germany*

Jae G. Song   *Department of Economics, University of Albany: SUNY, 1400 Washington Avenue, Albany NY 12222, USA*

Matthew Sutton   *Department of General Practice, University of Glasgow, 4 Lancaster Crescent, Glasgow, G42 0RR, UK*

Volker Ulrich   *Ernst-Moritz-Arndt-Universität Greifswald, Rechts- und Staarswissenschaftliche Fakultät, Lehrstuhl für Allgemeine Volkswirtschaftslehre, insb. Finanzwissenshaft, Postfach, 17487 Greifswald, Germany*

Frank Windmeijer   *Institute for Fiscal Studies, 7 Ridgemount Street, London WCIE 7AE, UK*

Adam Wagstaff   *Visiting Research Fellow, Human Development Network, Room G3-038, The World Bank, 1818 H Street NW, Washington CD 20433, USA*

Steven T. Yen   *Department of Agricultural Economics, 308-D Morgan Hall, 2621 Morgan Circle, University of Tennessee, Knoxville, TN 37996-4518, USA*

Preface

The purpose of this book is to give readers convenient access to a collection of innovative applications of econometric methods to data on health and health care. The contributions are selected from papers presented at the European Workshops on Econometrics and Health Economics which have been published in *Health Economics*. The Workshops were established in York, with meetings in 1992 and 1993. Since then they have taken place annually, with locations in eight different European countries. Publication of the present volume marks the tenth anniversary of the Workshop series, the overall aim of which is to provide a forum for the development and dissemination of econometric methods in health economics. When the Workshops were first established, there were relatively few European researchers at the frontiers of quantitative research in the area. Advances in quantitative techniques and the increased availability of datasets and computing technology had created the potential for large returns from attracting more researchers into health econometrics. There are indications that these returns are now being reaped. Over the years, there has been a steady rise in the quantity and general quality of submissions received for each Workshop.

We would like to thank everyone who has participated in the Workshop series, whether as an author or a discussant, and all of those who have reviewed papers for *Health Economics*. Our particular gratitude goes to the local organisers of the Workshops: Eddy van Doorslaer (Antwerp, 1994), Lise Rochaix (Paris, 1995), Guillem Lopez-Casasnovas (Barcelona, 1996), João Pereira (Lisbon, 1997), Unto Hakkinen and Miika Linna (Helsinki, 1998), Giacomo Pignataro and Ilde Rizzo (Catania, 1999) and Maarten Lindeboom and France Portrait (Amsterdam, 2000).

Introduction

ANDREW M. JONES[1] AND OWEN O'DONNELL[2]

[1]*University of York, UK and* [2]*University of Macedonia, Greece*

The volume and range of applied econometric work in health economics has increased dramatically over the past decade. This trend can be expected to continue and, probably, accelerate. The increasing emphasis on evidence based policy, the wide availability of individual level data and the recurring statistical issues of latent variables, unobservable heterogeneity, and nonlinear models combine to make health and health care a particularly rich field for the application of econometric analysis. In this context, it has become increasingly important for the applied researcher in health economics to have a good knowledge of relevant contemporary econometric techniques. This volume is intended to contribute toward such an understanding.

In terms of methodology, all the papers selected for this volume fall within the broad heading of 'microeconometrics'; econometric analyses of individual level data. This reflects the emphasis on microeconomic analysis in health economics generally. Analyses of individual level survey data require the use of a wide range of nonlinear models. Examples include binary responses, multinomial responses, limited dependent variables, integer counts and measures of duration. Such nonlinear models dominate health econometrics and applications can be found across the four parts of this volume. Given that the focus of the volume is on providing examples of good econometric practice in relation to issues arising with health and health care data, the papers have been grouped according to common econometric themes rather than by the subject matter of the applications. Hence, Part I deals with latent variables and selection problems, Part II with count data and survival models, Part III with flexible and semiparametric estimators and Part IV with panel data. The intention is to enable easy identification of papers which deal with data problems and econometric issues similar to those the reader might face in their own research.

A peculiarity of the field is that the variables of interest, such as health or quality of life, are often unobservable and may only be measurable with error, for example, through subjective reports. The estimation issues arising are dealt with by the papers included in Part I, which covers latent variables and selection problems. Modelling the number of visits to a physician and the number of medicine prescriptions received has been a major issue in the health econometric literature. Part II contains three papers on such count data models, as well as one on the related econometric problem of modelling survival duration. Analysis of expenditure data is complicated when there is a high proportion of observations with zero expenditure in the sample, as is likely to be the case with consumption of health care or cigarettes. The consistency of standard approaches to the problem rest on the validity of distributional assumptions. The papers included in Part III use flexible and non/semiparametric methods to weaken required distributional assumptions while dealing with the limited dependent variable problem. As in other fields, the use of longitudinal data is becoming increasingly prevalent in health economics research. The chapters which constitute Part IV all use panel data and, within this context, deal with important issues for research in health and health care such as dynamics, unobservable heterogeneity, endogeneity, binary response, censoring and survival.

The remainder of this introduction expands on some of the common econometric problems confronted when analysing data on health and health care and, by reference to the individual chapters, identifies appropriate techniques to deal with these problems.

Econometric Analysis of Health Data. Edited by Andrew M. Jones and Owen O'Donnell
© 2002 John Wiley & Sons Ltd.

LATENT VARIABLES AND SELECTION PROBLEMS

LATENT HEALTH

In health economics, empirical analysis is complicated by the fact that theoretical models often involve inherently unobservable (latent) concepts such as 'health' or 'quality of life'. This latent variable problem is central to models of the demand for health and to the construction of health status indices. Information from observable indicators, such as chronic illness or self-reported health status, must be used to proxy the latent concepts. However, there may be reason to suspect that the relationships between the latent variables and their observable indicators differ systematically with observable or unobservable factors, potentially leading to endogeneity problems. The papers included in Part I address these issues.

Few papers in the health economics literature have been more influential than Grossman's demand for health model [1]. However, empirical testing of the model is complicated by the fact that the central concept, 'health', is inherently unobservable and has to be proxied by indicator variables. The multiple indicators multiple causes (MIMIC) model, which can be estimated as linear structural relationships (LISREL), has been widely used to deal with the latent variable issue. This is the approach adopted by both Wagstaff (Chapter 1) and Erbsland, Reid and Ulrich (Chapter 2) to estimate Grossman-type demand for health models.

In general, a MIMIC model of latent health has the form,

$$H^* = X_1\beta_1 + \varepsilon_1 \tag{1}$$

$$HI_j = \gamma_j H^* + \varepsilon_{2j}, \quad j = 1\ldots J \tag{2}$$

where H^* is (latent) health capital, HI_j is observable health indicator j e.g. self-reported health (multiple indicators) and the X_1 are exogenous socioeconomic variables (multiple causes).

Identification requires some normalization of the parameter vector γ and restrictions on the covariances, such that the latent H^* is proxied by some linear combination of the health indicators. Assuming joint normality of the errors terms, estimation can be carried out by full information maximum likelihood (FIML). This general model might be used to estimate, for example, health production functions, as well as the demand for health model.

Application to the demand for health requires supplementation of Equations 1 and 2 with a demand for medical care equation,

$$M_k = \alpha_k H^* + X_{2k}\beta_{2k} + \varepsilon_{3k}, \quad k = 1,\ldots K \tag{3}$$

where M_k is medical care k e.g. physician visits and X_2 are exogenous socioeconomic factors. The latent health variable is endogenous in Equation 3 and exclusion restrictions on X_2 are required for identification.

Equations 1–3 represent the basic structure of the empirical models estimated by Wagstaff and Erbsland et al. The latter focus on the health impact of the environment, which is itself treated as a latent variable, proxied by indicators of noise and air pollution. Consequently, a measurement equation for quality of the environment, analogous to Equation 2, is added to the model. Latent environmental quality is included as a regressor in the latent health Equation 1, where it is treated as exogenous and found to have a significant positive effect.

Despite claims to the contrary, the links between the theoretical and empirical sections of applied econometric papers are often tenuous. This is not the case with the Wagstaff and Erbsland et al. papers, which both give careful consideration to the transition from Grossman's theoretical model to a feasible empirical specification of it. Indeed, this is the primary concern of Wagstaff, who argues that Grossman's empirical formulation, the basis of previous testing, fails to capture the dynamic character of the theoretical model and that this inconsistency may explain the apparent rejections of the model in earlier empirical work. The issue concerns the structural impact of health capital on the demand for medical care. From the optimality conditions, this marginal impact is negative for plausible values of the depreciation rate (Erbsland et al.). However, the restrictions imposed in order to arrive at an empirical specification result in health capital entering the structural demand for medical care equation with a parameter of positive unity. The empirical estimates presented in Chapters 1 and 2, as well as previous results obtained by Wagstaff [2], all support the theoretical predictions of the model but are inconsistent with the (Grossman) empirical specification. Wagstaff proposes an alternative empirical formulation, which results in health capital entering the structural demand for medical care equation with a negative parameter. In this respect, it is more consistent with the theory, although Erbsland et al. question whether the specification can be derived explicitly from the theoretical model. The formulation involves linear, rather than log-linear, specifications of the investment identity and the demand for health equation and relaxation of the neoclassical assumption of instantaneous adjustment of health stock to its desired level. As a result, dynamics are introduced to the empirical model.

In general, Wagstaff finds observable health indicators to be good proxies, latent health accounting for a minimum of 34% (functional limitations) and a maximum of 90% (self-assessed health) of the variance of the indicators. The proxies are less close in Erbsland et al.; for one indicator (duration of sick leave) only 11% of the variation is attributable to latent health and for two of the remaining three proxies, the majority of their variance is not attributable to latent health. Wagstaff's estimate of the variance in self-assessed health attributable to latent health is more than twice that of Erbsland et al. The source of such inconsistencies needs further attention before the MIMIC model can be used to identify the most reliable indicators of latent health. In both studies, a substantial amount of the variation in the observable health indicators cannot be attributed to latent health. This raises the question of what accounts for the unexplained variation and the possibility that such measurement error will create bias when observable indicators are used to proxy unobservable health.

Kerkhofs and Lindeboom (Chapter 3) take up this measurement error issue. As with Wagstaff and Erbsland et al., self-assessed health is treated as an indicator of unobservable health, but now allowance is made for the possibility that the relationship between the indicator and underlying latent concept varies with third factors. Their focus is on the possibility of state-dependent reporting errors arising from financial incentives and/or social pressures for non-workers to report ill health. This would create bias if, for example, self-assessed health were included as a regressor in a labour supply model or used to examine income-related health inequalities.

Correction for state-dependent reporting errors involves using an objective measure of health, H^0, in this case the Hopkins symptom checklist, plus socio-demographics, X_1, to instrument the latent variable, H^*. Identification of reporting behaviour relies on the assumption that, controlling for H^0 and X_1, employment status, S, contains no independent information on H^*. For example, there is no correlation between the unobservable determinants of employment and health, subject to the stated conditioning. Then, controlling for H^0 and X_1 any effect of S on self-assessed health, HI, can be attributed to reporting behaviour.

Both reported and objective health are categorical variables, which are assumed to be related to latent health as follows,

$$H^* = f(H^0) + X_1\beta + \varepsilon, \quad \varepsilon \sim N(0,1) \quad (4)$$

$$HI = i \ if \ \mu_{i-1} < H^* \leq \mu_i, \quad i = 1, \ldots m \quad (5)$$

$$\mu_i = g_i(S, X_2), \quad i = 1, \ldots m-1 \quad (6)$$

Reporting errors are allowed for through the dependence of the threshold values of the ordered probit, μ, on S and X_2. Comparison of Equations 4–6 with Equations 1 and 2 reveals that the basic structure of the models is the same.

The Kerkhofs and Lindeboom approach is more general in the sense that the parameters of the measurement equation are allowed to vary with observable characteristics.

Normalizing on the reporting behaviour of the employed, early retirees understate and the unemployed overstate their ill health to a moderate, but not significant, extent. Reporting behaviour is more distinct among those claiming disability insurance. Of the disability claimants who reported their health to be bad, one-third of them would not have done so had they been in employment, all else equal. There is no evidence that other exogenous characteristics – gender, age, marital status, education and religion – have an effect on misreporting. This latter result is reassuring for the health economics community which makes widespread use of the self-assessed health indicator, but the scale of the reporting biases deriving from disability status does give cause for concern.

A limitation of the approaches described above is that they treat health as a single latent concept and do not allow for its multidimensionality. For this reason, researchers might prefer to work directly with a range of health indicators, rather than attempt to compress these into a single latent index. So, it might be argued, that it is better to enter a range of health indicators directly into an utilization equation such as Equation 3. However, this approach leads to collinearity, degrees of freedom and interpretation problems when the number of indicators is large. This is typically the case when modelling health/ social care utilization by the elderly when the researcher may have a very large number of activities of daily living (ADL) indicators. Portrait, Lindeboom and Deeg (Chapter 15) measure health status by a method which compresses information from a large range of indicators but preserves the multidimensionality of the concept. The technique is the Grade of Membership (GoM) method of Manton and Woodbury [3]. Its application is considered in detail in an earlier paper by Portrait, Lindeboom and Deeg [4]. The technique takes information from a range of indicators and collapses these into different dimensions of health status, or pure types. Simultaneously, it estimates the degree to which an individual can be classified by each of the pure types. These 'Grades of Membership' are represented by a set of weights, summing to one for each individual across the different dimensions. For example, Portrait et al. are able to collapse 21 indicators of the health of a sample of the elderly into six pure types: chronic pulmonary disease and cancers, other chronic diseases, cognitively impaired, arthritis patients, cardiovascular diseases and a healthy group. An individual's health status is measured, continuously and in a multidimensional manner, by the set of weights indicating the extent to which they belong to each of the pure types.

For health applications, the GoM method has four main advantages over other data reduction methods, such as factor analysis or principal components. First, estimation of the dimensions and the individuals' attachments to these is carried out simultaneously. Second, it is nonparametric. Third, it respects the multidimensionality of health, in the sense that individuals are not classified to one type but are associated, to varying extents, with various types. Finally, it respects the dynamic nature of health, and so is suitable for longitudinal analysis, by producing a health measure, i.e. the weights, which is continuous. With such properties, the approach deserves further attention in the health economics literature.

SELECTION

Lahiri and Song (Chapter 4) focus on a single dimension of health – illness related to smoking. They recognize that individuals may, rationally, self-select into and out of smoking behaviour on the basis of their perception of their own risk of contracting a smoking related illness. Provided such perceptions are based on some true information, which may come from changes in health over time, failure to allow for self-selection will bias estimated health effects of smoking based on comparisons between the health of smoking and non-smoking samples.

Index functions for the decisions to start and stop smoking are specified from comparisons of lifetime utilities in respective states. These provide the means of correcting for selection in estimation of health outcome functions for non-smokers, ex-smokers and current smokers. Outcomes are binary – whether the individual has contracted a smoking-related disease. So, the model consists of a set of three binary switching regressions (probits), with sequential selection through the starting and stopping decision functions. Trivariate normality is assumed, facilitating estimation by FIML. The paper is instructive for anyone interested in estimating selection models by FIML. The authors describe how to go about testing for endogeneity (trivariate), normality and heteroskedasticity, as well as correcting for the latter. They also give useful tips on how to specify the likelihood to increase computational speed and aid convergence.

Evidence of substantial selection bias is found. The true mean risk factor for current smokers is estimated at around 20%, much higher than the observed risk factor in the sample for this group of 16%. Individuals who choose to continue smoking have a lower than average underlying disposition to contract a smoking-related illness and so the incidence of disease amongst this group is lower than would be found if there were random alloca-

tion to smoking. Given this, any estimation of the impact of smoking on health through comparison of the incidence of disease among smokers and non-smokers will be downward biased. This is an important finding calling for revision of previous estimates of the health costs of smoking.

COUNT DATA AND SURVIVAL ANALYSIS

COUNTS, HETEROGENEITY AND ZEROS

Count data regression is appropriate when the dependent variable is a non-negative integer-valued count, $y = 0, 1, 2, \ldots$. Typically these models are applied when the distribution of the dependent variable is skewed to the right, and contains a large proportion of zeros and a long right-hand tail. The most common examples in health economics are measures of health care utilization, such as numbers of physician visits or the number of prescriptions dispensed over a given period.

The basic approach to count data is to assume the probability of observing a count of y events over a fixed interval can be specified as a Poisson process. In order to condition the outcome, y_i, for observation i on a set of explanatory variables, X_i, it is usually assumed that,

$$E(y_i | X_i) = \lambda_i = \exp(X_i \beta) \qquad (7)$$

A peculiarity of the Poisson distribution is that both its mean and variance are equal to its one parameter, λ_i. Often, this restriction is inconsistent with data. In health care applications, for example, there is usually evidence of overdispersion, i.e. $E(y_i | X_i) < Var(y_i | X_i)$. One consequence can be under-prediction of the number of observations with zero counts; again, an empirical feature of many health care applications. Additional dispersion, due to unobservable heterogeneity, spreads the distribution out to the tails. In this sense, the phenomenon of excess zeros is no more than a symptom of overdispersion (see Mullahy [5]).

Although overdispersion can account for excess zeros, it may be that there is something special about zero observations *per se*, and an excess of zero counts may not be associated with increased dispersion throughout the distribution. Two approaches place particular emphasis on the role of zeros; zero-inflated models and hurdle, or two-part, models. The 'zero-inflated' or 'with zeros' model is a mixing specification which adds extra weight to the probability of observing a zero. This can be interpreted as a splitting mechanism which divides individuals into non-users and potential-users; that is, one treats the observations as being of fundamentally different types in relation to their demand for health care.

In contrast, the hurdle, or two-part, models, tend to be motivated by a representation of the patient–doctor relationship as one of principal and agent. This makes a distinction between patient-initiated decisions, such as the first contact with a general practitioner (GP), and decisions that are influenced by the doctor, such as repeat visits, prescriptions, and referrals (see for example, Pohlmeier and Ulrich [6]). The consequence, in statistical terms, is a hurdle model which allows the participation decision, $(0, 1)$, and the positive count, $(1, 2, 3 \ldots)$, to be generated by separate probability processes. The two-parts of the model can be estimated separately as a binary process, e.g. probit, and a truncated at zero count process.

Grootendorst (Chapter 5) provides an empirical comparison of two-part and zero-inflated specifications. The study uses data from the 1990 Ontario Health Survey to analyse the impact of copayments on the utilization of prescription drugs by the elderly, exploiting the fact that individuals become eligible for zero copayments on their 65th birthday. Neither zero-inflated nor two-part models (TPM) are parsimonious, often doubling the number of parameters to be estimated. Since more complicated models may be prone to over-fitting, Grootendorst uses out-of-sample forecasting accuracy to evaluate their performance. The models are estimated on a random sample of 70% of the observations. The estimated models are used to compute predictions for the remaining 30% (the forecast sample). Models are then compared on the basis of the mean squared error for the forecast sample. In addition to the split-sample analysis, Voung's non-nested test is computed. The TPM outperforms the other specifications on all of the criteria.

Deb and Trivedi [7] introduce a different approach to the zero count issue. Health care survey data are not usually specific to a period of illness but to a period of calendar time, during which the first recorded visit is not necessarily the initial one in a course of treatment. In this context, it is argued, a TPM specification cannot be justified by appeal to a principal–agent characterization of the data generating process. Their alternative approach is based on the argument that observed counts are sampled from a mixture of populations which differ in respect of their underlying (latent) health, and so demands for health care. That is, there may be severely ill individuals, who are high frequency users, at one extreme and perfectly healthy individuals, who are non-users, at the other. This characterization of the data can be captured by latent class models, for example, the finite mixture model (FMM) which postulates that each observation of a random variable is drawn from a super-population which is itself an additive mixture of C distinct sub-populations, j, which appear in proportions, π_j (Heckman and Singer

[8]). That is, the density of a C-point FMM takes the form,

$$P(y_i | \cdot) = \sum_{j=1}^{C} \pi_j P_j(y_i | \cdot), \quad 0 \le \pi_j \le 1, \sum_{j=1}^{C} \pi_j = 1 \qquad (8)$$

This density can serve as an approximation to any true but unknown distribution. In this sense, the approach is semiparametric. Specifying each of the $P_j(y_i | .)$ as a separate negbin process, gives the negbin FMM. Estimation is carried out by maximum likelihood, with the π_j's being estimated simultaneously with the other parameters of the model.

Deb and Trivedi [7] not only argue that their approach is more consistent with the data generating process than the TPM but that the zero-inflated models are a special case of the general FMM with unobservable heterogeneity. That is, in the zero-inflated models, the zero counts alone are presumed to be sampled from a mixture of two sub-populations (non-users and potential users).

Deb and Holmes (Chapter 6) apply both a count and continuous version of the FMM to mental health care visits and expenditure data from the US National Medical Expenditure Survey. In each case, appealing to evidence from Deb and Trivedi [7], they argue that two points of support, i.e. $C = 2$, are sufficient to approximate the underlying distribution. In addition to dealing with the 'zeros' issue, they argue the FMM is better suited to representing the behaviour of high frequency users, who account for a large fraction of mental health care. While the TPM distinguishes between non-users and users, it makes no further distinction across the users. The FMM, on the other hand, allows users to be comprised of a variety of population types, one of which might be severely ill, high-dependency cases. Deb and Holmes seek a model which can be used for capitation-based funding and so are particularly concerned with a achieving a good fit with the data, not only in respect of representing the means of health care use among sub-populations but also capturing the full distributions of use. The performance of the count version of the FMM is compared with the negbin hurdle model for mental health care visits, while the continuous FMM is compared with the censored lognormal regression for (positive) expenditures. Comparison is based both on in-sample model selection criteria (Akaike and Bayesian information criteria) and goodness-of-fit, plus out-of-sample forecasting to check for over-parameterization. Both the in-sample and out-of-sample comparisons consistently find in favour of the FMM for both the count and continuous models. The FMM appears to be particularly successful in representing high intensity use.

Taking the results of Grootendorst and of Deb and Holmes together, one might conclude that while the TPM can out-perform a restricted version of the mixing model, i.e. the zero-inflated model, this is no longer true when the restriction on the mixing model is relaxed. However, one should be cautious about drawing such conclusions given the two studies differ not only in the specifications compared but in the types of health care and countries examined. Jimenez, Labeaga and Martinez-Granado (Chapter 7) provide further valuable evidence on the relative performance of the TPM and FMM specifications. They estimate (reduced form) demand for health care equations for 12 European countries using three waves of data from the *European Community Household Panel*, distinguishing between utilization of GPs and specialists.

The TPM and FMM estimated are the same as those adopted by Deb and Holmes. Model selection is based on Akaike and Bayesian information criteria. For GP visits, the results suggest the FMM is more consistent with the data than the TPM. This is true both when parameter homogeneity is imposed across countries and for the vast majority of comparisons on a country-by-country basis. For specialists, a different picture emerges, for the homogeneous parameter specification, the TPM is favoured and this is true for six of the 12 individual country comparisons. Aggregating the information criteria across countries also favours the TPM.

Jimenez *et al.* rationalize the difference in the preferred specification for GP and for specialist visits on the basis that multiple spells of illness/treatment are likely to be observed for GP visits but the survey data for specialist visits are more likely to represent a single spell. Given this, the TPM, with its rationalization through the principal–agent story, should be more suited to representing specialist visit data than GP visit data. This is an important warning against the idea that there is one econometric specification waiting to be discovered that is best suited to modelling all types of health care utilization data. The appropriate method can be expected to vary with, for example, the type of health care, the nature and length of the survey and the nature of the health care system. Despite finding in its favour with respect to GP visits, Jimenez *et al.* express some apprehension about the latent class approach. It is somewhat of a statistical black-box, the specification not being derived from an economic theory of health care demand. The large number of parameters to be estimated can also lead to problems of non-convergence of the likelihood and over-parameterization.

The primary motivation of Jimenez *et al.* is not to compare econometric specifications but to examine heterogeneity in the demand for health care across European countries. They examine both the extent to which the behavioural response of health care utilization to certain factors, such as health and income, varies across countries and the impact of health system characteristics on utilization. There are significant differences across countries, the restriction of parameter homogeneity being rejected. However, there are also similarities in the effect of variables such as the health stock, income or family structure on utilization. Health system characteristics do have significant effects on utilization. For example, a GP gatekeeper system increases frequency of visits to GPs and reduces those to specialists. Fee-for-service payment has the opposite effect on the relative demand for GPs and specialists, a finding consistent with induced demand theory. Total health care expenditure, and the fraction accounted for by the public sector, have no impact on GP use but do raise demand for specialist visits.

EVALUATION OF TREATMENT EFFECTS

Evaluation is central to the health economics literature. The goal of many researchers is to identify the impact of some treatment on outcomes and compare this with the cost of the treatment. The core of the problem is the identification of the treatment effect. This is made difficult by the fact that it is impossible to observe the counterfactual. That is, we can observe the outcome for some individual, i, with treatment, y_{1i}, but it is impossible to observe the outcome *for the same individual*, without treatment, y_{0i}. Hence, individual specific treatment effects, $y_{1i} - y_{0i}$, are inherently unidentified. A way out is to estimate a particular aspect of the distribution of treatment effects; of which, the most popular choice is the average treatment effect (ATE), given by $E(y_{1i} - y_{0i})$. This is convenient because the linearity of the expectations operator allows the statistic to be estimated through comparison of the two marginal means, i.e. $E(y_{1i} - y_{0i}) = E(y_{1i}) - E(y_{0i})$. Confounding factors can be controlled for either experimentally, by randomization, or statistically, by suitable regression methods.

The ATE is, however, only one of many possible summary statistics of the distribution of treatment effects. While it is likely to be of great policy interest, other statistics may also be informative. Lee and Kobayashi (Chapter 8) introduce two mean-based 'proportional' treatment effects which are particularly suitable when the outcome variable is a count, to be modelled by an exponential regression function. The problem with using the ATE in such a regression framework is that determinants of the outcome which are common across the treatments do not cancel out as they do with a linear regression. Lee and Kobayashi's solution is to define a proportional ATE, i.e. $E(y_{1i} - y_{0i})/E(y_{0i})$, which removes the nuisance terms irrespective of whether the regression function is linear or exponential. This can be calculated both conditional and unconditional on third factors which interact with treatment. Lee and Kobayashi suggest estimating the latter, which can be thought of as the marginal treatment effect and may be of central importance, by the geometric average, across the sample, of their proportional ATE which can be calculated by evaluating this statistic at the means of the data. Confidence intervals are derived for this marginal effect.

The outcome variables in the Lee and Kobayashi study are physician visits and hospital days and the 'treatment' is physical exercise. Two waves of the US Health and Retirement Survey are used allowing the potential endogeneity of exercise to be dealt with by first differencing. This raises a potential problem of identification if the treatment effects were to be a function of any time invariant parameters. Foreseeing this, the authors interact exercise, which is time varying, with all of the control variables. Light exercise has a positive short-run effect on health care use and a negative long-run effect. Vigorous exercise has a negative effect in both the short and long run. However, none of the estimated treatment effects are significantly different from zero.

DURATION ANALYSIS AND HETEROGENEITY

Count data models are, in general, dual to duration models. This duality applies to particular parametric models: if the count is Poisson, the duration is exponential; if it is negative binomial, the duration is Weibull. By using more information – the continuous variation in durations – duration models offer efficiency gains over count models. In health economics, obvious applications of duration analysis, or survival analysis as it is known in the epidemiology and biostatistics literature, are to lifespan, mortality rates and length of hospital stay.

For example, let length of stay be a random variable M with a continuous probability density function $f(m)$, where m is a particular realization of M. The probability of a length of stay of at least m is given by *the survival function*,

$$S(m) = 1 - F(m) = 1 - \int_0^m f(t)dt = P(M \geq m) \qquad (9)$$

A related concept is the *hazard rate*,

$$\lambda(m) = \lim_{\Delta m \to 0} \frac{P(m < M \leq m + \Delta m \mid M \geq m)}{\Delta m}$$

$$= \frac{f(m)}{S(m)} \qquad (10)$$

which, in this example, is the rate of discharge after a length of stay of m, given a length of stay of at least m.

In a variety of contexts, there may be considerable interest in the behaviour of the hazard rate over time. If the hazard rate is increasing (decreasing) with time, there is said to be positive (negative) duration dependence. Disentangling duration dependence from the effects of unobservable heterogeneity is a central problem in the literature. To illustrate, imagine that length of stay data is sampled from two groups, a 'very ill' group and a 'less ill' group, which differ in respect of their health status. The hazard rates are constant (time invariant) for each group but their magnitudes differ. As time goes by, the sample will contain a higher proportion of those with the lower hazard rate; as those with the higher hazard will have been discharged. If the heterogenity is unobserved, this will lead to a spurious estimate of negative duration dependence.

Unobservable heterogeneity can be incorporated by adding a general heterogeneity effect v and specifying the survival function as,

$$S(m) = \int_v S(m \mid v)g(v)dv \qquad (11)$$

where the unknown distribution $g(v)$ can be modelled parametrically using a variety of distributions, the gamma being a popular choice. Alternatively, returning to the latent class model discussed above, the Heckman and Singer [8] nonparametric approach can be adopted by approximating the distribution of v by a discrete distribution, characterized by mass-points and probabilities, that are estimated along with the other parameters of the model.

Duration models can also be extended to allow for multiple destinations, or competing risks. Hamilton and Ho's (Chapter 9) study of the surgical volume–outcome relationship for hip fractures in Québec provides an example that combines competing risks, unobservable heterogeneity, and fixed effects. They use 3 years of hospital discharge data. The longitudinal nature of the data allows control for quality of providers through hospital specific fixed effects, while analysing within-hospital volume–outcome relationships. As a result, they can discriminate between the 'practice makes perfect effect' and 'selective referral effect' (that hospitals with good outcomes will get more referrals).

Their competing risks specification allows for a correlation between the two outcomes; post-surgery length of stay and inpatient mortality. This is important, *ceteris paribus*, a death in hospital is more likely for a patient with a longer length of stay. With two exhaustive and mutually exclusive destinations for discharges, alive (*a*) or dead (*d*), the probability of exit to state *r*, after a length of stay *m*, for patient *i*, in hospital *h*, at period *t*, with observable characteristics *X*, is,

$$f_r(m_{iht} \mid X_{iht}) = \lambda_r(m_{iht} \mid X_{iht})$$

$$\prod_{k \in a,d} \exp\left[-\int_0^{m_{iht}} \lambda_k(u \mid X_{iht}) \mathrm{d}u \right], \quad r = a, d$$
(12)

This is a variant on Equation 10, rewritten with the exit probability rather than the hazard rate on the left-hand side. The first term on the right-hand side is the transition intensity, the equivalent of the hazard rate in single destination models and the second term is the survivor function. A functional form for the transition intensity must be chosen. Hamilton and Ho use the proportional hazards specification, with a log-logistic distribution for the baseline transition intensity. The distribution of unobservable heterogeneity (frailty) is approximated using the Heckman-Singer nonparametric approach. Three mass points are used (*C* = 3), the interpretation being that the distribution is made up of three types of patients, and their associated probabilities, π_j, are estimated along with the other parameters.

The results of the study show that when hospital fixed effects are added to the model the coefficient on volume, measured by the logarithm of live discharges, declines substantially and becomes insignificant with respect to live discharges. Volume does not have a significant effect on inpatient deaths with or without hospital fixed effects, although cruder models without unobservable heterogeneity and with fewer controls for co-morbidities do show a significant effect. Allowance for hospital fixed effects and individual unobservable heterogeneity is therefore important in testing the 'practice makes perfect' hypothesis.

FLEXIBLE AND SEMIPARAMETRIC ESTIMATORS

FLEXIBLE ESTIMATORS

In health survey data, measures of continuous dependent variables such as alcohol, tobacco or medical care expenditures invariably contain a high proportion of zero observations and limited dependent variable techniques are required. The Tobit model is the most basic of such techniques. In this approach, both the participation (e.g., whether to start or quit smoking) and levels (e.g., how much to spend on cigarettes) decisions are represented by the same linear function of observables and unobser-

vables. The double hurdle approach is less restrictive, in that the determinants of participation and of consumption are allowed to differ. However, a limitation of the standard double hurdle specification is that it is based on the assumption of bivariate normality for the error distribution. Empirical results will be sensitive to misspecification, and maximum likelihood (ML) estimates will be inconsistent if the normality assumption is violated. This may be particularly relevant if the model is applied to a dependent variable that has a highly skewed distribution, as is often the case with the applications mentioned above.

A flexible generalization of the double hurdle model is proposed by Yen and Jones (Chapter 10). The Box–Cox double hurdle model allows explicit comparisons of a wide range of limited dependent variable specifications that have been used in the health economics literature. As in the standard double hurdle model, the conditional distribution of the latent variables is assumed to be bivariate normal, permitting stochastic dependence between the two error terms. Unlike the standard model, the observed variable is related to the underlying latent variable by a Box–Cox transformation. This relaxes the normality assumption on the conditional distribution of *y*. This flexibility is at the price of making greater demands on the data and care should be taken to check for evidence of over-fitting.

Yen and Jones derive the log-likelihood function for a sample of independent observations and show that the general model can be restricted to give various special cases:

1. The Box–Cox double hurdle with independent errors.
2. The standard double hurdle with dependence.
3. The generalized Tobit model with log(*y*) as dependent variable in the regression part of the model. Then, assuming independence between the two error terms, gives the special case of the two-part model in which normality is assumed and the equations are linear.

The Box–Cox double hurdle model is applied to data on the number of cigarettes smoked in a sample of current and ex-smokers from the British Health and Lifestyle Survey. The estimated Box–Cox parameter (λ) is significantly different from both zero and one, indicating rejection of both the standard double hurdle and the generalized Tobit models.

SEMIPARAMETRIC ESTIMATORS

The Box–Cox model is a flexible specification in the sense that, up to a point, the data are allowed to determine the functional form, with linearity and log-linearity available as special cases to be tested, rather than imposed. However, it remains parametric, requiring the imposition of particular distributional assumptions. In recent years, the econometrics literature has seen an explosion of theoretical developments in nonparametric and semiparametric methods, which relax functional form and distributional assumptions. These are beginning to be used in health economics, with the applications of the finite mixture model in Chapters 6, 7 and 9, discussed above, providing good examples.

Many non- and semiparametric methods are founded on the Rosenblatt–Parzen kernel density estimator. This method uses appropriately weighted local averages to estimate probability density functions of unknown form; in effect, using a smoothed histogram to estimate the density. The kernel function provides the weighting scheme; its bandwidth determines the size of the 'window' of observations that are used, and the height of the kernel function gives the weight attached to each observation. This weight varies with the distance between the observation and the point at which the density is being estimated. Variants on this basic method of density estimation are also used to estimate distribution functions, regression functionals, and response functions (see e.g., Pagan and Ullah [9]).

Blundell and Windmeijer (Chapter 11) provide an example of the use of a semiparametric estimator to deal with sample selection bias. The context for their analysis is the design of a regression-based formula for the allocation of resources across geographic areas to hospitals in the English NHS. Differences in average waiting times for elective surgery are used to identify the determinants of the demand for acute hospital services. The equilibrium waiting time framework is used, but in order to identify the impact of need variables on the demand for services the analysis selects areas with low waiting times. This creates the possibility of sample selection bias and, to add robustness to the analysis, the standard Heckit two-step estimator is compared to a semiparametric selection model. This relies on the fact that the sample selection model can be written as a 'partially linear model' (Robinson [10]),

$$y_i = X_i\beta + g(\eta_i) + \varepsilon_i \tag{13}$$

where η_i is the linear index from a (probit) selection equation.

Estimation of the partially linear model is handled by taking the expectation of Equation 13 conditional on η and then differencing to give,

$$y_i - E(y_i | \eta_i) = [X_i - E(X_i | \eta_i)]\beta + \varepsilon_i \tag{14}$$

given the conditional moment conditions

$E(\varepsilon | \eta) = E(\varepsilon | X, \eta) = 0$. The conditional expectations $E(y_i | \eta)$ and $E(X_i | \eta)$ can be replaced by nonparametric regressions of y and each element of X on an estimate of η. Then ordinary least squares (OLS) applied to Equation 14 gives $\sqrt{n}$-consistent and asymptotically normal estimates of β, although the asymptotic approximation may perform poorly in finite samples and bootstrap methods are preferable.

Parkin, Rice, and Sutton (Chapter 12) examine age, time and cohort effects on GP utilization and reported morbidity with data from the British General Household Survey (GHS). These relationships are likely to be highly nonlinear and be subject to sampling variability. A standard regression approach can deal with the latter problem but cannot capture the nonlinearity well through a linear specification or even polynomial generalizations. On the other hand, simple histograms of, for example, GP use against birth, age or survey years confound the nonlinearity with the sampling variability. Underlying patterns may be obscured by data which are overly 'rough' because of noise associated with adjacent year fluctuations.

The starting point for their analysis is a general relationship between GP utilization (y) and age (X),

$$y_i = g(X_i) + \varepsilon_i \tag{15}$$

The relationship is presented graphically using a plot of the lowess estimator. This is a kernel-based method that extends the Nadaraya–Watson estimator by fitting local polynomials. However most of the analysis uses an alternative method, roughness penalized least squares (RPLS). This method minimizes a penalized sum of squares and is implemented by replacing the 'continuous' variable, age, by a full set of binary indicators for each year of age. Simply regressing y on these dummy variables gives a nonparametric regression estimate in the form of a (highly discontinuous) step-function. The method of RPLS imposes smoothness on this regression through the penalty function. This puts restrictions on the coefficients for adjacent years of age, in order to penalize large values of the second derivative g''. The degree of smoothing is determined by the weight given to the penalty function and this is chosen by cross validation. The basic model can be extended by adding a linear function of other variables (Z),

$$y_i = Z_i\beta + g(X_i) + \varepsilon_i \tag{16}$$

so that the model takes the partially linear form discussed above. Again estimation is done by RPLS. Parkin et $al.$'s results show that linear age specifications are rejected for all models and evidence of time heterogeneity is found in one of the morbidity measures, limiting long-standing illness, and in GP utilization.

CLASSIC AND SIMULATION METHODS FOR PANEL DATA

UNOBSERVABLE HETEROGENEITY IN NONLINEAR MODELS

Applied work in health economics frequently has to deal with both the existence of unobservable individual effects, that are often likely to be correlated with observed explanatory variables, and with the need to use nonlinear models to deal with qualitative and limited dependent variables. The combined effect of these two problems creates difficulties for the analysis of longitudinal data, particularly if the model includes dynamic effects such as lagged adjustment or addiction.

Consider a nonlinear model, in which there are repeated measurements ($t = 1,\ldots, T$) for a sample of n individuals ($i = 1,\ldots, n$), for example, a binary choice model based on the latent variable specification,

$$y^*_{it} = X_{it}\beta + v_i + \varepsilon_{it},\qquad(17)$$

where $y_{it} = 1$ if $y^*_{it} > 0$, and v_i is an unobservable time invariant individual effect. Then, assuming that the distribution of ε_{it} is symmetric with distribution function $F(.)$,

$$P(y_{it} = 1 \mid X_{it}, v_i) = P(\varepsilon_{it} > - X_{it}\beta - v_i) = F(X_{it}\beta + v_i)\qquad(18)$$

This illustrates the 'problem of incidental parameters', that arises if the v_i's are treated as parameters, or 'fixed effects', to be estimated along with the β's. As $n \to \infty$ the number of parameters to be estimated (β, v) also grows. In linear models β and v are asymptotically independent, which means that taking mean deviations or differencing allows the derivation of estimators for β that do not depend on v. In general, this is not possible in nonlinear models and the inconsistency of estimates of v carries over into estimates of β (an exception to this general rule is the conditional logit estimator).

Assuming that v and ε are normally distributed and independent of X_{it} gives the random effects probit model (REP). In this case v can be integrated out to give the sample log-likelihood function,

$$\ln L = \sum_{i=1}^{n} \ln \int_{-\infty}^{\infty} \prod_{t=1}^{T} \Phi[d_{it}(X_{it}\beta + v)]f(v)dv \qquad(19)$$

where $d_{it} = 2y_{it} - 1$. This expression contains a univariate integral which can be approximated by Gauss-hermite quadrature (Butler and Moffitt [11]). This model is widely used in applied work, but it relies on the maintained assumptions that v is normal and uncorrelated with the regressors. Lopéz (Chapter 13) applies methods that relax the assumption that the effects and regressors are uncorrelated while Deb (Chapter 14) introduces a semiparametric method, based on finite mixtures, that relaxes the assumption of normality.

An approach to dealing with individual effects that are correlated with the regressors is to specify $E(v \mid X)$ directly. For example, in dealing with a random effects probit model, Chamberlain [12] suggests using,

$$v_i = X_i\alpha + u_i, u_i \sim iid\, N(0, \sigma^2) \qquad(20)$$

where $X_i = (X_{i1},\ldots, X_{iT})$. Then, by substituting Equation 20 into Equation 17, the distribution of y_{it} conditional on X_i but marginal to v_i has the probit form,

$$P(y_{it} = 1) = \Phi[(1 + \sigma^2)^{-\frac{1}{2}}(X_{it}\beta + X_i\alpha)] \qquad(21)$$

The model could be estimated directly by ML, but Chamberlain suggests a minimum distance estimator. This takes the estimates from reduced form probits on X_{it}, for each cross-section, and imposes the restrictions implied by Equation 21 to retrieve the parameters of interest (β, σ). Bover and Arellano [13] and Labeaga [14] develop and apply the Chamberlain approach to deal with situations that combine a dynamic model and limited dependent variables. Bover and Arellano show that the problem can be formulated in terms of an asymptotically efficient GMM estimator. They also propose a less efficient, but computationally convenient, two-step within-groups estimator. This applies the standard within-groups estimator, using the fitted values of the latent variables from each of the T reduced forms.

López (Chapter 13) makes use of the within-groups approach to estimate the demand for medical care using the Spanish Continuous Family Expenditure Survey. The dependent variable measures expenditure on non-refundable visits to medical practitioners, for which 60% of households make at least one purchase during the eight quarters that they are measured. This leads López to use an infrequency of purchase specification, which allows a separate hurdle for non-participation, identified as no purchases during all eight quarters. In specifying the demand for medical care López combines the logarithmic version of the Grossman model with the partial adjustment model used by Wagstaff (Chapter 1). The estimates, for the impact of age, education, and the log(wage), show that controlling for censoring and unobservable individual effects does influence the results. This is to be expected, as unobservable heterogeneity is likely to be a particular problem in the use of expenditure survey data, which do not contain any direct measures of morbidity.

Deb (Chapter 14) develops a random effects probit model in which the distribution of the individual effect is approximated by a discrete density. This is another example of the finite mixture model, as applied to count data regressions by Deb and Holmes (Chapter 6). In this case the sample log-likelihood is approximated by,

$$\ln L = \sum_{i=1}^{n} \ln \left\{ \sum_{j=1}^{C} \pi_j \prod_{t=1}^{T} \Phi[d_{it}(X_{it}\beta + v_j)] \right\},$$

$$0 \le \pi_j \le 1, \sum_{j=1}^{C} \pi_j = 1 \tag{22}$$

Monte Carlo experiments are used to assess the finite sample properties of the estimator. These show that only three to four points of support are required for the discrete density to mimic normal and χ^2 densities sufficiently well so as to provide unbiased estimates of the structural parameters and the variance of the individual effect. An empirical application, to data from the 1996 US Medical Expenditure Panel Survey, shows that both observed family characteristics and unobserved family-level heterogeneity are important determinants of the demand for preventive care.

SIMULATION METHODS

The random effects probit model, as described in Equation 19, only involves a univariate integral. More complex models, for example where the error term ε_{it} is assumed to follow an AR(1) process, lead to sample log-likelihood functions that involve higher order intergrals. Monte Carlo simulation techniques can be used to deal with the computational intractability of nonlinear models, such as the panel probit model and the multinomial probit (see e.g., Hajivassiliou [15]). Popular methods of simulation-based inference include classic maximum simulated likelihood (MSL) estimation, as used by Portrait et al. (Chapter 15), and Bayesian Markov Chain Monte Carlo (MCMC) estimation, as used by Hamilton (Chapter 16).

The principle behind MSL estimation is to replace population expectations with a sample analogue. As a simple illustration, consider the example of the random effects probit model. An individual's contribution to the sample likelihood function can be written in the form,

$$L_i = \int_{-\infty}^{\infty} \{h(v)\}\phi(v)dv = E_v h(v) \tag{23}$$

where $\phi(v)$ denotes the standard normal pdf. Then the individual contribution to the corresponding simulated likelihood function is,

$$L_i = (1/R) \sum_{j=1}^{R} h(v_j) \tag{24}$$

where the v_j's are draws from a standard normal and the simulated likelihood is the average of $h(v_j)$ over R draws. The MSL estimator finds the parameter values that maximize the simulated likelihood function.

Portrait et al. (Chapter 15) use the Longitudinal Ageing Study Amsterdam (LASA) to analyse long-term care utilization by the Dutch elderly. They specify a model of the need for long-term care, the use of informal care, formal care at home, institutional care and attrition due to mortality between the two waves of the panel. The use of these care alternatives is modelled jointly, and stochastic dependence is allowed between the various care options. This requires the evaluation of higher order integrals and the model is estimated by MSL. The results show strong effects of health status, gender, socioeconomic variables, and prices on utilization of long-term care services.

Hamilton (Chapter 16) uses a Bayesian panel data Tobit model of Medicare expenditures for recent US retirees, that allows for deaths over the course of the panel. A Tobit model is used because the individual data on monthly medical expenditures from the New Beneficiary Survey contains a high proportion of zeros. This is combined with a probit equation for mortality to give a simultaneous equations LDV model. Hamilton argues that estimation can be conveniently handled by Bayesian MCMC methods.

Bayesian MCMC provides an alternative to the high dimensional integration required for classical ML methods. The posterior density function of the parameters of the model is simulated by taking repeated draws from it, using Monte Carlo simulation methods. Under appropriate conditions, a Markov chain, in which draws are conditional on the previous iteration, should converge to a stationary distribution that is independent of the initial values. Gibbs sampling simplifies this process when the joint posterior density can be decomposed into full conditional densities for sub-sets of parameters. A further attraction of the MCMC method, in the context of LDV models, is the use of data augmentation. This means that the observed values of the LDV (y) can be replaced by the simulated values of the latent variable (y^*) and standard estimators for linear models can be used. In Hamilton's model the system of equations is estimated by seemingly unrelated regression (SURE). The model is implemented using a multivariate t distribution, rather than normality, to allow for heavy tails in the distribution of medical expenditure. The results suggest that survival effects are important, with a higher probability of mortality associated with higher medical expenditure in the last year of life.

CONCLUSION

As pointed out at the beginning of this introduction, there have been substantial developments in the use of econometrics to analyse health and health care over the last decade. The papers included in this volume demonstrate the rich potential of the field and will hopefully encourage its further development over the next decade. We hope the volume will be instructive for existing contributors to health econometrics and inspire others to join the field. In this introduction we have aimed to highlight some of the common econometric problems which arise with health and health care data and, through reference to the applications contained in the individual chapters, demonstrate techniques available to confront these problems.

REFERENCES

1. Grossman, M. On the concept of health capital and the demand for health. *Journal of Political Economy* 1972; **80**: 223–255.
2. Wagstaff, A. The demand for health. Some new empirical evidence. *Journal of Health Economics* 1986; **5**: 195–233.
3. Manton, K.G. and Woodbury, M.A. A new procedure for analysis of medical classification. *Methods of Information in Medicine* 1982; **21**: 210–220.
4. Portrait, F. Lindeboom, M. and Deeg, D.J.H. Health and mortality of the elderly: the grade of membership method, classification and determination. *Health Economics* 1999; **8**: 441–457.
5. Mullahy, J. Heterogeneity, excess zeros, and the structure of count data models. *Journal of Applied Econometrics* 1997; **12**: 337–350.
6. Pohlmeier, W. and Ulrich, V. An econometric model of the two-part decision making process in the demand for health care. *Journal of Human Resources* 1995; **30**: 339–360.
7. Deb, P. and Trivedi, P.K. Demand for medical care by the elderly: a finite mixture approach. *Journal of Applied Econometrics* 1997; **12**: 313–336.
8. Heckman, J.J. and Singer, B. A method of minimizing the distributional impact in econometric models for duration data. *Econometrica* 1984; **52**: 271–230.
9. Pagan, A. and Ullah, A. *Nonparametric Econometrics*. Cambridge: Cambridge University Press, 1999.
10. Robinson, P. Root-N-consistent semiparametric regression. *Econometrica* 1988; **56**: 931–954.
11. Butler, J.S. and Moffitt, R. A computationally efficient quadrature procedure for the one-factor multinomial probit model. *Econometrica* 1982; **50**: 761–764.
12. Chamberlain, G. Panel data. In Griliches, Z. and Intrilligator, M., eds., *Handbook of Econometrics*. Amsterdam: Elsevier, 1984; 1247–1318.
13. Bover, O. and Arellano, M. Estimating dynamic limited-dependent variable models from panel data, *Investigaciones Económicas* 1997; **21**: 141–165.
14. Labeaga, J.M. A double-hurdle rational addiction model with heterogeneity: estimating the demand for tobacco. *Journal of Econometrics* 1999; **93**: 49–72.
15. Hajivassiliou, V.A. Simulation estimation methods for limited dependent variable models. In Maddala, G.S., Rao, C.R. and Vinod, H.D., eds., *Handbook of Statistics*, Vol. 11. Amsterdam: Elsevier, 1993; 519–543.

Section I

Latent Variables and Selection Problems

1

The Demand for Health: an Empirical Reformulation of the Grossman Model

ADAM WAGSTAFF

The World Bank, Washington DC, USA

Despite the acclaim with which *The Demand For Health* [1] was greeted following its publication 20 years ago, Grossman's model of health capital accumulation has been the subject of surprisingly few empirical tests. Of course, many empirical studies of the demand for health care and the demand for and production of health do refer to Grossman's ideas, but since very few actually set up and test an empirical counterpart to Grossman's model, it is hard to tell just how far the results of these studies support the predictions of the model.

The few studies that have been based on Grossman's formal model give conflicting results. All closely follow Grossman's own empirical formulation and employ double logarithmic demand functions for health and health care. The main difference between the studies is to be found in the specification of the demand-for-health-care equations: Grossman and Muurinen [2] estimated reduced-form equations, while the author in an earlier study [3] estimated both reduced-form and structural equations. The reduced-form estimates of all three studies were broadly consistent with the predictions of Grossman's model, but the structural parameters of the author's earlier study were invariably the wrong sign. This suggested that, in contrast to what was implied by Grossman's and Muurinen's work, the available empirical evidence did not, in fact, support Grossman's theoretical model.

The purpose of this paper is to examine the various reasons for the apparent rejection by the data of the Grossman model. To what extent is the rejection more apparent than real? In other words, might the rejection be due to the introduction of inappropriate assumptions in moving from the theoretical model to the empirical model? Might the apparent rejection be due, for example, to an inappropriate specification of the demand-for-

health-care equation? Another line of enquiry concerns the possibility that the apparent rejection may be due to inappropriate assumptions in the theoretical model. Might the result be due, for example, to a failure to take into account in the theoretical model that adjusting to the desired stock of health capital may not be instantaneous?

GROSSMAN'S MODEL

In Grossman's theoretical model, individuals are assumed to inherit a stock of health capital H_0. Thereafter their health stock evolves according to the relationship

$$H_t - H_{t-1} = I_{t-1} - \delta_{t-1}H_{t-1}, \qquad (1.1)$$

where H_t is health stock at the beginning of period t, I_{t-1} is gross investment during the period $t-1$ and δ_{t-1} is the rate of depreciation in operation during the same period. In Grossman's formulation – the formulation adopted in the present paper – δ depends only on the individual's age and is hence exogenous. The individual's utility and income are both increasing functions of the stock of health capital, and in selecting the optimal time path of H_t, the individual bears these benefits in mind, along with the costs of 'holding' health capital. The latter comprise interest costs, depreciation costs and any offsetting capital gains. All are increasing in the cost of new investment. Formally, the equilibrium stock of health capital is defined by the condition

$$\tau_t + a_t = \{r + \delta_t - \tilde{\pi}_{t-1}\}\pi_t, \qquad (1.2)$$

where τ_t is the pecuniary marginal benefit of health capi-

Econometric Analysis of Health Data. Edited by Andrew M. Jones and Owen O'Donnell

tal, a_t is the non-pecuniary marginal benefit, r is the rate of interest, π_t is the marginal cost of investment and $\tilde{\pi}_{t-1}$ is its percentage change.

Although it is the time profile of health that the individual selects, the means by which this is achieved is, of course, the investment profile. If the individual wishes to increase his health stock from one period to the next, or if he wishes it to decrease by less than the amount of depreciation, he must undertake some health investment. Since health capital cannot be sold, investment cannot be negative. The model is 'neoclassical' in that stocks are assumed to adjust instantaneously to their new equilibrium values. The predictions of the effects on health and investment of changes in the model's parameters are derived from Equations 1.1 and 1.2.

PREVIOUS EMPIRICAL WORK

Following Grossman, the approach to date in empirical work has been to derive a double-logarithmic demand-for-health and demand-for-health-care equations from Equations 1.1 and 1.2.

The demand-for-health equation is derived by specifying functional forms for τ_t (or a_t), δ_t and π_t, and by assuming that $r - \tilde{\pi}_{t-1}$ is either zero or some function of time. In the case of the pure investment model, for example, the estimating equation has the form

$$\ln H_t = \alpha_1 \varepsilon \ln w_t - \alpha_1 \varepsilon \ln P_t^m - \alpha_2 \varepsilon t_t + \alpha_3 \varepsilon E, \qquad (1.3)$$

where $\varepsilon(0 \leqslant \varepsilon \leqslant 1)$ is the elasticity of the MEC schedule (the schedule relating τ_t to H_t), w is the wage rate, P^m is price of medical care, t is age and E is education. The parameter α_1 reflects the productivity of medical care in the production of health investments and – given the Cobb Douglas production technology – ought to be positive but not larger than one. The parameter α_2 reflects the effect of aging on depreciation and ought therefore to be positive. The parameter α_3 reflects the productivity of education in health production and is hypothesized to be positive.

To obtain the demand-for-health-care equations, the investment identity is log-linearized to obtain

$$\ln I_{t-1} = \ln H_{t-1} + \ln \delta_{t-1} + \ln[(\tilde{H}_t/\delta_{t-1}) + 1]. \qquad (1.4)$$

The term in square brackets is assumed to be zero (Grossman), invariant across the sample (Muurinen), or randomly distributed across the sample (Wagstaff). The demand-for-health-care equation proper is then obtained by combining Equation 1.4 with the investment production function (a Cobb-Douglas technology is assumed)

and the cost-minimization condition for gross investment. The structural demand-for-medical-care equation thus has the form

$$\ln M_t = \ln H_t + (1 - \alpha_1)\ln w_t - (1 - \alpha_1)\ln P_t^m + \alpha_2 t_t - \alpha_3 E, \qquad (1.5)$$

where the coefficient of plus one on the log of health capital reflects the derived demand hypothesis (an increase in the desired stock of health capital ought to increase health care utilization). Note that the signs of coefficients are exactly the opposite of those in demand-for-health equation. Thus the coefficient on education in this equation reflects solely the productivity effect; i.e., holding health constant, the better educated ought to demand less health care, since they are more efficient producers of health. Rather than estimate Equation 1.5 directly, Grossman and Muurinen estimate instead a reduced-form demand-for-health-care equation, obtained by substituting Equation 1.4 in Equation 1.5:

$$\ln M_t = [\alpha_1(\varepsilon - 1) + 1]\ln w_t - [\alpha_1(\varepsilon - 1) + 1] \\ \ln P_t^m + \alpha_2(\varepsilon - 1)t_1 + \alpha_3(\varepsilon - 1)E \qquad (1.6)$$

In this equation, as in the demand-for-health equation, the coefficients reflect not only the parameters of the technology, but also the demand elasticity, ε.

Broadly speaking, the parameter estimates obtained to date for the demand-for-health and the reduced-form demand-for-health-care equations lend support to Grossman's model. In the author's earlier study, for example, education entered these two equations with positive and negative signs respectively, which is consistent with education-efficiency hypothesis and with the demand elasticity being less than one.

The parameter estimates of the structural demand-for-health-care equation reported in Wagstaff [3] tell a different study, however. The coefficient on health was negative, which is inconsistent with the derived demand hypothesis, and education had a positive coefficient in this equation, contrary to what is predicted by theory. These results, coupled with the reduced-form parameter estimates, imply that the demand elasticity is outside the admissible range, so that the two wrong signs when multiplied together give the right sign for the reduced-form parameter. Similar results are obtained for other variables.

PROBLEMS WITH PREVIOUS EMPIRICAL WORK

Two possible responses to these results seem possible. The first is that the theoretical model has not been tested properly due to the introduction of inappropriate assumptions in moving from the theoretical model to the empirical model. The second is that the theoretical model *has* been tested properly and has been found to be wanting, suggesting that modifications might be in order.

The obvious weakness in Grossman's empirical formulation lies in the derivation of the demand-for-health-care equation. The assumption that $\tilde{H}_t/\delta_{t-1}$ is zero is particularly weak. It is at odds with the theoretical model and eliminates entirely the inherently dynamic character of the net investment identity. The implications of this assumption can be most easily seen if instead of converting Equations 1.1 and 1.2 to log-linear equations, one retains the inherently linear nature of the net investment identity and adopts a linear specification of the demand-for-health equation. Thus let the latter be of the form

$$H_t = \beta X_t + u_t, \tag{1.7}$$

where X_t is a vector of variables reflecting the arguments of the first-order condition (i.e. Equation 1.2), such as age and education, and β is a vector of coefficients. Substituting Equation 1.7 into Equation 1.1 and rearranging yields

$$I_{t-1} = \beta X_t - (1 - \delta_{t-1})H_{t-1} + u_t. \tag{1.8}$$

In terms of the variables included, Equation 1.8 is very similar to the structural demand-for-health-care equation implied by Grossman's empirical formulation: in both equations measures of investment are expressed as functions of the arguments of the demand-for-health equation and the stock of health capital, albeit lagged capital stock in the case of Equation 1.8. The interpretation of the parameters is, however, quite different. In contrast to those in the structural equation, the coefficients on the X-variables in Equation 1.8 ought to have the same sign as their counterparts in the demand-for-health equation. Moreover, the sign of the coefficient on health stock in Equation 1.8 ought to be negative, whereas the coefficient on (contemporaneous) health ought to be positive in Grossman's structural equation. Equation 1.8 suggests, therefore, that the observed negative coefficient on health stock in structural demand-for-health-care equations and the positive coefficients on variables such as education in these equations may, after all, be quite consistent with Grossman's theoretical model. The implication is, then, that it is Grossman's empirical formulation of his model which is to be rejected, not the theoretical model itself.

An alternative line of enquiry is that it is the theoretical model which requires some reformulation. One possibility, suggested by the author in his earlier paper, is that the apparent inconsistency between the theory and the empirical results may be due to a failure to recognize that individuals are unable to adjust their health stocks instantaneously. Although the assumption of instantaneous adjustment may well be unwarranted, it would appear, on reflection, that it is unlikely to be the source of the apparent inconsistency between the data and the model. To see why, suppose that instead of assuming instantaneous adjustment, we assume a partial adjustment framework. Thus assume that desired health stocks are generated according to the process

$$H_t^* = \beta X_t + u_t, \tag{1.9}$$

where H_t^* are desired stocks, and that a fraction $\mu(0 \leqslant \mu \leqslant 1)$ of the gap between desired and actual stocks is closed each period. Thus

$$H_t - H_{t-1} = \mu(H_t^* - H_{t-1}), \tag{1.10}$$

so that if $\mu = 1$, adjustment is instantaneous and actual and desired stocks coincide, as in Grossman's formulation. Combining Equations 1.1, 1.9 and 1.10 yields

$$I_{t-1} = \mu\beta X_t - (\mu - \delta_{t-1})H_{t-1} + \mu u_t. \tag{1.11}$$

Examination of Equation 1.11 reveals that although the signs of the coefficients on the X-variables are unaffected by less-than-instantaneous adjustment, the sign of the coefficient on lagged health stock could actually be positive (i.e., if $\mu < \delta$). Thus recognizing non-instantaneous adjustment does not actually help to explain the negative coefficient on health stocks in the structural demand-for-health-care equation. On the contrary, non-instantaneous adjustment makes a negative coefficient *less* likely.

AN ALTERNATIVE EMPIRICAL FORMULATION OF GROSSMAN'S MODEL

The above suggests that any empirical test of Grossman's model ought to acknowledge the inherently linear character of the net investment identity and should not therefore involve a long-linearization of this equation. Since any empirical model will need to include a demand-for-health equation as well as an investment equation, this implies that the former ought to be intrinsically linear. In what follows it is assumed that it is actually linear, although clearly this assumption could be relaxed in future work to allow for squared, cubed and cross-product terms and hence for a more flexible functional form. Since non-instantaneous adjustment seems highly plausible, it also seems desirable to allow for this in the empirical model.

Equations 1.1, 1.9 and 1.10 would therefore seem to be a more sensible starting point for a test of the Grossman model. The demand-for-health equation for this empirical formulation of the model is found by combining Equations 1.9 and 1.10 to obtain

$$H_t = \mu\beta X_t + (1 - \mu)H_{t-1} + \mu u_t, \qquad (1.12)$$

so that, in contrast to Grossman's formulation, lagged health stocks affect the current demand for health. Grossman's model is the special case where $\mu = 1$. Note that the coefficients on the X-variables in Equation 1.12 ought to be equal to those in Equation 1.11: testing this restriction provides a test of the derived demand hypothesis.

Suppose, for the moment, that δ is invariant across individuals. Then if health stocks and investment were observable, one could proceed directly and estimate Equations 1.11 and 1.12. This would generate estimates of μ and δ. Of course, unrestricted estimation would leave β and the variance of u_t over-identified, since the two equations would give two different sets of estimates of these parameters. The answer to this is to impose the appropriate cross-equation equalities in the estimation process, which, if the derived demand hypothesis is tenable, ought to be accepted by the data.

This leaves the problem that δ is unlikely to be invariant across the sample. If it is assumed that δ is affected only by the person's age, so that all other 'environmental' variables affect the efficiency of health production, the answer would seem to be estimate separate models for different age groups. If δ were the only parameter which is thought to vary with age, the appropriate cross-group equalities ought to be imposed to ensure that parameters other than δ are the same for all age groups. In fact it seems more plausible to assume that both δ and μ vary with age, since it seems likely that the elderly find it harder than the young to adjust their health stocks to their desired levels.

All this assumes that health stocks and investment are observable. Of course, in reality they are not, but their unobservability can be overcome using a Multiple Indicator Multiple Cause (MIMIC) latent variable model [4]. The unobservability of health capital can be overcome by introducing health indicators and specifying additional equations linking these to the stock of health capital. Obvious indicators include responses to questions such as 'Do you suffer from any long-standing health problem?' and 'Do you consider your health to be excellent, good, fair or poor?' The unobservability of health investment can be overcome by introducing demand-for-health-care equations. As theory requires, these equations condition on health investment, as well as on other arguments of the demand function for health care, such as

education (if education affects the efficiency of health production), prices (including time prices) and possibly supply factors (such as the availability of the relevant facilities).

In what follows it is assumed that the answers to the same survey questions on health are available at two points in time. These two vectors of variables – denoted below by y_t and y_{t-1} – are assumed to be linearly related to H_t and H_{t-1} respectively according to the health indicator equations

$$\begin{bmatrix} y_t \\ y_{t-1} \end{bmatrix} = \begin{bmatrix} \cap_t & 0 \\ 0 & \cap_{t-1} \end{bmatrix} \begin{bmatrix} H_t \\ H_{t-1} \end{bmatrix} + \begin{bmatrix} \varepsilon_t \\ \varepsilon_{t-1} \end{bmatrix} \qquad (1.13)$$

where $\cap_t$ and $\cap_{t-1}$ are coefficient vectors and ε_t and ε_{t-1} are vectors of error terms. To ensure identification, a normalization is introduced into each of the coefficient vectors; to ensure that H_t and H_{t-1} are measured in the same units, the same normalization is introduced in both $\cap_t$ and $\cap_{t-1}$. Ideally one would allow for the possibility that ε_t and ε_{t-1} are correlated, but identification problems were encountered when this was attempted. It is also assumed that information on health care utilization is available for the intervening period. Denote by M_{t-1} the vector of health care utilization variables and by Z_{t-1} the vector of variables other than gross investment which influence the demand for health care. Then, if the demand-for-health-care function is linear, in addition to Equation 1.10, we have

$$M_{t-1} = BI_{t-1} + \Gamma Z_{t-1} + e_{t-1} \qquad (1.14)$$

where B and Γ are a vector and matrix of coefficients respectively, and e_{t-1} is a vector of error terms. Again, in order to ensure identification, one normalization is introduced into the vector B. It is also assumed that some rows of Γ are empty, i.e. that utilization of some types of health care does not depend on the Z-variables.

DATA AND VARIABLE DEFINITIONS

The model consists of the demand-for-health equation (Equation 1.12), the health investment equation (Equation 1.11), the health indicator equations (Equation 1.13), and the demand-for-health-care equations (Equation 1.14). Data are required therefore on each of the variables in each of these equations.

The data for the present empirical exercise are taken from the *Danish Health Study* [5] (DHS). This followed some 1000 households (1752 adults) over a period of 12 months, beginning October 1982. Data on health and background variables (such as education) were obtained at the beginning and end of year, and detailed information on morbidity and use of health services was obtained for each week of the study by means of a diary. The rate of attrition is relatively low (76% of households interviewed at the start of the study completed the 12 months), although there is evidence that the probability of completing the study was related to age, education and initial health status [5].

Of the numerous health indicators available in the DHS, three were selected for the present exercise:

- FUNLIM, a question relating to functional limitations, defined as a dummy variable taking a value of one in the year in question if the health of the person limited them from doing anything they wanted to do:
- PAH, a question relating to physician-assessed health, defined in terms of categorical responses to the statement 'According to the doctors I have seen my health is now excellent', with the value 1 corresponding to 'agree entirely', the value 2 to 'agree', the value 3 to 'don't know', the value 4 to 'disagree' and the value 5 to 'disagree entirely'; and
- SAH, a question relating to self-assessed health, defined in terms of categorical responses to the statement 'My health is excellent', with values of 1 to 5 defined as in PAH.

The values of these variables for 1982 are denoted below by FUNLIM82, PAH82 and SAH82, and those for 1983 by FUNLIM83, PAH83 and SAH83. The two FUNLIM variables have been chosen for the normalizations: the relevant elements of $\cap_t$ and $\cap_{t-1}$ have been set equal to -1.0, thus ensuring that the unobservable health variables are both increasing in good health.

The empirical model has been estimated for all adults, irrespective of whether or not they are in paid employment. Four variables have been included in the X-vector:

- EQFAMINC, equivalent household pre-tax monthly wage income in October 1982. The equivalence scale is that discussed by Buhmann *et al.* [6], with a household size elasticity of 0.5. It is regrettable, but no information is available on household wage income at the end of the study or on non-wage income at either date. EQFAMINC will thus substantially understate the pre-tax incomes of pensioners, and will understate – but presumably to a lesser extent – the incomes of households containing social security recipients:
- SCHOOL, the level of schooling attained, converted into years of schooling. Measures of post-school education were also included, but were found to be insignificant:
- MALE, a dummy taking a value of one for males;
- AGE, the individual's age in years.

In Grossman's pure investment and pure consumption models, the relevant elements of β are expected to be positive and negative for SCHOOL and AGE respectively. In the pure consumption model, the relevant element of β for EQFAMINC ought to be positive if EQFAMINC is viewed as a proxy for the marginal utility of initial wealth.

The indicators of health investment that have been used are all measures of health care utilization. Other forms of health investment have been excluded in the present analysis. The indicators used include:

- GPCONS, the number of consultations over the year with a general practitioner (GP). All consultations have been included, irrespective of whether they were face-to-face or telephone consultations, and irrespective of where they occurred;
- HOSPDAYS, the number of days as an inpatient in hospital over the year;
- SPCONS, the number of consultations over the year with a specialist;
- PHYSIO, the number of sessions with a physiotherapist;
- OUTPATIENT, the number of outpatient visits during the year;
- ACCEMER, the number of visits to a hospital accident and emergency department.

It is assumed that the last two indicators depend only on the amount of investment undertaken, and do not depend on other factors.

Variables included in the Z-vector include SCHOOL, but also several variables reflecting the availability of health care facilities, as well as distance to GP:

- GP/1000, the number of GPs per 1000 population in the individual's district (*kommune*);
- SP/1000, the number of community specialists per 1000 population in the individual's district;
- BEDS/1000, the number of hospital beds per 1000 population in the individual's district;
- PHYS/1000, the number of physiotherapists per 1000 population in the individual's district;
- DIST-GP, distance in km from the individual's home to his or her GP.

The first and last are assumed to affect only GPCONS. The second is assumed to affect only SPCONS, BEDS/1000 is assumed to affect only HOSPDAYS and PHYS/1000 is assumed to affect only PHYSIO.

EMPIRICAL RESULTS

To take into account the possibility that δ varies according to age, the sample (consisting entirely of adults) was split into two sub-samples of roughly equal size, the first comprising the under-41s ($N = 707$, after listwise deletion) and the second comprising the over-41s ($N = 655$). The most restrictive model is where only $\mu - \delta$ varies across the two age groups (and therefore only δ varies, since $(1 - \mu)$ is invariant) and where the coefficients on the X-variables are constrained to be equal in the demand-for-health and investment equations. The least restrictive model is that in which all parameters – including $\cap_t$ and $\cap_{t-1}$ – vary across the two age groups and the equality constraints across the demand-for-health and investment equations are not imposed.

Parameters were estimated using the computer program LISREL [7]. Since the health indicators are all ordinal variables and the health care utilization variables are heavily concentrated around zero, the best estimation strategy would be to explicitly recognize that the health indicators are ordinal variables and treat the utilization variables as censored variables. This can in principle be done with LISREL by using Weighted Least Squares (WLS) to analyse a matrix of polychoric correlations (i.e., estimates of the correlation in the latent bivariate normal distribution representing the two ordinal variables), with the asymptotic variances and covariances of the polychoric correlations as weights. In the present case this proved infeasible: the program PRELIS [8] – which accompanies LISREL and computes the correlation and covariance matrices required by LISREL – was unable to compute the asymptotic covariance matrix. Instead, the polychoric correlation matrix was analysed by means of Maximum Likelihood (ML), since, of the various estima-

tion methods available in LISREL, this tended to give the best fit (i.e., the smallest chi-squared value).

Tables 1.1 and 1.2 present the parameter estimates of the least restrictive model. The lack of t-statistics for FUNLIM82 and FUNLIM83 in Table 1.1 and for OUT-PAT in Table 1.2 reflects the fact that these indicators have been used to scale the three latent variables, H_{t-1}, H_t and I_{t-1}.

Since all three health indicators are likely to be decreasing in good health it is reassuring to find negative coefficients in both sets of health indicator equations. It is also reassuring to find that the latent health variables explain a substantial proportion of the variation in the health indicators. The same is not true of the investment variable. Although all utilization measures are increasing in health investment, the Z-variables and health investment combined account for a relatively small proportion of the variation in the utilization variables, except in the case of out-patient visits, where the R^2 is fairly high. It is, of course, not uncommon to find low R^2 values in microeconometric health care utilization equations. But the implication for the Grossman model is that health care utilization may be a poor indicator of health investment. This probably explains – at least in part – why the R^2 of the investment equation in both sub-samples is very low.

Turning to the parameter estimates of the equations in Table 1.2, the coefficients of the demand-for-health equations have the expected sign, except in the case of the coefficient on AGE in the under-41s equation. Although this is not significant, the signs in the two sub-sample

Table 1.1a   ML estimates of health indicator equations for under 41s

	FUNLIM82	PAH82	SAH82	FUNLIM83	PAH83	SAH83
H_{t-1}	-1.000	-1.385 (16.18)	-1.622 (16.39)			
H_t				-1.000	-1.264 (17.53)	-1.310 (17.72)
R^2	0.342	0.656	0.900	0.427	0.684	0.736

Note: t-values in parentheses.

Table 1.1b   ML estimates of health indicator equations for over 41s

	FUNLIM82	PAH82	SAH82	FUNLIM83	PAH83	SAH83
H_{t-1}	-1.000	-1.183 (20.75)	-1.257 (21.55)			
H_t				-1.000	-0.998 (23.56)	-1.071 (25.62)
R^2	0.520	0.727	0.821	0.673	0.671	0.775

Note: t-values in parentheses.

Table 1.2a ML estimates of structural equations for under 41s

	H_t	I_{t-1}	OUTPAT	ACCEMER	GPCONS	HOSPDAYS	SPCONS	PHYSIO
H_{t-1}	0.687	−0.265						
	(11.03)	(4.18)						
I_{t-1}			1.000	0.189	−0.442	−0.752	0.222	0.342
				(3.14)	(6.58)	(8.42)	(3.66)	(5.37)
EQFAMINC	0.032	0.030						
	(1.43)	(0.86)						
SCHOOL	0.072	0.005			0.014	−0.054	0.025	−0.071
	(3.01)	(0.13)			(0.38)	(1.49)	(0.66)	(1.93)
MALE	0.000	−0.089						
	(0.02)	(2.55)						
AGE	0.023	−0.009						
	(0.98)	(0.25)						
GP/1000					0.077			
					(2.12)			
SP/1000							0.027	
							(0.72)	
BEDS/1000						0.012		
						(0.37)		
PHYS/1000								−0.057
								(1.57)
DIST-GP					−0.037			
					(1.03)			
$\mathrm{cov}(u_1, u_2)$	−0.074							
	(3.57)							
μ	0.313							
δ	0.048							
R^2	0.394	0.096	0.591	0.021	0.122	0.335	0.031	0.076

Note: t-values in parentheses. $\mathrm{Cov}(u_1, u_2)$ is covariance of error terms of first two equations.

equations suggest the possibility of a non-linear effect of age. The coefficients on H_{t-1} suggest that, contrary to what is assumed in Grossman's model, individuals do not adjust instantaneously to their desired health stocks. The results suggest, unsurprisingly, that the elderly adjust more slowly to their desired stocks than do the young. Turning to the investment equation, the results suggest that in both samples $\mu > \delta$, but surprisingly the implied value of δ is smaller for the over-41s than for the under-41s. Moreover, the value of δ is actually *negative* for the former group. One possible explanation of this is that δ has in effect been specified in two different ways in the model: as a linear function of age in the X vector and as a step function of age when $(\mu - \delta)$ in Equation 1.7 is allowed to vary with age. A more consistent treatment (with the effect of age specified as a step function in both cases) might yield more sensible results.

The coefficients on the X-variables in the investment equation all have the expected sign, except that on EQFAMINC in the over-41s sub-sample, but this is not significant. As noted above, the derived demand hypothesis can be tested by testing the restriction that the coefficients on the X-variables are the same in the demand-for-health and investment equations. In the LISREL program, this can be accomplished by comparing the model's chi-squared values with and without the restrictions imposed. The relevant value is 18.58 with 8 degrees of freedom, which compare with tabular values at the 1% and 5% levels of 20.09 and 15.51. The restriction implied by the derived demand hypothesis is therefore rejected at the 5% level but not at the 1% level. This contrasts with the decisive rejection of the hypothesis in the author's earlier empirical work using Grossman's own empirical formulation.

Turning to the demand-for-health-care equations, it is apparent that, again in contrast to the author's earlier empirical work, the results also lend some support to the education-efficiency hypothesis. Holding the quantity of investment constant, education tends to reduce the demand for health care, as the Grossman model predicts. Moreover, the negative sign of the coefficients on GP-DIST lends support to the time-price hypothesis. The availability of facilities also appears to have some effect on utilization, with greater availability increasing utilization except in the case of physiotherapy.

As indicated above, a chi-squared test does not reject

Table 1.2b ML estimates of structural equations for over 41s

	H_t	I_{t-1}	OUTPAT	ACCEMER	GPCONS	HOSPDAYS	SPCONS	PHYSIO
H_{t-1}	0.849	−0.253						
	(15.98)	(4.68)						
I_{t-1}			1.000	0.246	0.526	0.763	0.279	0.513
				(4.66)	(9.63)	(12.68)	(5.29)	(9.35)
EQFAMINC	0.074	−0.016						
	(2.51)	(0.36)						
SCHOOL	0.005	0.109			−0.102	−0.100	−0.045	0.012
	(0.19)	(2.73)			(2.75)	(2.81)	(1.11)	(0.33)
MALE	0.004	−0.117						
	(0.17)	(3.17)						
AGE	−0.061	−0.005						
	(2.15)	(0.13)						
GP/1000					0.097			
					(2.68)			
SP/1000							0.137	
							(3.41)	
BEDS/1000						−0.020		
						(0.60)		
PHYS/1000								−0.048
								(1.31)
DIST-GP					−0.068			
					(1.90)			
cov(u_1, u_2)	−0.16							
	(6.56)							
μ	0.151							
δ	−0.102							
R^2	0.595	0.077	0.703	0.043	0.210	0.408	0.072	0.189

Note: t-values in parentheses. Cov(u_1, u_2) is covariance of error terms of first two equations.

the cross-equation restrictions implied by the derived demand hypothesis. A further set of restrictions of interest are the equality restrictions across the two age groups. Are the data consistent, in other words, with only δ varying across age groups? The relevant chi-squared statistic is 113.22, with 30 degrees of freedom. (The cross-equation restrictions implied by the derived demand hypothesis are imposed in both models.) The cross-group restrictions are thus rejected by the data, suggesting that there are parameters other than δ which also vary across age groups.

DISCUSSION

This paper has argued that the empirical formulation of the Grossman model used in previous tests of the theoretical model is inappropriate, since it fails to take into account the inherently dynamic character of the health investment process. The fact that the author's earlier structural equations estimates were inconsistent with the predictions of the theoretical model may not therefore

necessarily be a cause for concern. Indeed, the alternative formulation of the empirical model proposed in the present paper appears to be more consistent not only with Grossman's theoretical model but also with the data. In contrast to the author's earlier results obtained using Grossman's own empirical formulation, the results in the present paper lend support to the derived-demand and education-efficiency hypotheses. They also suggest, however, that, contrary to what is assumed in Grossman's theoretical model, individuals do not adjust their health stocks instantaneously.

It remains to be seen, of course, whether these empirical results can be replicated on other data-sets. The results reported in van Doorslaer [9], suggest that such replications might well be successful. The equations estimated there are different from those estimated in the present paper, being health investment production functions rather than demand equations, but there are similarities. Van Doorslaer's results add weight, for example, to the finding that adjustment of health capital stocks is non-instantaneous.

ACKNOWLEDGEMENTS

This paper was written whilst I was a Visiting Research Fellow at the Centre for Health Economics (CHE) at the University of York. I am grateful to CHE for financing the visit and to Terkel Christiansen for making the Danish Health Study data available and for translating the variable names and labels. The paper has benefited from helpful comments from Michael Grossman, Andrew Jones, an anonymous referee and participating at the European Workshop on Modelling and Econometrics in Health Economics held at York in July 1992. I alone am responsible for any errors.

REFERENCES

1. Grossman, M. *The Demand for Health: a Theoretical and Empirical Investigation*. New York, NBER, 1972.
2. Muurinen, J.M. *An economic model of health behaviour – with empirical applications to Finnish health survey data*. Unpublished DPhil Dissertation, York, University of York, 1982.
3. Wagstaff, A. The demand for health: some new empirical evidence. *Journal of Health Economics* 1986; **5**: 195–233.
4. Jöreskog, K.G. and Goldberger, A.S. Estimation of a model with multiple indicators and multiple causes of a single latent variable. *Journal of the American Statistical Association* 1975; **70**: 631–639.
5. Bentzen, N., Christiansen, T. and Pedersen, K.M. *The Danish Health Study*. Odense, Odense University, 1988.
6. Buhmann, B., Rainwater, L., Schmaus, G. and Smeeding, T. Equivalence scales, well-being, inequality and poverty: sensitivity estimates across 10 countries using the Luxembourg Income Study database. *Review of Income and Wealth* 1988; June: 115–142.
7. Jöreskog, K.G. and Sörbom, D. *LISREL 7: A Guide to the Program and Applications*, 2nd edn. Chicago IL, SPSS Inc., 1989.
8. Jöreskog, K.G. and Sörbom, D. *PRELIS: A Program for Multivariate Data Screening and Data Summarization. A Preprocessor for LISREL*. Mooresville IA, Scientific Software Inc., 1986.
9. Van Doorslaer, E.K.A. *Health, Knowledge and the Demand for Medical Care: an Econometric Analysis*. Maastricht and Wolfeboro NH, van Gorcum, 1987.

2

Health, Health Care, and the Environment: Econometric Evidence from German Micro Data

MANFRED ERBSLAND,[1] WALTER RIED[2] AND VOLKER ULRICH[3]

[1]*Fachhochschule Neubrandenburg, Neubrandenburg, Germany,* [2]*University of Mannheim, Mannheim, Germany and* [3]*Ernst-Moritz-Arndt-Universität Griefswald, Griefswald, Germany*

In developed countries a substantial amount of the resources available is devoted to health care. Indeed, the provision of a broad range of high quality health care services can safely be taken to play a major role in maintaining and promoting the health of a given population. While there is evidence for the significance of a sophisticated system of health care, the potential importance of other determinants of individual health must not be overlooked. Among the first to observe this was Sir William Petty in his investigations on 'Political Arithmeticks'. As early as the seventeenth century, he was able to demonstrate the considerable influence of sanitary conditions on human mortality. From the point of view of allocation theory, non-medical determinants of health are important mainly with respect to the following two issues. First, what is their specific contribution to the attainment of health targets? And, second, to what extent is it possible, by relying more on those other determinants, to reduce consumption of health care?

Our paper investigates the influence of several variables on both individual health and consumption of medical care in the Federal Republic of Germany. In the course of our empirical analysis, we focus on the impact of the quality of the environment since this is often hypothesized to be an important factor affecting health in industrialized countries. This observation notwithstanding, with the exception of a paper by Cropper [1], the interactions between environmental conditions, health and health care have failed, in our view, to receive much attention in the literature. Given that the quality of the environment cannot be observed directly, we proceed by modelling it as a latent variable which may be described by means of suitable indicators. A major aim of our paper is to provide answers to the questions raised above in the context of the specific data set considered below. In as much as environmental quality affects individual health and/or consumption of medical care, this has implications for environmental policy as well. More precisely, any policy geared at improving the quality of the environment needs to be evaluated with respect to its side effects on health care.

The conceptual framework of our paper is given by the notion, due to Mushkin [2], that an individual's health may usefully be considered as a capital stock which, in the course of time, provides services to its owner. At the same time, it is possible to augment this stock of capital by means of gross investment which encompasses, among other inputs, consumption of medical care. Thus, while his stock of health represents the ultimate objective of a rational individual, his demand for medical care can be derived from it. One of the advantages of this approach is to provide a clear distinction between health on the one hand and use of medical care on the other. This enables us to analyse the effects of the quality of the environment on both variables separately.

Our paper is organized as follows. In section two we present the basic Grossman model which formalizes Mushkin's ideas within the context of an intertemporal utility maximization problem. From this we derive a sub-model of much simpler structure which also provides the background for our empirical specification. Section three contains a brief description of the database underlying our empirical analysis. Furthermore, we combine the structural model of section two with a measurement

Econometric Analysis of Health Data. Edited by Andrew M. Jones and Owen O'Donnell
© 2002 John Wiley & Sons Ltd. Previously published in *Health Economics*, Vol. 4; pp. 169–182 (1995). © John Wiley & Sons Ltd

model in order to account for the latent variables considered. Section four gives estimation results where we also provide an interpretation for the more important parameter estimates. In particular, we discuss our results with respect to the impact of the quality of the environment. Finally, section five contains our conclusions while also offering several suggestions for future research.

THE GROSSMAN APPROACH

In this section, we present the theoretical model introduced by Grossman [3] as well as a submodel constituting a special case of it from a theoretical point of view. On the one hand, this will help to bring out clearly those additional restrictions which underlie our empirical analysis. On the other hand, this provides a convenient opportunity to characterize fully the main equations of the model and the dynamics of the stock of health capital. In our view, the literature up to now has failed to take those latter two aspects adequately into consideration.

While, more recently, the Grossman model or generalizations thereof have been presented mainly in continuous time [1,4,5], we have chosen, following Grossman, to work in discrete time. This implies a period analysis which, among others, offers the advantage of being better suited to empirical data referring to intervals of time. The latter holds, for example, for the data collected by the German Socio-economic Panel (SOEP), which supplies the data base for our empirical analysis.

In his model Grossman combines both life cycle and household production theory with the concept of health as a capital stock which is subject to depreciation but can be augmented by means of gross investment. In every period, this health capital stock provides services accruing as 'healthy time' which the individual is free to use either as labour supply or as an input to his household production.

More specifically, we consider an individual whose decision problem is to choose, for the remainder of his lifetime, time paths for his health capital as well as for consumption of commodities in an optimal way. The terminal time of this optimization problem is determined endogenously, it is reached as soon as the stock of health capital is equal to or falls below a given lower bound. Some constraints of this problem are technological, this concerns, in particular, the output from household production activities. Further restrictions on the set of feasible solutions are given by an intertemporal budget constraint, a flow equation for the stock of health capital and an upper bound on the uses of time given by the length of the period under consideration.

The starting point for the individual's decision problem

is given by an intertemporal utility function U as follows:

$$U = \sum_{t=0}^{n} m_t u_t \qquad (2.1)$$

$$u_t = u(h_t, Z_t) \qquad (2.1a)$$

u_t refers to utility in period t as generated by the pair (h_t, Z_t), with h_t representing the services of the health capital (H_t) stock and Z_t the commodities produced by the individual. As Equation 2.1 illustrates, total intertemporal utility is given by a weighted sum of the utilities u_t. Essentially, the weights m_t are determined by the individual's rate of time preference. Moreover, Equation 2.1 implies intertemporal separability of the utility function U, which, in effect, leads to rather simple solutions in the optimization problem considered below [6].

For the services of the health capital stock as measured in units of healthy time, assume

$$h_t = h(H_t); \quad \frac{\partial h}{\partial H_t} > 0, \qquad (2.2)$$

with the derivative expressing the positive influence of health on healthy time.

The production of commodities takes place by transforming consumption goods purchased in the marketplace with the help of an additional time input. For the sake of simplicity, we focus on a single aggregate commodity whose production depends on an aggregate consumption good G_t and a time input T_t. In addition, the output of production activity is taken to be affected by an exogenous parameter X_t:

$$Z_t = Z(G_t, T_t; X_t) \qquad (2.3)$$

X_t denotes the level of education of the individual, i.e. his stock of human capital (excluding his health capital stock). We assume the production function Z to be linear homogenous with respect to (G_t, T_t) which implies constant marginal costs of the production of commodities in every period.

The change in the stock of health capital over time is given by netting out gross investment I_t with depreciation of the existing stock:

$$\Delta H_{t+1} = H_{t+1} - H_t = I_t - \delta_t H_t, \qquad (2.4)$$

where δ_t denotes the rate of depreciation taken to be constant within a period. The individual is capable of producing gross investment by combining medical care M_t and a time input TH_t in the following way:

$$I_t = I(M_t, TH_t; X_t) \qquad (2.5)$$

Just like the production of commodities, this household production function exhibits parametric dependence on X_t. Furthermore, we assume I to be linear homogeneous in (M_t, TH_t). Therefore, in any period, production of gross investment takes place at a constant marginal cost.

In addition, it is necessary to observe another restriction relating work income, expenditures on both the aggregate consumption good and medical care to the change in the individual's wealth position. With respect to period t, the budget constraint is given by

$$V_{t+1} = (1 + r)(V_t + W_t TW_t - P_t^M M_t - P_t^G G_t), \qquad (2.6)$$

with V_t denoting financial wealth, r the rate of interest (taken to be constant over time), W_t the wage rate, TW_t working time and P_t^M (P_t^G) the price of medical care (of the aggregate consumption good), all for period t. For the present value change in financial wealth, one obtains the following flow equation:

$$\frac{V_{t+1}}{(1 + r)^{t+1}} - \frac{V_t}{(1 + r)^t} = \frac{W_t TW_t - P_t^M M_t - P_t^G G_t}{(1 + r)^t}. \qquad (2.6a)$$

Finally, in every period, by definition the total time budget Ω will be exhausted by healthy time h_t on the one hand and sick time TL_t on the other:

$$\Omega = h_t + TL_t. \qquad (2.7)$$

In the following, we assume h_t to be spent exclusively on the three uses of time already mentioned above. In other words, h_t covers either working time or the individual's time input to household production. Thus, we have:

$$\Omega = TW_t + TH_t + T_t + TL_t. \qquad (2.7a)$$

Now the individual's intertemporal optimization problem can be stated as a problem of discrete optimal control [7]. The objective is to maximize

$$U = \sum_{t=0}^{n} m_t u[h(H_t), Z_t]$$

subject to the restrictions given by Equations 2.3, 2.4, 2.5, 2.6a and 2.7a. The stock of health capital and the present value of financial wealth represent state variables whose values at time $t = 0$ constitute additional restrictions. Moreover, a terminal condition – e.g., non-negativity – will have to be met for financial wealth, while the terminal time of the optimization problem is determined endogenously by the time path of health capital according to:

$$n = \min\{i \in N | H_t \leqslant H_{\min}\} \qquad (2.8)$$

with N denoting the set of natural numbers and $H_{\min}$ representing a lower bound on the stock of health capital.

As for the set of control variables, its composition will, in general, depend on which specific problem one intends to study. In what follows, we shall focus on M_t and Z_t. Therefore, suppose an 'interior solution' holds for these two variables and for TW_t as well. Then, after performing some algebraic manipulation, one obtains four necessary conditions representing the core of the model:

$$\left(\frac{m_t(1 + r)^t}{\lambda_0^v} \frac{\partial u}{\partial h_t} + W_t\right)\frac{\partial h}{\partial H_t} = \pi_{t-1}^I(1 + r) - \pi_t^I(1 - \delta_t) \qquad (2.9)$$

$$\frac{m_t(1 + r)^t}{\lambda_0^v} \frac{\partial u}{\partial Z_t} = \pi_t^Z \qquad (2.10)$$

$$V_0 + \sum_{t=0}^{n} \frac{W_t h_t - \pi_t^I\left(\frac{\partial \pi_t^I}{\partial P_t^M}\right)^{-1} M_t - \pi_t^Z Z_t}{(1 + r)^t} = 0 \qquad (2.11)$$

$$\Delta H_{t+1} = H_{t+1} - H_t = \left(\frac{\partial \pi_t^I}{\partial P_t^M}\right)^{-1} M_t - \delta_t H_t \qquad (2.12)$$

λ_0^V is a time invariant costate variable which gives the marginal utility of the present value of financial wealth, while π_t^I (π_t^Z) represents marginal costs of gross investment (the commodity) in period t. In Equations 2.11 and 2.12, we have replaced I_t because, due to the assumption of an interior solution with respect to M_t – which implies an interior solution with respect to I_t as well – one has, according to Shepard's lemma:

$$M_t = \frac{\partial \pi_t^I}{\partial P_t^M} I_t, \qquad (2.13)$$

building on the homogeneity property of the production function I.

Now suppose conditions sufficient for a maximum are fulfilled. Then, the system of Equations 2.9 to 2.12 not only determines an optimal value for λ_0^V but also optimal time paths for the stock of health capital H_t, the commodity Z_t, and the demand for medical care M_t. In this general case, Equations 2.9 and 2.10 contain H_t, Z_t and λ_0^V as endogenous variables, while the intertemporal budget constraint Equation 2.11 gives an equation in H_t, Z_t and M_t. Finally, Equation 2.12 implicitly is an equation in all endogenous variables. This can be made explicit by approximating ΔH_{t+1} by an appropriate expression which has been obtained by taking first differences of Equations 2.9 and 2.10.

It is important to see that Equation 2.9 describes the optimality condition for health capital in period t. If the individual wishes to increase H_t by a marginal unit without modifying the remainder of the corresponding time path, gross investment in period $(t-1)$ will need to be increased by a marginal unit as well. At the same time, I_t can be reduced by $(1-\delta_t)$ because a higher stock of health capital in period t allows for lower gross investment given that H_{t+1} does not change. The costs associated with this move are given by the right hand side of Equation 2.9. The left hand side depicts the benefits associated with a marginally higher H_t resulting from an increase in healthy time. The first term represents the benefit due to a higher consumption of h_t, while the second term captures the benefit relating to the productive use of the additional time, either as working time or as an input to household production. Although this choice of terminology is not entirely satisfactory, it is customary to describe these effects as the consumption and the investment benefit, respectively, of a marginal increase in the stock of health capital. To sum up, Equation 2.9 characterizes the optimal time path of health capital by equilibrating marginal benefits and marginal cost for every element H_t.

For an empirical analysis, it is useful to simplify the rather complicated structure of the model given by Equations 2.9 to 2.12. Following Grossman, the literature has focussed mainly on the analysis of two sub-models, each taking into account only part of the marginal benefits of health capital. As their names suggest, the pure consumption model deals exclusively with the consumption benefit, while the pure investment model emphasizes the investment benefit. It can be shown, however, that the pure consumption model, by neglecting any investment benefit, generates a number of extremely implausible implications. In particular, it takes the individual's marginal product of healthy time devoted to gross investment to be no higher than zero while he derives no utility from leisure at the margin [8]. Thus, the pure consumption sub-model implies the individual to be satiated with respect to leisure at an intertemporally optimal position. This surely limits its usefulness in any applied work. Therefore, in what follows we shall rely on the pure investment model.

In the investment sub-model, the consumption benefit of health – at the optimum position – is taken to be zero. In other words, suppose:

$$\frac{\partial u}{\partial h_t} = 0. \tag{2.14}$$

This assumption is not quite as restrictive as it may

appear at first sight. In particular, any benefit derived from the use of additional healthy time, either in household production or in labour supply, is already accounted for.

Utilizing condition Equation 2.14 helps to simplify the Grossman model considerably. The optimality condition for the stock of health capital now reads:

$$W_t \frac{\partial h}{\partial H_t} = \pi_{t-1}^I(1+r) - \pi_t^I(1-\delta_t). \tag{2.9a}$$

Since it contains no other endogenous variables, this equation alone determines the optimal stock of health capital in period t. This implies that the change in health capital, ΔH_{t+1}, will not depend on any other endogenous variable. Hence, in the pure investment sub-model, both the stock of health capital and consumption of medical care are determined by Equations 2.9a and 2.12 alone.

If one is interested only in the development of health capital H_t and medical care M_t, the structure of the pure investment model makes it possible to restrict the analysis to Equations 2.9a and 2.12. This holds because the optimal time paths for H_t and M_t are determined independently of both λ_0^V and the optimal time path for Z_t. For this reason, in what follows we will neglect Equations 2.10 and 2.11.

As regards comparative static analysis, it is useful to distinguish between two categories of effects. In order to see this, look at Equation 2.12 and let us investigate the effects of a change in a parameter which determines the stock of health capital according to Equation 2.9a. Since any parameter affecting health capital is contained in Equation 2.12 as well, the change under consideration gives rise to two effects. First, there is a direct influence on the demand for medical care, which captures the effect on M_t for a given stock of health capital. It is customary to describe this effect as the *direct effect* of the parameter variation. Apart from this, another effect operates through the influence on the individual's health. The corresponding change in M_t represents the *indirect effect* of the parameter variation which is brought about solely through its effect on H_t. The *total effect* on the demand for medical care is given by the sum of both effects, direct and indirect.

On the way to a version of the model given by Equations 2.9a and 2.12 which can be estimated empirically, we still need to address two issues. First, both equations exhibit a structure which is partly additive, and partly multiplicative. Since we intend to estimate the model by means of a linear approach, we shall introduce additional assumptions such that the multiplicative structure 'prevails'. Second, for some variables such as, e.g., the rate of depreciation we need to give functional specifications describing the influence of exogenous variables. In both instances, we will follow previous work by Grossman, Cropper and Wagstaff to a considerable degree, although our approach is slightly different [1,3,5].

Taking natural logarithms of Equation 2.9a yields:

$$\ln W_t + \ln \frac{\partial h}{\partial H_t} = \ln[\pi_{t-1}^I(1 + r) - \pi_t^I(1 - \delta_t)]. \qquad (2.9b)$$

Following Grossman, we choose as functional form for the function h measuring the services provided by the stock of health capital in units of healthy time:

$$h_t = \Omega - \alpha_1 H_t^{-\alpha_2}; \alpha_1 > 0, \alpha_2 > 0. \qquad (2.18)$$

This implies a concave h, i.e., decreasing marginal productivity of health capital.

Transforming the right hand side of Equation 2.9b by factoring out the product of the rate of depreciation and the marginal cost of gross investment yields:

$$\ln[\pi_{t-1}^I(1 + r) - \pi_t^I(1 - \delta_t)]$$

$$= \ln \pi_t^I \delta_t + \ln\left[1 + \frac{\pi_{t-1}^I\left(r - \frac{\Delta\pi_t^I}{\pi_{t-1}^I}\right)}{\pi_t^I \delta_t}\right]. \qquad (2.19)$$

The difference

$$\left(r - \frac{\Delta\pi_t^I}{\pi_{t-1}^I}\right)$$

compares the rate of return on an asset with the normalized capital gains component of gross investment I_{t-1}. We assume that this term or, more precisely, the whole expression

$$\pi_{t-1}^I\left(r - \frac{\Delta\pi_t^I}{\pi_{t-1}^I}\right)(\pi_t^I \delta_t)^{-1}$$

is close to zero. In addition, we take the corresponding deviation to be distributed randomly over individuals. Hence, the second term on the right hand side of Equation 2.19 may be interpreted as a stochastic error term.

Furthermore, let us suppose the production function for gross investment is of the Cobb-Douglas type. Thus, the logarithm of marginal cost can be expressed as a weighted sum of the logarithms of factor prices, if one takes into account the parametric influence of X_t:

$$\ln \pi_t^I = \alpha_3 \ln W_t + (1 - \alpha_3)\ln P_t^M + \alpha_4 X_t; 0 < \alpha_3 < 1. \qquad (2.20)$$

If the individual's level of education as measured by X_t exerts a positive influence on his investment productivity, we should expect a negative sign for α_4.

Finally, following Cropper, suppose the logarithm of the rate of depreciation to be given by:

$$\ln \delta_t = \ln \delta_0 + \alpha_5 t + \alpha_6 Y_t, \qquad (2.21)$$

with Y_t representing a vector of parameters other than the age factor that affect depreciation of health capital. In particular, this vector contains an element describing environmental conditions. Given that we are going to easure the quality of the environment negatively, we should expect a positive sign for the corresponding element of the parameter vector α_6.

With these assumptions, one obtains for Equation 2.9b, solving for $\ln H_t$:

$$\ln H_t = \frac{1}{\alpha_2 + 1}[k_1 + (1 - \alpha_3)\ln W_t - (1 - \alpha_3)\ln P_t^M$$

$$- \alpha_4 X_t - \alpha_5 t - \alpha_6 Y_t + u_t] \qquad (2.9c)$$

where

$$k_1 = \ln \alpha_1\alpha_2 - \ln \delta_0$$

and

$$u_t = -\ln\left[1 + \frac{\pi_{t-1}^I\left(r - \frac{\Delta\pi_t^I}{\pi_{t-1}^I}\right)}{\pi_t^I \delta_t}\right]$$

hold.

In order to get an estimable equation for the consumption of medical care, take natural logarithms of Equation 2.12:

$$\ln M_t = \ln \frac{\partial \pi_t^I}{\partial P_t^M} + \ln(\delta_t H_t + \Delta H_{t+1}). \qquad (2.12a)$$

Utilizing the specification for the marginal cost of gross investment, one obtains:

$$\ln \frac{\partial \pi_t^I}{\partial P_t^M} = \ln(1 - \alpha_3) + \ln \pi_t^I - \ln P_t^M$$

and, after replacing $\ln \pi_t^I$:

$$\ln \frac{\partial \pi_t^I}{\partial P_t^M} = \ln(1 - \alpha_3) + \alpha_3 \ln W_t - \alpha_3 \ln P_t^M + \alpha_4 X_t \quad (2.22)$$

Furthermore, the second term on the right hand side of

Equation 2.12b can be transformed as follows:

$$\ln(\delta_t H_t + \Delta H_{t+1}) = \ln \delta_t H_t + \ln\left(1 + \frac{\Delta H_{t+1}}{\delta_t H_t}\right). \quad (2.23)$$

The fraction

$$\frac{\Delta H_{t+1}}{\delta_t H_t}$$

measures the change in health capital ΔH_{t+1} relative to depreciation occurring in period t. If, firstly, the exogenous variables determining the stock of health capital change only slightly over time and, secondly, the rate of depreciation is sufficiently bounded away from zero, then this fraction will be close to zero. We follow Wagstaff in assuming that the deviations of this fraction from zero are distributed in a random manner over individuals [5]. Hence, the second term on the right hand side of Equation 2.23 may be interpreted as an error term. Consequently, one arrives at the following specification for the logarithm of the demand for medical care:

$$\ln M_t = k_2 + \alpha_3 \ln W_t - \alpha_3 \ln P_t^M$$
$$+ \alpha_4 X_t + \alpha_5 t + \alpha_6 Y_t + \ln H_t + v_t, \quad (2.12b)$$

where

$$k_2 = \ln(1 - \alpha_3) + \ln \delta_0 \text{ and } v_t = \ln\left(1 + \frac{\Delta H_{t+1}}{\delta_t H_t}\right)$$

hold.

Apart from a minor aspect, the task of providing an empirical specification appropriate for linear analysis has been accomplished. As can be seen from Equation 2.12b, our specification implies the logarithm of health capital to influence the logarithm of medical care with a coefficient equal to one. In contrast to physical capital, for example, it is characteristic of the stock of health capital, however, that it cannot be observed directly but needs to be captured by using appropriate health indicators. In general, approaches to the measurement of health supply values which are determined only up to some kind of (e.g., monotonic) transformation. In this sense, any empirical measurement of health is subject to a certain degree of arbitrariness. Therefore, it seems sensible not to determine the coefficient on $\ln H_t$ on *a priori* grounds.

Thus, our final equation for the logarithm of consumption of medical care reads as follows:

$$\ln M_t = k_2 + \alpha_3 \ln W_t - \alpha_3 \ln P_t^M$$
$$+ \alpha_4 X_t + \alpha_5 t + \alpha_6 Y_t + \alpha_7 \ln H_t + v_t, \quad (2.12c)$$

where we expect a positive sign for α_7.

THE FULL EMPIRICAL MODEL

Since it is neither directly observable nor measurable, we have chosen to model the stock of health capital as a latent variable. The same is true for the other variable we are primarily interested in, i.e., the quality of the environment. Due to the availability of only limited information on this variable, it enters our empirical model as a latent variable, too. Thus, the structural model outlined above contains two latent variables. While health capital is determined endogenously, environmental pollution is treated as a latent exogenous variable which reflects its role as a potential determinant of health.

The basic idea, therefore, is to supplement the structural model with a measurement model in which each latent variable is described by means of a set of indicators. For the stock of health capital, four indicators are available (HI). These are the degree of handicap, self-rated health status, the duration of sick leave, and information on chronic complaints, all as reported by the individual. As regards the quality of the environment, we have been forced to rely on only two indicators (EI). These are given by the degree of noise pollution and the degree of air pollution, as perceived by the individual. As it happens, both these indicators measure the quality of the environment negatively. Thus, it is really environmental pollution that is reflected by our indicators. In what follows, therefore, we shall refer to environmental pollution bearing in mind that this is related to the quality of the environment in an obvious way (i.e., inversely). For further information on the range of the indicators of our measurement model consult Table 2.1.

Our full empirical model is as follows:

$$\ln HI_i = \lambda_{hi} \ln H^* + \varepsilon_i, i = 1, 2, 3, 4, \quad (2.24)$$

$$EI_j = \lambda_{ej} E^* + \delta_j \quad j = 1, 2, \quad (2.25)$$

$$\ln H^* = \gamma_{11} E^* + \gamma_{12} Z + \zeta_1 \quad (2.26)$$

and

$$\ln M_k = \beta_k \ln H^* + \gamma_{k1} E^* + \gamma_{k2} Z + \zeta_k, \quad k = 2, 3, 4 \quad (2.27)$$

where we have used an asterisk to denote latent variables and the vector Z contains all those exogenous variables other than environmental pollution which may influence individual health. Figure 2.1 depicts the model given by Equations 2.24 to 2.27 in terms of a path diagram.

Our data source is given by the third wave of the West German Socio-economic Panel (SOEP), collected in 1986

Table 2.1 Descriptive statistics $(N = 3317)$[1]

Variable	Definition	Mean	Standard deviation
Environmental indicators			
CH07	noise pollution 1–5	2.0678	1.1010
CH08	air pollution 1–5	2.0932	1.0906
Health indicators			
ln CP69	handicapped individual 1–3	0.2828	0.3872
ln CP70	chronic complaints	0.2140	0.3203
ln CP0101	self-rated health 1–11	1.9903	0.4033
ln CP7302	duration of sick leave (days)	1.5382	1.5278
Demand for health services			
ln CP7102	number of visits to a general practitioner	0.7595	0.7176
ln FARZT	number of visits to a specialist	0.9155	0.8523
ln CP7203	hospital days 1985	0.3695	0.9658
Z-variables			
ln CP5202	net monthly income	7.4279	0.5442
CP8801	sex	0.4169	0.4931
CP8802	age in years	39.0865	11.6048
CPNAT	nationality	0.2819	0.4500
CPSBIL	education 1–3	2.0422	0.4692
CP0903	doing sports 1–4	2.0389	1.2742
CP6204	private insurance	0.0868	0.2816
CGGK	community size 1–7	4.4540	1.7997
CH0603	accessibility of resident physician 1–4	1.8478	1.085

[1] Employees only; third wave of the Socio-economic Panel (SOEP); the variable names CH07, CH08, CP69, CP70, CP0101, CP7302, CP7102, CP7203, CP8801, CP8802, CPNAT, CPSBIL, CP0903, CP6204, CGGK, and CH0603 correspond to the original description of the reference manual (cf. Deutsches Institut für Wirtschaftsforschung 1993); ln in front of a variable denotes the natural logarithm. If a zero value is possible for a variable, we have added one before performing the log transformation.

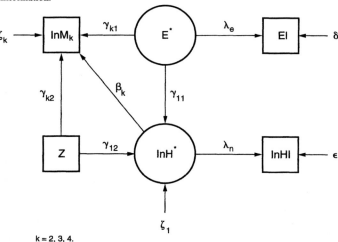

$k = 2, 3, 4.$

Figure 2.1. Path diagram of the model

[9–11]. Apart from standard questions which are repeated on a yearly basis, this particular wave additionally contains self-rated information on environmental conditions. In order to comply fully with the theoretical analysis of the Grossman model, our sample is restricted to those individuals who exhibit a positive demand for health services. Since our empirical analysis includes three demand variables, a positive demand for health services is equivalent to at least one positive entry in any of these components. In addition, we confine the analysis

Table 2.2   Estimation results: measurement equations

Indicators	Latent variables		R^2
	Environmental pollution (E^*)	Health capital ($\ln H^*$)	
Noise pollution (CH07)	0.7539		0.5623
Air pollution (CH08)	0.8318 (4.1045)		0.6920
Duration of sick leave (ln CP7302)		-0.3308 (-13.4703)	0.1094
Handicapped individual (ln CP69)		-0.8140 (-23.8913)	0.6627
Self-rated health (ln CP0101)		0.6273	0.3936
Chronic complaints (ln CP70)		-0.6493 (-22.2958)	0.4217

Total number of observations: 3317; t-values in brackets, based on robust standard errors. The coefficient of determination R^2 is one minus the ratio of error and variable variance. The latter is equal to one in the standardized model.

Table 2.3   Estimation results: structural equations

Explanatory variables	Dependent variables			
	Health capital ($\ln H^*$)	Number of visits to a general practitioner ($\ln$ CP7102)	Number of visits to a specialist ($\ln$ FARZT)	Hospital days ($\ln$ CP7203)
Health ($\ln H^*$)		-0.2557	-0.2977	-0.2640
		(-10.3470)	(-11.6480)	(-8.3756)
Environmental pollution (E^*)	-0.0909	-0.0001	-0.0018	-0.0567
	(-3.5654)	(-0.0052)	(-0.0766)	(-2.8219)
Income (ln CP5202)	0.0591	-0.0708	0.0485	-0.0145
	(2.2741)	(-3.5549)	(2.4051)	(-0.7330)
Sex (CP8801)	-0.0188	-0.0823	0.1377	-0.0352
	(-0.8103)	(-4.2424)	(6.9292)	(-1.7756)
Age (CP8802)	-0.2961	0.0513	-0.0876	-0.0465
	(-13.2913)	(2.6955)	(-4.8428)	(-2.2985)
Nationality (CPNAT)	0.0206	0.0578	-0.0661	0.0385
	(0.9317)	(2.9759)	(-3.3930)	(1.8505)
Education (CPSBIL)	0.0727	-0.0323	0.0338	0.0027
	(3.2325)	(-1.7002)	(1.8240)	(0.1451)
Doing sports (CP0903)	0.1075	-0.0281	0.0739	0.0026
	(5.3503)	(-1.6082)	(4.2965)	(0.1436)
Private insurance (CP6204)	0.0163	-0.0343	0.0273	
	(0.8596)	(-2.0653)	(1.6408)	
Community size (CGGK)	-0.0412	-0.1519	0.1431	-0.0227
	(-2.1259)	(-8.7691)	(8.4429)	(-1.3164)
Accessibility of resident physician (CH0603)	-0.0666	-0.0132		
	(-3.3909)	(-0.7890)		
R^2	0.1383	0.1243	0.1284	0.0676

Total number of observations: 3317; t-values in brackets, based on robust standard errors. The coefficient of determination R^2 is one minus the ratio of error and variable variance. The latter is equal to one in the standard model.

to the working population, since the use of the duration of sick leave as health indicator makes sense only for working individuals. This leaves us with an actual sample of 3317 observations for our estimation. Table 2.1 summarizes the basic descriptive statistics of the variables used in our study.

In order to scale the dimension of the latent variables H^* and E^* we have restricted the parameters λ_{h3} and λ_{e1}. This implies that the corresponding indicators act as reference indicators for the respective latent variable. While this constitutes a necessary precondition for identification, identification is obtained by imposing a number of additional zero-restrictions on the parameters of our model which can be read off from Tables 2.2 and 2.3.

The disturbances are assumed to be independently normally distributed with zero expectation. These assumptions enable us to estimate Equations 2.24 to 2.27 by Full Information Maximum Likelihood using the GAUSS-module LINCS. Developed by Schoenberg and Arminger [12], LINCS (Linear Covariance Structures) is a program written in GAUSS which allows for flexible programming and provides, for instance, heteroskedasticity-consistent estimates of the standard errors.

Since in most applications the assumption of multivariate normality of the data cannot be maintained, the precondition for MLE no longer holds. Given that this is true, e.g., for the dependent variables of our measurement model, the validity of our estimation procedure may be questioned. As Gouriéoux *et al.* point out [13], ML-estimates based on the false distributional assumption should more accurately be referred to as 'Pseudo Maximum Likelihood Estimates'. More importantly, they have shown that ML-estimates obtained under the erroneous assumption of multivariate normality are not meaningless, however, since they minimize the Kullback information criterion and can be interpreted as 'Minimum-Ignorance-Estimators' [14]. While the consistency of the parameter estimates may hold, estimates of the corresponding standard errors using the false distributional assumption are no longer valid. Thus, it is necessary to use heteroskedasticity-consistent standard errors which can be computed according to White's proposal, given the consistency of parameter estimates. More detailed information on this correction may be found in the literature [12,15].

RESULTS

Tables 2.2–2.4 present the estimation results based on the standardized solution. This implies that all variances are equal to one [12,16]. While Tables 2.2 and 2.3 contain our estimates of the measurement sub-model and of the direct effects of the structural sub-model, respectively, Table 2.4 provides information on both indirect and total effects of the exogenous variables on the demand for medical services.

Turning to the measurement sub-model first, it is reassuring to find that none of the coefficients is of the 'wrong' sign. As inspection of the coefficient of determination (R^2) reveals, the latent variable environmental pollution explains quite a substantial part of the variance of each indicator. With respect to the stock of health capital, the corresponding figures turn out to be lower, the exception being the indicator 'degree of handicap', 66.2 percent of

whose variance is explained by variations in individual health. On the other hand, health capital explains around 11 percent of the variation in the 'duration of sick leave'. The reason may be that this indicator is more likely to reflect the individual's satisfaction with his working conditions rather than pointing to a specific illness.

Turning to the structural sub-model, our results are broadly as follows. As for the health capital equation, most of the coefficients are both of the correct sign and statistically significant. With respect to the demand for health care equations, however, our estimation results are less satisfactory.

In particular, we obtain a negative coefficient on the stock of health capital which is found to be significant in all three equations. While this finding is in line with the results of other studies, it clearly disagrees with our empirical specification. It is tempting to conclude that, given this discrepancy, the corresponding structural parameters are of the 'wrong' sign [17]. This, however, would be premature. Looking at Equation 2.12, it is straightforward to show that the impact of a marginal increase in health capital on the demand for health care is given by

$$\frac{\partial M_t}{\partial H_t} = -\frac{\partial \pi_t^I}{\partial P_t^M}(1 - \delta_t). \quad (2.28)$$

If one takes reasonable values for δ_t to be restricted by $0 < \delta_t < 1$, then the Grossman model obviously implies a negative influence of health on consumption of medical care. Thus, while our empirical results certainly disagree with our empirical specification, they do not provide evidence against the Grossman model.

In a more recent paper, Wagstaff proposed a different empirical specification of the Grossman model which yields a negative sign for the coefficient on health capital in the demand for health care equation [18]. Moreover, his formulation also reverses the signs of the coefficients on the exogenous variables in this equation which, again, is in line with the results of most empirical studies. Thus, although it is not quite clear how his specification can be derived from the theoretical model, Wagstaff's approach surely represents a very interesting alternative for the purpose of empirical research.

As expected, the latent variable environmental pollution E^* exerts a negative impact on the stock of health capital H^*. Increasing environmental pollution goes along with a higher rate of depreciation and, hence, induces a decrease in the stock of health capital. Contrary to the prediction of our theoretical model, we find a negative relationship between environmental pollution and health care demand. However, the direct effects on the number of GP visits and on specialist visits are not significant.

Table 2.4 Indirect and total effects on the demand for health services

	Demand for health services					
	Number of visits to a general practitioner (ln Cp7102)		Number of visits to a specialist (ln FARZT)		Hospital days (ln CP7203)	
Explanatory variables	Indirect effect	Total effect	Indirect effect	Total effect	Indirect effect	Total effect
Environmental pollution	0.0232	0.0231	0.0271	0.0253	0.0240	−0.0327
(E*)	(3.4068)	(1.0989)	(3.4750)	(1.1410)	(3.3614)	(−1.3718)
Income (ln CP5202)	−0.0151	−0.0859	−0.0176	0.0309	−0.0156	−0.0301
	(−2.2360)	(−4.1845)	(−2.2913)	(1.5316)	(−2.2339)	(−1.5257)
Sex (CP8801)	0.0048	−0.0775	0.0056	0.1433	0.0050	−0.0302
	(0.8046)	(−3.9031)	(0.8083)	(7.0917)	(0.8083)	(−1.5179)
Age (CP8802)	0.0757	0.1270	0.0881	0.0005	0.0782	0.0317
	(7.8333)	(7.1818)	(9.2857)	(0.0769)	(7.2222)	(1.6250)
Nationality (CPNAT)	−0.0053	0.0525	−0.0061	−0.0722	−0.0054	0.0331
	(−0.9333)	(2.6551)	(−0.9280)	(−3.6069)	(−0.9286)	(1.5480)
Education (CPSBIL)	−0.0186	−0.0509	−0.0216	0.0122	−0.0192	−0.0165
	(−3.0870)	(−2.6141)	(−3.1440)	(0.6377)	(−3.0153)	(−0.8715)
Doing sports (CP0903)	−0.0275	−0.0556	−0.0320	0.0419	−0.0284	−0.0258
	(−4.8438)	(−3.1616)	(−4.9767)	(2.3932)	(−4.5745)	(−1.4130)
Private insurance (CP6204)	−0.0042	−0.0385	−0.0049	0.0224	−0.0043	−0.0043
	(−0.8548)	(−2.2581)	(−0.8647)	(1.3114)	(−0.8506)	(−0.8506)
Community size (CGGK)	0.0105	−0.1414	0.0123	0.1554	0.0109	−0.0168
	(2.1000)	(−7.9437)	(2.0714)	(8.9634)	(2.0714)	(−0.6702)
Accessibility of resident	0.0170	0.0038	0.0198	0.0198	0.0176	0.0176
physician	(3.2432)	(0.2250)	(3.2549)	(3.2549)	(3.2115)	(3.2115)

Number of observations: 3317; t-values in brackets, based on robust standard errors.

The corresponding indirect effects of environmental pollution on the three health care demand variables are both positive and significant, i.e. the increased rate of depreciation implies a higher consumption of medical services (see Table 2.3). In this case, medical consumption may be interpreted as a gross investment which tends to compensate for the higher rate of depreciation.

With respect to the class of Z-variables, the coefficients on the variables income, age, and education display the theoretically expected impact on the latent variable health capital H^*. As for their influence on the consumption of medical care, our results are mixed. High income earners consult a general practitioner less frequently, but have more contacts with a specialist. If the general practitioner treats only minor health problems, opportunity costs might play an important part. There are controversial opinions on the sign of the income variable. Van de Ven and van der Gaag [19] report a negative effect of income on the demand for medical services. On the one hand, a high income results in a high demand (direct effect), but, on the other hand, this leads to a higher level of health capital which reduces consumption (indirect

effect). *A priori* the total effect is undetermined. Our estimation results indicate that with regard to GP visits the direct and the indirect effect are both significant and point in the same direction, resulting in a negative total effect (see Table 2.4). The direct and the indirect effect of income on the number of specialist visits are of opposite signs, while the resulting total effect is not significant.

The binary variable for the type of medical insurance is only significant for visits to a general practitioner. Individuals that are privately insured pay fewer visits to a general practitioner. This result reflects mainly the institutional setting of Germany, where the GP has no gatekeeper function for privately insured patients. Unlike a patient insured in the statutory health insurance, a privately insured patient can choose his physician(s) without any restriction.

As expected, the age variable exerts a negative impact on the stock of health capital. Puzzling are the direct effects of age on the demand for health services, which turn out to be both negative and significant as far as the number of specialist visits and hospital days are concerned. One explanation of this finding might be the way

Table 2.5 Results of the specification tests

Model part to be analyzed	Test statistics[1]
Value of the Hausman-type specification test when analyzing structural parameters only	HTST = 0.11
	DG = 44
	Pr = 1.0
Value of Hausman-type specification test for all parameters	HTST = 1238.61
	DG = 55
	Pr = 0.00

[1]HTST = Test statistic of the Hausman-type specification test; DG: degree of freedom; Pr: Probability-level.

we have modelled the age effect. More precisely, we consider only a linear age term although it is well known that age possesses a convex relationship with respect to health care demand. The latter implies that the number of physician consultations and hospital days first decreases and then increases with age. Nevertheless, the total effect of age on each component of health care demand has the expected positive sign and is statistically significant for both GP and specialist consultations.

Doing sports has a positive effect on the stock of health capital. More ambiguous is the relationship between sports and the consumption of medical services. The direct effect in Table 2.3 is only significant for vists to specialists and the positive sign indicates the consequences of sport injuries. This result contrasts with the indirect effects, which operate through the stock of health capital and reduce the demand for health services (see Table 2.4). Only for the number of specialist visits, the resulting total effect is significant at the 5 percent level. This increased demand for specialist services can be interpreted as gross investment which is to compensate for the hazards potentially associated with doing sports.

Between community size and the number of specialist consultations we find a positive direct effect which may reflect the overproportional supply of specialists in larger communities. In addition, the corresponding coefficient in the GP equation is negative, indicating that GP services are substituted by specialist services in larger communities and cities.

Finally, consider the impact of the accessibility of the general practitioner. Since this variable measures the distance to his physician, it is an important determinant of the individual's time costs associated with the consumption of medical care. Given that the actual money prices of medical care – with only minor exceptions – are fully covered by health insurance, the 'accessibility of the general practitioner' therefore can be expected to act as a proxy for the user price of medical care. This is confirmed by its coefficient in the health capital equation which is

both negative and statistically significant. However, the corresponding effect in the demand for GP consultations equation fails to be significant.

In order to test for the consistency of our parameter estimates, we apply a Hausman-type specification test. In this modified Hausman-test proposed by Schoenberg and Arminger [12], the FIML-estimator which is consistent and efficient under the null hypothesis but inconsistent and inefficient under the alternative, is compared to a weighted estimator which is consistent but inefficient under both alternatives. The weights are introduced to increase the power of the test. They are chosen such that observations in which the endogenous variables are poorly predicted get a higher weight than observations that predict the endogenous variables well [12,20]. A sufficiently well specified model should result only in small differences between the two estimates. The test statistic of the Hausman-type specification test has a χ^2-distribution.

Table 2.5 summarizes the results of the specification tests. Note that there is no evidence of misspecification of the structural model, while the overall specification of our model has to be rejected. An explanation for the strong discrepancies in the test results might be the extremely parsimonious specification of the covariance structure of the disturbances.

CONCLUSION

Our analysis indicates that the quality of the environment as measured negatively by the level of environmental pollution is an important determinant of individual health. On the other hand, the relationship between environmental pollution and the demand for health care is not clear-cut. We have found a negative direct effect on health care demand but this is statistically significant only in the case of hospital days. In contrast, the corresponding indirect effect on all three demand variables is both positive and significant, i.e., a higher level of environmental pollution as it operates through the stock of health capital implies a higher consumption of medical services.

These results suggest that any policy directed at improving the quality of the environment is likely to generate benefits in the field of health care as well. More precisely, due to its positive effect on health, a higher quality of the environment *ceteris paribus* enables the individual to enter any given period with a higher stock of health capital. In this sense, then, any such environmental policy can be interpreted in terms of preventive medicine, too.

It is important to bear in mind that our primary intention has been to estimate the overall impact of the quality of the environment on both health capital and the demand for health care. In essence, this provides the main reason for our focussing on the latent variable environmental pollution. For the purpose of policy analysis, it will usually make more sense to investigate the influence of individual components of environmental pollution, i.e., one will be interested in the effects of, say, the level of air pollution on the stock of health capital and the consumption of medical care. This can be done without changing the substance of the analysis presented above.

Finally, let us briefly comment on the results of the Hausman-type specification test. While we find no evidence for misspecification of the structural model, the overall specification of our model has been rejected. We suspect this may be due primarily to the limitations of our measurement model. Unfortunately, household surveys like the Socio-Economic Panel do not contain much information on environmental factors. Thus, it is not possible to achieve a satisfactory description of the quality of the environment.

In this vein, we take our results to indicate two further aspects for future research on the relationship between health, health care and the environment. First, an attempt should be made to map latent variables by means of indicators more accurately. Furthermore, in our view the application of panel data is of special interest to cope with the impact lag which characterizes the influence of environmental pollution on both health and health care demand.

ACKNOWLEDGEMENT

We are grateful to participants at the Third European Workshop on Econometrics and Health Economics held at Antwerp, in particular Adam Wagstaff and Eddy van Doorslaer, for a number of helpful suggestions. Of course, responsibility for any errors that remain is ours.

REFERENCES

1. Cropper, M. Measuring the benefits from reduced morbidity. *American Economic Review* 1981; **71**: 235–240.
2. Mushkin, S.J. Health as an investment. *Journal of Political Economy* 1962; **70**: S129–S157.
3. Grossman, M. *The demand for health: a theoretical and empirical investigation.* Occasional paper 119. National Bureau of Economic Research. New York and London, 1972.
4. Muurinen, J.-M. Demand for health. A generalized Grossman model. *Journal of Health Economics* 1982; **1**: 5–28.
5. Wagstaff, A. The demand for health. Some new empirical evidence. *Journal of Health Economics* 1986; **5**: 195–233.
6. Killingworth, M.R. *Labour supply.* Cambridge, 1983.
7. Léonard, D. and van Long, N. *Optimal control theory and static optimization in economics.* Cambridge, 1992.
8. Ried, W. *On the benefits of additional healthy time: the Grossman pure consumption model revisited.* Mannheim: mimeo, 1994.
9. Deutsches Institut für Wirtschaftsforschung, (ed.), *Das Sozio-ökonomische Panel. Benutzerhandbuch.* Vol. I u. II. Berlin, 1993.
10. Projektgruppe Sozio-ökonomisches Panel. Zehn Jahre Sozio-ökonomisches Panel (SOEP). *DIW, Vierteljahresheft* 1993: 27–42.
11. Burkhauser, R.V. *An Introduction to the German Socio-economic Panel for English speaking researchers: Cross national studies in ageing.* Program Project Paper No. 1. All-University Gerontology Center, The Maxwell School. Syracuse University, 1990.
12. Schoenberg, R. and Arminger, G. *LINCS2.0 (Linear Covariance Structures). A computer program for the analysis of linear models incorporating measurement error disturbances as well as structural disturbances.* User's guide. RJS Software, Kent, WA, 1989–90.
13. Gouriéroux, C., Monfort, A. and Trognon, A. Pseudo maximum likelihood methods: Theory. *Econometrica* 1984; **52**: 681–700.
14. Gouriéroux, C. and Monfort, A. *Statistique et modeles econometriques. Vol. 1 – Notions générales, Estimation, Prévision, Algorithmes.* Paris, 1989.
15. Arminger, G. and Müller, F. *Lineare Modelle zur Analyse von Paneldaten.* Opalden, 1990.
16. Jöreskog, K.G. and Sörbom, D. *LISREL 7. A guide to the program and applications.* 2nd edition. Chicago, 1989.
17. Leu, R.E. and Gerfin, M. Die Nachfrage nach Gesundheit – ein empirischer Test des Grossman-Modells. In Oberender, P. (ed.), *Steuerungsprobleme im Gesundheitswesen.* Baden-Baden: Nomos, 1992.
18. Wagstaff, A. The demand for health: an empirical reformulation of the Grossman model. *Health Economics* 1993; **2**: 189–198.
19. Van de Ven, W. and van der Gaag, J. Health as an unobservable. A MIMIC-model of the demand for health care. *Journal of Health Economics* 1982; **1**: 157–183.
20. Krämer, W. and Sonnberger, H. *The linear regression model under test.* Heidelberg and Wien, 1986.

3

Subjective Health Measures and State-Dependent Reporting Errors

MARCEL KERKHOFS[1] AND MAARTEN LINDEBOOM[2]

[1] *Tilburg University, Tilburg, the Netherlands and* [2] *Free University, Amsterdam, the Netherlands*

INTRODUCTION

While life expectancy increased and working conditions and the quality of health care improved in the past decades, participation rates of elderly workers declined dramatically in most OECD countries. One is tempted to relate this decline to the expansion of social security systems over the same period. Yet the majority of non-participating elderly report that health rather than financial incentives was the primary consideration in their retirement behaviour. And indeed, inclusion of subjective health measures in retirement models generally led to large and dominant effects of health, and relatively small effects of financial incentives on retirement behaviour. This phenomenon generated a large number of contributions to the retirement literature, trying to explain the dominant health effects, and propose solutions to the problem (see for instance Lambrinos [1], Parsons [2], Anderson and Burkhauser [3], Bazzoli [4], Butler *et al.* [5], Stern [6] and Bound [7] for retirement models, or Bartel and Taubman [8], Lee [9] and Chiricos and Nestel [10] for earnings equations). The central argument is that health should be treated as an endogenous variable in retirement models. Health may be endogenous in the 'classical' sense that it is correlated with unobserved factors – such as the rate of time preference – that affect retirement behaviour [11]. Others expect a causal relationship to run from participation to health; for example through work-related injuries and stress, or the other way round: 'retirement *per se* causes bad health via boredom' (Sickless and Taubman) [12]. Additionally, the endogeneity of health measures may result from systematic misreporting. It is argued that responses to questions concerning health will be biased due to economic incen-

tives or that responses are adapted to conform to social norms. Reporting health as the main reason for inactivity is socially more accepted than expressing a relatively strong preference for leisure. Furthermore, eligibility conditions for some Social Security Allowances – notably Disability Insurance Benefits – are contingent upon bad health. Respondents may be worried about the confidentiality of their answers or about political consequences of the findings of the survey. Reporting errors may therefore depend on the respondent's labour market status. In retirement models, this reversed causality will typically lead to biased parameter estimates and misleading conclusions.

In the absence of state dependent reporting errors, the endogeneity problems boil down to standard problems for which solutions are readily available. So in a way the main issue in the empirical analysis of the 'Retirement-Health Nexus' (cf. Anderson and Burkhauser [3]) is the state dependence of responses to health questions. The objective of this paper is to assess the relative importance of state dependent reporting errors in health measures.

In order to eliminate the subjective nature of responses to questions about health, various authors have used measures that are believed to be more objective, for instance observed future death of respondents in the sample [2,3], or sickness absenteeism records [13]. As pointed out by Bazzoli [4] and Bound [7] the variable of interest is the extent to which health impedes working and parameter estimates in retirement models are subject to errors in variable bias if these objective measures are not perfectly correlated with work related health. The use of lagged responses to health questions or an instrumental variable method as proposed by Stern [6] or Aarts and de Jong [14] are also of little help, since the state dependent reporting errors are not eliminated. Bound [7] elegantly shows how in the context of a labour supply model in which financial variables affect health-reporting, each of the solutions proposed in the literature leads to different biases. The use of mortality information as a proxy will tend to underestimate the effects of health and overestimate the effects of financial variables, whereas if it is used to instrument subjective health measures the impact of health is correctly estimated, but the effect of economic variables is underestimated. On the other hand the sign of the biases is ambiguous if subjective health measures are used.

The objective of our model is to provide more insight into the state dependence of self-reported health measures. In section 3 we state a condition that enables us to determine systematic response errors from the comparison of subjective and objective health measures across four different groups of respondents: the employed, the unemployed, the disabled and the early retired. The procedure is attractive as it is relatively simple and does not require the specification of a complete model of participation or retirement decisions. This is an advantage, as results obtained in previous analyses of the endogeneity of health variables were sensitive to misspecification of the participation, retirement or earnings equations. Furthermore, our model of self-reported health may be embedded in a more complete retirement model.

The way in which we identify the state dependence of reporting errors is related to the analysis by Butler *et al.* [5]. They compare two dichotomous arthritis measures: one subjective measure based on a direct question and an objective measure derived from a more detailed list of symptoms and indicators. The relation between these two variables is investigated by running a regression of a measure of the degree of association between the two variables on a set of socio-economic variables. Their results indicate that the relationship between the measures is significantly stronger for employed respondents than for the others.

Although the motivation for this analysis is to study the impact of endogenous reporting errors in health measures that are typically used in labour-supply studies – work-related health indicators – corresponding objective measures are less readily available than for an individual's general health status. In the empirical application we will therefore limit our scope to the analysis of subjective general health measures. An individual's response is modelled as a function of a latent (true) health indicator, based on an objective measure and several other controls. The ordered response model that translates this latent variable into the observed categorical response is allowed to differ across the four labour market states mentioned above. In this way, the response distortions may be differ-

ent for the disabled than for the retired, employed or unemployed. Explicitly modelling reported health as a deviation from some underlying true health indicator allows us to generate health measures free of state dependent reporting errors.

In section 3 we present the model and discuss the assumption underlying our approach. For the empirical application we use data from a Dutch survey held in 1993 among approximately 4700 households of Dutch elderly. The dataset is comparable in structure and contents to the HRS of the University of Michigan Research Center, and contains detailed information on health and retirement issues. This dataset is discussed in section 4. Section 2 presents some information about the Dutch disability allowance system. It is generally recognized that this system has increasingly been used as a lay-off/quit route that is financially attractive to both employers and employees. One would therefore expect misreporting to be a particularly serious problem in Dutch data. Although the model was not developed for that purpose, the estimates provide some information as to the extent to which the disability allowance was used inappropriately. In section 5 we present the statistical model and the empirical implementation. Section 6 discusses the results, and section 7 concludes.

THE DUTCH DISABILITY INSURANCE SYSTEM

The Dutch disability insurance system consists roughly speaking of two programs: a general disability fund called AAW that provides a disability benefit at a minimum level and an additional program, WAO, that supplements the disability allowance for private sector workers to 80% of the gross wage they earned in their last job. For public sector employees a similar supplementary allowance is provided by the public sector pension fund. The philosophy of these allowances is to insure workers against losses in their earnings capacity that result from illness or injury. A worker who has been on sickness-leave for a period of 12 months can apply for a DI-allowance. Depending on the severity of the disability one may receive a full or a partial allowance. The DI-system is a pay-as-you-go system that is funded by contributions from employers (AAW) and workers (AAW and WAO).

The assessment of the degree to which a worker is disabled is performed by a central medical service called GMD. In determining the loss of earnings capacity the GMD doctors have to take the applicant's labour market opportunities into account as well as the fact that it is in general extremely difficult for partially disabled to find a job. Because of this difficulty and the fact that the organizations of employers and the labour unions manage the institutions that administer the allowances, the application procedures and the admittance criteria, it has become common practice to treat partially disabled unemployed as if they were fully disabled. In recent years it has become clear that employers and workers have used the DI-system as a financially attractive way of ending labour contracts with mutual consent. The employee receives the DI-benefit for an indefinite period, whereas unemployment benefits run out after one year. In practice, employers have made the regulation even more attractive by offering to supplement the DI-benefit to a higher percentage of previous earnings. Especially for older workers the DI-allowance appears to have served as an unofficial early retirement scheme.

The growing popularity of the DI-programs can be seen from the development of the number of recipients over the previous decades: from 215 400 in 1970, 657 100 in 1980 to 880 800 in 1990 (the Dutch labour force was 5.7 million in 1990). Since 1983 the economic recovery has led to a growth of the number of jobs and a steady decline in the number of unemployed, but over these years the number of DI-recipients continued to grow at a constant speed. The unrealistically high number of disabled and the costs associated gave rise to a parliamentary inquiry in 1993. The conclusion of this inquiry was that the DI-system has become overly generous. As a direct consequence the GMD has started reexamination procedures, reconsidering the applications of DI-recipients under 40. In June 1994, 8684 benefits of DI-recipients younger than 35 had been reexamined. Only 50% of these allowances was confirmed. In 7% of the cases the allowance was reduced and 43% was rejected completely. It may be expected that the percentage of rejections would be much higher for DI-recipients of 50 years and older.

Some indirect evidence of this claim may be found in the CERRA-data, that are used in the empirical application of the model. The respondents were asked whether their health severely or totally restricted them to perform

Table 3.1 Percentage of affirmative responses to the proposition 'health restricts me severely or totally in performing my job'

	Age			
	43–47	48–52	53–57	58 +
Employed	4.7	4.2	6.6	9.4
Self-employed	2.4	8.5	12.0	13.0
Early retired	—	—	5.3	14.2
Disabled	94.3	95.4	92.2	89.0
Unemployed	17.7	17.4	19.7	19.7
Others	—	—	13.0	26.2

Source: CERRA-I, October 1993.

their job. Although the answers to this question are expected to suffer from systematic mis-reporting the general pattern is clear. Table 3.1 contains the percentage of affirmative answers for subsamples according to age and labour market status. For all categories health problems increase with age, except for the disabled. Of the group of disabled aged 58 and older 11% admit that their health does not seriously impede their ability to work. It therefore seems reasonable to expect reporting errors in self-reported health measures to be a serious problem in Dutch surveys from the period considered.

MODELLING REPORTING BEHAVIOUR

In modelling subjective health measures we will introduce a latent variable representing the true value of the health measure. The reported health measure will be denoted by H^s and the corresponding latent true health is denoted by H^*. In the empirical application H^s and H^* will refer to an individual's general health status, such as the answer to a survey question like 'How good would you rate your health? Very good, good, fair, sometimes good/sometimes bad, or bad'. Rather than one measure, H^* could refer to a set of health measures. For ease of exposition we will restrict ourselves to single measures. Reporting errors will be analyzed by comparing the subjective health measure to an objective measure of the same health variable, denoted by H^o. A physician-diagnosed report would be the ideal objective measure of a respondent's general health condition. However, a professional diagnosis is typically not available in survey data and we have to rely on other sources of (more) objective health information.

With respect to a respondent's general health status a more objective measure may be derived from an extensive questionnaire on various health problems, diseases and health-related impediments in performing a large number of everyday activities. One such questionnaire is the Hopkins Symptom Checklist (HSCL). A score from that list will be used in the empirical application in section 6. It may be argued that this measure will probably still be subject to systematic mis-reporting, but for our purposes it is likely to be a sufficiently objective benchmark to which the all-in answer H^s can be compared. If H^o also suffers from state-dependent reporting errors our model will only provide a lower bound to the extent of mis-reporting. Alternative 'objective' measures that could be used are observed mortality rates (in a panel) or the number of visits to a doctor in the previous year. Both of these measures are clearly objective, but are too specific to serve as a measure for general health H^*.

The health variables H^s and H^* may also refer to more specific aspects of an individual's health. For applications in labour supply and retirement models a work-related measure should be used, denoting the restrictions an individual perceives in performing his job. As it will be more difficult to find objective measures that sufficiently account for an individual's work conditions, we will as a first application use the model to analyze a general health measure. Even then, the objective measure H^o may be an imperfect instrument for H^*. For that purpose an additional set of exogenous variables X_1 is used to describe H^*. Typically, X_1 will contain variables such as age and education. The role of these variables is to provide complementary information in order to describe H^* sufficiently well. If H^o and H^* are more dissimilar, the role of the exogenous variables in X_1 becomes more important. In the model of the general health status, with the HSCL-score as H^o, one may expect a minor role for X_1. Modelling work-related health measures the role of X_1-variables will gain in importance.

In the introduction two types of endogeneity problems were mentioned. First of all H^* may be related to the individual's labour market status S (S = employed, unemployed, disabled or early retired). This relation can be a direct causal relationship: health problems caused by work or inactivity. Alternatively, the relation between H^* and S could be indirect – the 'classical' endogeneity problem – when S and H^* depend on common unobservables. One way in which this type of endogeneity emerges is if one's health status and one's career are considered to result from simultaneous investment decisions regarding education, work and health. We will refer to this kind of dependence of H^* on S as type I endogeneity. Secondly, H^s and S will be related due to state dependent reporting errors. This kind of endogeneity will be denoted as type II endogeneity. In a complete model of retirement decisions both types of endogeneity have to be modelled explicitly. In this analysis we are specifically interested in type II endogeneity. We will therefore make an assumption about the relationship between H^* on the one hand and H^o, X_1 and S on the other. This assumption allows us to abstract from type I endogeneity.

Assumption 1 *the conditional probability distribution of H^* conditional on H^o, X_1 and S is independent of S. Denoting the conditional probability density by pdf(.):*

$$\text{pdf}(H^* | H^o, X_1, S) \equiv \text{pdf}(H^* | H^o, X_1).$$

Essentially this assumption states that the objective health measure H^o – if necessary assisted by the control variables X_1 – is a sufficient statistic for the impact of S on H^*. Put differently: type I endogeneity can be ruled out by conditioning on H^o and X_1. This simply means that, added to H^o and X_1, S provides no further information

about the latent true health variable H^*. Any effect of the current employment status S on H^* (type I endogeneity) is assumed to be sufficiently captured by the objective measure H^o and additional exogenous variables. As, by the assumption, pdf($H^* | H^o, X_1, S$) is identical for all respondents irrespective of their value of S, any effect of S on H^s – controlling for H^o and X_1 – represents 'reporting behaviour'.

Although we specifically concentrate on the effect of the labour market status S on reporting behaviour, other exogenous variables may also affect reporting behaviour. If a respondent with a university degree states that his health is 'good' he may not mean the same as a non-skilled respondent filling out the same box. This sort of differences of expression or language will be captured by a set of exogenous variables X_2. These exogenous variables are assumed to affect H^s and not H^*. Reformulating the above assumption accordingly:

$$\text{pdf}(H^* | H^o, X_1, S, X_2) \equiv \text{pdf}(H^* | H^o, X_1).$$

We can now specify the model as follows:

$$H^* = f_1(H^o, X_1, \varepsilon_1; \theta_1) \tag{3.1}$$

$$H^s = f_2(H^*, S, X_2, \varepsilon_2; \theta_2). \tag{3.2}$$

The variables ε_1 and ε_2 are random disturbances, f_1 describes the relationship between true health and its instruments and f_2 represents reporting behaviour. Bound [7] and Stern [6] model reporting errors as a relationship between H^s and the wage rate rather than the labour market status S. In the Netherlands the unemployment benefits, early retirement income and disability allowances are closely linked to previous earnings. We assume that the labour market state S sufficiently describes the income one receives relative to previous earnings. Only disability allowances are contingent on the health status. We may therefore expect the unemployed, early retired and pensioners to respond in a manner similar to the employed. This assumption will however not be imposed in the model we estimate. Rather we will specify separate functions for each state:

$$H^s = f_{2,S}(H^*, X_2, \varepsilon_2; \theta_2). \tag{3.3}$$

In this way we also take account of the fact that financial motives are not the only cause of reporting biases. Using S rather than the wage rate allows for these other sources of state-dependent reporting. Early retired might find it important to stress that they did not drop out and can still do the work they used to. They may therefore exaggerate their health status. As we do not think that the wage rate (capturing the financial motives for systematic mis-reporting) adds much to the effect of S, we do not explicitly include it in f_2. Any role would be as an element of X_2.

The role of exogenous variables in this model triggers the question whether an exogenous variable such as one's gender or level of education should be in X_1 or in X_2. The null-hypothesis that education affects true health rather than reporting behaviour can clearly be tested. The opposite hypothesis that education effects represent reporting behaviour – people of different education levels speaking different languages – and not real health differences is fundamentally untestable as the effect of the variables in X_2 on H^s is more flexible than that of the X_1-variables. (Notice that even if no effect of education on H^s is found, it may be that significant health differences are cancelled out by differences in reporting behaviour.) Determining the role of the exogenous variables is important when it comes to correcting for subjective reporting. For that purpose X_2-variates have to be treated in a way similar to S.

If necessary we may for a specific health measure have to use more than one objective measure or additional exogenous variables X_1. If, on the other hand, the objective measure is sufficiently good f_1 could be an identity. In that case estimation of this model is only of theoretical interest, as H^o could be used in the retirement model instead of H^s. In general this will not be so or we cannot be sure if it is the case. We will then have to use this model of individual response behaviour in conjunction with the retirement model or use the response model to correct the subjective measures.

To correct for state-dependent reporting errors we do not have to determine who tells the truth and who lies. As far as our model is concerned everyone lies or rather, speaks a different language. The only thing we have to do in order to correct for state dependence effects is to decide upon a common language for all respondents. It may for example be that early retirees are overly positive about their health. Translating the subjective measures of respondents in the other labour market states to the response he or she would have given had he been early retired, cleanses the subjective measure of state dependent reporting errors. In section 6 we will use the employed as the reference group. For the exogenous variables in X_2 the health measure can be corrected in a similar way.

DATA

We use data from the first wave of a Dutch panel survey called CERRA-I (Centre for Economic Research on Retirement and Aging, wave I). The survey was developed specifically for the analysis of retirement issues. In structure and content it resembles the Health and Retirement Survey (HRS) of the Michigan Survey Centre. The dataset consists of approximately 4700 households in which the head of the household was between 43 and 63 years of age. In each household both the head and – if available – his or her partner were interviewed in October 1993. This resulted in about 8000 individual records with extensive information on labour market status, (sources of) income, labour market history, housing, health status and a variety of socio-economic variables. For the present purposes we excluded the partners and the self-employed, and focused on breadwinners that are Employed (E), Unemployed (U), Disabled (D) or Early Retired (ER). This leaves about 4300 observations. We distinguish between the four labour market states mentioned, rather than between workers and non-workers, because we expect the three non-work states to be very different with respect to biases in health reporting. A Dutch worker is eligible for disability benefits if the worker is incapable of performing any commensurate employment. Hence eligibility of Disability Insurance is contingent upon bad health. To obtain Unemployment Insurance benefits a worker has to be involuntary unemployed and must – prior to the unemployment spell – have been gainfully employed for at least 39 consecutive weeks. An unemployment benefit can only be received for a limited period, the length of which depends on the work history. Eligibility conditions for the Early Retirement schemes differ among industries, but are in general a function of tenure and age. In each labour market state, health reporting is therefore affected by a different combination of financial incentives and social pressure. The differences between these combinations may be used to disentangle the various sources of reporting errors.

After exclusion of incomplete and inconsistent records 3859 individuals remained for which we used the information on health to construct various health measures. For the current analysis we define H^s and H^o as referring to general health. H^s is defined as the answer to the question: 'How good would you rate your health? very good (1), good (2), fair (3), sometimes good sometimes bad (4), bad (5)'.

The health measure H^o is constructed using the Hopkins Symptom Checklist (HSCL). The HSCL is a validated objective test of general health used in the medical sciences to assess the psychoneurotic and somatic pathology of patients (respondents). The test, consisting of 57 items, is known to have an excellent rate of internal consistency: the test results are highly correlated with objective medical reports on the patient's health status. The answers to these 57 items result in a mental score, a physical score and a total health score. For the analysis we use the score results on total health, ranging from very good (1) to very bad (7). Crosstabulations of the health measures controlling for labour market states are given in Table A1 in the appendix. From this table it can be seen that for Employed, Unemployed and Early Retired the bulk of the responses to H^s is concentrated in the left tail of the distribution (low values of H^s, denoting good health), whereas for the Disabled the distribution is skewed to the right. A similar picture emerges for the variable H^o, the Disabled seem to be less health than others. On the other hand, a lot of Disabled with low scores for H^o seem to be in bad health according to H^s. Finally the relationship between the two health measures can be seen to be fairly similar for the Employed, Unemployed and Early Retired.

STATISTICAL MODELS AND EMPIRICAL IMPLEMENTATION

The health measures H^s and H^o are categorical variables defined on different scales. It is therefore a natural choice to use an ordered response framework. The specification of f_1, and f_2 in section 3 will be along the lines of an ordered probit model, but in order to account for differences in response behaviour, the threshold levels are allowed to depend on S and X_2. More specifically, the latent health variable takes on the role of the index variable:

$$H^* = f(H^o) + X_1'\beta + u, \quad u \sim \mathcal{N}(0,1). \quad (3.4)$$

The health response H^o is now defined as

$$H^S = i \Leftrightarrow c_{i-1} < H^* \leqslant c_i, \quad i = 1,\ldots,n, \quad (3.5)$$

where n is the number of answer categories and the threshold levels c are allowed to be different for different values of S and X_2:

$$c_i = g_i(S, X_2), \quad i = 1,\ldots,N-1, \quad (3.6)$$

($c_0 = -\infty$ and $c_n = \infty$). Various specifications of g_i are possible. Two specifications proved to be particularly useful:

$$g_i(S, X_2) = \delta_{s,i} + X_2'\gamma_i$$

and

$$g_i(S, X_2) = X_2'\gamma_{s,i}.$$

In the first specification the threshold levels are shifted by

the exogenous variables X_2 and by S independently. The second more flexible specification allows the effect of X_2 on the threshold levels to be different for different labour market states (the first specification is a special case of the second in which only the intercepts may differ with S). To limit the number of parameters it may be convenient to assume $\gamma_{S,i} = \gamma_S$. In that case the exogenous variables shift the threshold levels by the same amount, but the shifts are allowed to differ over the labour market states. For the disabled the threshold levels are expected to lie to the left of those of employed respondents. Individuals with identical true health H^* will in that case respond with a higher value of H^s if they are disabled than if they are employed.

$f(H^o)$ consists of a dummy variable for each level of H^o. In order to identify the parameters we make the arbitrary assumption that the parameter of the dummy for '$H^o = 1$' is zero. The usual normalization in ordered probit models is to set c_1 equal to zero. In this model that would clearly be too restrictive. As was pointed out in section 3 exogenous variables may play very different roles in this model depending on whether they are in X_1 or in X_2. The X_1 variables are part of the index model (determining the true health status), but we can rewrite the definition of H^s as follows:

$$H^s = i \Leftrightarrow g_{i-1}(S, X_2) - X_1'\beta < f(H^o)$$
$$+ u \leqslant g_i(S, X_2) - X_1'\beta. \quad (3.7)$$

This formulation makes clear that we can never reject the hypothesis that an exogenous variable should be in X_2 rather than in X_1. The opposite hypothesis that an exogenous variable such as gender does not affect response behaviour and only affects the true health status H^* is more restrictive and can be tested. An exogenous variable that should be in X_1 (and to emphasize the role of state-dependence we would like this to hold for all exogenous variables) will, when included in X_2, shift all threshold levels in the same way and the effect will be identical for all labour market states. If one of these properties fails to hold, the exogenous variable is at least to some extent responsible for reporting errors.

A related problem was mentioned by Wagstaff and van Doorslaer [15]. They find significant effects of education on (reported) health. One would like to know if the observed health differences between subsamples stratified by the education level may be interpreted as differences in health rather than differences in language or differences in perception. In terms of the notation we adopt here one would like to know whether education is in X_1 or in X_2. Wagstaff and van Doorslaer conclude that objective health measures are called for and this is essentially the way in which we identify reporting errors in this model. It can always be argued that education affects reporting behaviour (this hypothesis is not testable), but if the effect of education is independent of S and identical for each threshold, the effect on reporting behaviour would be of a very specific type and the alternative interpretation (education having a real effect on health) may be adopted.

The fact that some exogenous variable has to be in X_2 rather than in X_1 may be undesirable or counterintuitive but it never threatens the heart of our model. This is different for H^o. The role of H^o – be it a single variable or a vector of health indicators – determines the interpretation of the index H^* as the true value of the health measure. This variable is therefore firmly positioned in the index-equation and should not affect the reporting behaviour (just as S only affects reporting behaviour and not H^*). Like in the case of the exogenous variables, we may therefore test whether H^o should be in X_2 or not. If H^o affects the thresholds differently or interacts with S the specification of the model is not satisfactory.

Two further comments are in order before we turn to the estimation results. Firstly, unlike other studies we do not include replacement ratios and or wages in the set of exogenous variables. In the Netherlands only the eligibility conditions of Disability Insurance require poor health. Hence, for those out of work, financial motives are only part of the multiple sources of the reporting errors. Furthermore, our model is a partial model, explaining observed responses conditional on labour market state $S \in \{E, ER, U, D\}$. Conditional on S, there is no reason to believe that there exists an independent effect of the replacement ratio on the probability to report with error.

Secondly, it may be tempting to include job characteristics in the set of exogenous variables. There are reasons to believe that responses concerning health may typically depend on the kind of (previous) work. It is however likely that responses, on (self-reported) job characteristics are subject to the same biases as the subjective health variable H^s. Non-working respondents may be inclined to respond towards bad job characteristics. As a consequence inclusion of such variables will bias the estimation results.

ESTIMATION RESULTS

The model was estimated by the maximum likelihood method. The typical likelihood contribution is:

$$\Phi(g_i(S, X_2) - f(H^o) - X_1'\beta) \\ - \Phi(g_{i-1}(S, X_2) - f(H^o) - X_1'\beta), \quad (3.8)$$

where $\Phi(.)$ is the standard normal distribution function. Table 3.2 reports estimation results for three model specifications (absolute t-values are in brackets). The esti-

mates in the first column do not use the latent health measure ($H^* = u$). Effectively, a separate ordered probit model was estimated for each of the subsamples, with $S \in \{E, ER, U, D\}$. The threshold levels for the disabled are systematically lower than for the other categories, implying that the reported health status of the disabled is on average worse than for the employed, the unemployed and the early retired. Ranking the other three groups, the thresholds are lowest for the unemployed, followed by the employed and the early retired respectively. The differences between these groups are however much smaller.

From these estimates we cannot deduce whether the observed differences account for differences in true health or for different reporting behaviour. For this purpose we have to introduce H^o as a more objective benchmark. These estimates are in the second column of Table 3.2. The changes in $\hat{c}_1$ result from the shift in the sample average of H^* (due to the normalization restriction that the parameter for '$H^o = 1$' is equal to zero). Introduction of H^o moves the threshold levels of the four subsamples closer together, but the disabled are still systematically more negative in their health evaluation than the others. The change in the value of the logarithm of the likelihood indicates that the role of H^o in this model is vital. Notice that the H^o-dummies are highly significant and determine a monotonously increasing relation between H^* and H^o. H^o was constructed from the Hopkins Symptom Checklist as a discrete variable with values on a scale from 1 to 7. More flexible transformations of the HSCL-score – using higher order Legendre polynomials – have been considered, but these did not significantly improve or change the estimates.

In the third set of estimates in Table 3.2, age, gender, education, marital status and religion are included in the specification of the health index (through X_1). Only the education level is statistically significant (and has a very high t-value). The negative sign of that parameter indicates that more education corresponds to lower values of H^* and therefore a better health. Education is measured on a scale from 1 to 7. Although this is an awkward way of modelling the impact of the level of education, it proved not to be significantly worse than models in which each education level had dummies of their own. Moreover, the estimated parameters in these more flexible models were very close to the linear specification. Because education is the prime candidate for inclusion in X_2, we have chosen the more restrictive specification in order to keep the number of parameters manageable. Though not significant at the 5% level, the parameter estimates of age and marital status are substantial. Apparently, one's general health condition deteriorates with age. More surprisingly, married individuals are *ceteris paribus* less healthy. The introduction of the exogenous variables in X_1 alters the

Table 3.2 Estimation results, exogenous variables in X_1

	I		II		III	
H^o						
1			—	—	—	—
2			0.37	(7.1)	0.38	(7.2)
3			0.66	(12.7)	0.67	(12.6)
4			0.97	(14.6)	0.98	(14.6)
5			1.10	(11.5)	1.09	(11.3)
6			1.32	(16.1)	1.35	(16.0)
7			1.91	(19.4)	1.93	(19.2)
Exogenous variables (β)						
age					0.006	(1.6)
female					−0.008	(0.1)
education					−0.072	(7.7)
married					0.084	(1.4)
religious					−0.038	(0.8)
Threshold levels						
Employed						
c_1	−0.60	(21.9)	−0.18	(4.2)	−0.05	(0.2)
$c_2 - c_1$	1.59	(44.7)	1.72	(45.0)	1.74	(41.2)
$c_3 - c_2$	0.69	(15.8)	0.77	(16.7)	0.78	(16.5)
$c_4 - c_3$	0.67	(8.8)	0.75	(8.8)	0.76	(9.0)
Early Retired						
c_1	−0.62	(14.3)	−0.25	(4.5)	−0.05	(0.2)
$c_2 - c_1$	1.82	(29.0)	1.95	(28.7)	1.96	(25.5)
$c_3 - c_2$	0.74	(7.1)	0.81	(8.6)	0.82	(8.3)
$c_4 - c_3$	0.82	(3.5)	0.93	(3.7)	0.95	(3.7)
Unemployed						
c_1	−0.81	(14.3)	−0.27	(3.7)	−0.10	(0.4)
$c_2 - c_1$	1.39	(20.5)	1.56	(21.6)	1.58	(20.5)
$c_3 - c_2$	0.66	(9.8)	0.77	(11.0)	0.78	(11.1)
$c_4 - c_3$	0.83	(5.6)	0.95	(7.2)	0.95	(7.2)
Disabled						
c_1	−1.84	(19.6)	−1.10	(10.5)	−0.89	(3.4)
$c_2 - c_1$	1.36	(14.7)	1.51	(15.0)	1.55	(14.9)
$c_3 - c_2$	0.79	(18.1)	0.89	(16.8)	0.90	(16.7)
$c_4 - c_3$	0.91	(14.9)	1.03	(15.5)	1.04	(15.5)
Log likelihood	−4448.99		−4165.57		−4132.25	

average value of H^* and the threshold levels shift accordingly. Apart from this shift, the parameter estimates of the coefficients of H^o and the steps between the thresholds $\hat{c}_i - \hat{c}_{i-1}$ are robust.

The next step is to investigate whether education and other exogenous variables should be in X_2 rather than X_1. The estimates for that more general model are in Table 3.3. The latent health index is now equal to $f(H^o) + u$ and the exogenous variables are all in X_2. The effects of S and X_2 are allowed to interact, but have an identical effect on each threshold:

$$g_i(S, X_2) = c_{S,i} + X_2' \gamma_S.$$

Estimates with separate γ-vectors for each threshold (γ_i or $\gamma_{S,i}$) were very similar to the ones in Table 3.3. The specification with $\gamma_{S,i}$ was rejected by a likelihood ratio test. The estimates of $f(H^o)$ are close to those in Table 3.2. The education variable has a significantly negative parameter for all four subsamples. The only other significant exogenous variable is age of the employed: older age corresponding to more positive health reporting. This variable may refer to age patterns, but also to a cohort effect. The likelihood ratio test comparing specification III in Table 3.2 to the estimates in Table 3.3 is in favour of the more restrictive specification. The test-statistic is 15.48 whereas the 5% critical value for 15 restrictions

Table 3.3 Estimation results, exogenous variables in X_2

H^o			E		ER		U		D	
1	—	—								
2	0.37	(6.9)								
3	0.67	(12.5)								
4	0.97	(14.4)								
5	1.09	(11.0)								
6	1.35	(15.9)								
7	1.93	(18.6)								
Threshold levels		E		ER		U		D		
Exogenous variables (γ)										
age	0.0096	(1.9)	0.021	(1.0)	0.01	(0.8)	−0.014	(1.4)		
female	−0.011	(0.1)	0.34	(1.6)	0.044	(0.2)	−0.026	(0.2)		
education	−0.073	(5.7)	−0.047	(2.0)	−0.064	(2.3)	−0.11	(4.8)		
married	0.000	(0.0)	0.059	(0.4)	0.29	(1.6)	0.13	(1.1)		
religious	−0.049	(0.7)	0.017	(0.2)	0.046	(0.3)	−0.10	(1.0)		
Intercepts ($\delta_{S,i}$)										
c_1	0.036	(0.3)	0.96	(0.7)	0.23	(0.4)	−2.17	(3.8)		
$c_2 - c_1$	1.74	(40.9)	1.97	(25.4)	1.58	(20.0)	1.58	(14.6)		
$c_3 - c_2$	0.78	(16.2)	0.83	(8.2)	0.77	(10.6)	0.91	(16.7)		
$c_4 - c_3$	0.76	(8.8)	0.96	(3.7)	0.93	(7.1)	1.05	(14.8)		
Log likelihood	−4121.825									

equals 25.0. The hypothesis that the exogenous variables should be in X_1 instead of X_2 can therefore not be rejected. This leaves the labour market status as the only variable that significantly affects health reporting. This surprisingly strong result may to some extent be caused by the particularities of the Dutch DI-system at the time of the interview. The next wave in the CERRA-panel is planned for October 1995. Whether the specific circumstances of the Dutch DI-system are responsible for the outcomes will become clear from estimates using those data. Nevertheless, the idea of financial motives and strong preferences for leisure as the driving forces behind state-dependent health reporting originated in the US. It would be interesting to see whether the model holds out with data from other countries, the US in particular.

As a final check on the validity of the model, we allow H^o to interact with S. The estimates of this model are in Table 3.4. The other parameters are hardly affected by this change and the likelihood ratio tests against the models in Table 3.3 and Table 3.2 (III) reject the interaction. The LR-statistics are 16.36 and 31.82 with critical values of 28.9 and more than 43.8 respectively.

Based on the likelihood ratio tests the preferred specification is model III of Table 3.2: the model with state-dependent thresholds and the other exogenous variables working through the latent health index only. To further examine the fit of the model an appropriate coefficient of variation would be useful. McKelvey and Zavoina [16] proposed an R^2 for the ordered probit model. This measure is not suitable for the model in this paper be-

cause the threshold levels depend on exogenous variables, notably the labour market situation. The goodness of fit may be judged by comparing likelihood values between the various specifications. Introduction of the exogenous variables significantly improved the estimated model. The corresponding value of the likelihood ratio test is 66.64 with a 5% critical value of 11.07, using the estimates we can predict the response for each individual. Two such predictors are the median and mode predictors. The mode predictor selects the cell with the largest probability, while the median predictor sets ε equal to zero. Using either predictor 54.1% of the values of H^s are predicted correctly. For 94.3% of the respondents the median prediction differs at most 1 from the actual response. The corresponding percentage is 93.0% for the mode predictor. Percentages as high as these are common in models for polychotomous variables in which the response frequencies are unevenly distributed. In such a situation the frequency distribution of predicted responses is typically much more centred than the distribution of actual responses. Point predictions do little justice to the probabilistic nature of the ordered response model. In fact, an ordered response model defines for each individual the probability that a specific response will be given. Averaging these estimated probabilities over subsamples, we are able to see whether the model can reproduce the conditional sample distributions of the responses. The results for subsamples based on a respondent's labour market situation are depicted in Figure 3.1. The diagram shows for each subsample and for each

Table 3.4 Estimation results, H^o and the exogenous variables in X^2 ($H^* \equiv 0$)

Threshold levels	E		ER		U		D	
H^o								
1	—	—	—	—	—	—	—	—
2	0.34	(4.9)	0.27	(2.4)	0.55	(3.5)	0.60	(3.0)
3	0.66	(9.3)	0.58	(4.9)	0.89	(5.7)	0.73	(4.1)
4	1.02	(10.5)	0.69	(3.7)	1.17	(6.7)	1.03	(5.5)
5	1.11	(7.5)	0.76	(2.8)	1.38	(5.4)	1.15	(5.2)
6	1.38	(9.8)	1.36	(4.3)	1.85	(8.0)	1.28	(6.8)
7	2.06	(9.7)	2.27	(5.4)	2.24	(9.2)	1.85	(9.2)
Exogenous variables (γ)								
age	0.0096	(1.9)	0.024	(1.2)	0.012	(1.1)	−0.015	(1.6)
female	−0.015	(0.1)	0.94	(1.8)	0.037	(0.2)	−0.014	(0.1)
education	−0.073	(5.6)	−0.046	(2.8)	−0.060	(2.2)	−0.11	(4.7)
married	0.003	(0.0)	0.070	(0.4)	0.33	(1.8)	0.113	(0.9)
religious	−0.046	(0.6)	0.022	(0.2)	0.048	(0.3)	−0.089	(0.8)
Intercepts ($\delta_{s,i}$)								
c_1	0.033	(0.1)	1.04	(0.8)	0.58	(0.9)	−2.17	(3.7)
$c_2 - c_1$	1.75	(40.2)	1.95	(24.8)	1.63	(19.4)	1.57	(14.6)
$c_3 - c_2$	0.79	(16.2)	0.83	(8.2)	0.79	(10.4)	0.90	(16.6)
$c_4 - c_3$	0.76	(8.8)	1.00	(3.7)	0.95	(7.1)	1.03	(15.1)
Log likelihood	−4114.08							

response category a cluster of 2 or 3 bars. The first of these corresponds to the sample distribution of the actual responses H^s. The second bars stand for the average predicted probabilities mentioned above. The predicted and actual sample distributions are very similar and show no evidence of misspecification.

The estimates in Table 3.2 (III) are used to compute so called cleansed health-measures. For each individual we have computed what their response would have been had they been employed. This counterfactual simulation is performed to gain more insight into the relative importance of state-dependent reporting errors. The predictions are conditional on the exogenous variables, as well as on the value of H^s. For employed – being the reference category – the cleansed measure is identical to the actual response. For the other three subsamples the frequency distributions of the cleansed measures are represented by the third bar in each cluster in Figure 3.1. In order to compute the cleansed measures one may again use point predictions or predicted response probabilities. The percentages used in Figure 3.1 (b) to (d) are computed as average predicted probabilities. Roughly speaking, the early retirees would be somewhat more negative about their health, while unemployed would become more positive in their health reporting. The differences are small however. Especially when compared to the results for the disabled. Controlling for the effect of the labour market status on reporting behaviour, the frequency distribution of the responses of the disabled would severely shift to the

left. Although the resulting distribution still shows that disabled are less healthy than other respondents, the relative frequencies in categories 3, 4 and 5 fall considerably, leading to a sharp increase of the probability of $H^s = 1$ or 2. Of the disabled respondents rating their health as 'bad' ($H^s = 5$) only one third would give the same answer if they would have been employed, other things being equal.

CONCLUDING REMARKS

The estimation results in the previous section bear strong evidence of the presence of state-dependent reporting errors. While other exogenous variables are not found to have a statistically significant mis-reporting effect, the labour market status – mainly the disabled relative to the other categories – has a significant and robust effect on reported health measures. Relative to a (more) objective health measure this effect prevails, whereas no significant difference between the reporting behaviour of employed, unemployed and early retired respondents is found. If the more objective measure is subject to the same type of systematic reporting errors, the reporting errors found in our estimates provide a lower bound of the actual extent of mis-reporting. In contrast to this finding, the other exogenous variables do not have a significant effect on reporting behaviour. The only exogenous variable that significantly effects reported health measure is the level of education. The hypothesis that this effect is a real health

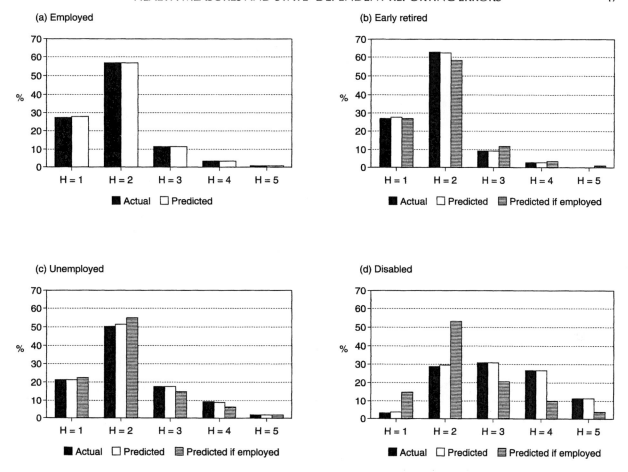

Figure 3.1. Frequency distributions of reported, predicted and cleansed health measures for each labour market state

effect and does not reflect differences in perception or language cannot be rejected.

Although the results from this analysis are more satisfactory than could be expected, the analysis in this paper remains a first attempt. The motivation for this analysis was the use of health measures in retirement and labour supply models. For those models more specific health measures have to be used. These kind of work-related health measures will be subject to reporting errors similar to those investigated in this paper, but objective measures will be more difficult to find. This entails a stronger role for additional control variables (X_1). First applications of the model to work-related health measures confirm the results of this paper. The exogenous variables in X_1 gain in importance, but the labour market status is the only significant variable related to reporting errors.

Apart from these applications the model has to be applied to data from different countries to see if the strong evidence of state dependent health reporting only holds for the Dutch data and the period of time considered in this analysis. Apart from this, the use of alternative objective health measures and control variables has to be investigated. Another subject for further study is the stochastic specification of the model. Although the results in this paper provide no reason to suspect specification problems, in the application to more specific health measure it is expected that heteroskedasticity may become important. The same holds for the assumed linear dependence of H^* on the exogenous variables. More rigorously, semi-parametric estimation techniques provide an alternative to maximum likelihood estimation. One alternative approach would be to extend the maximum score estimator to the ordered probit model with variable thresholds that was used in this paper.

Finally, the model should be used for what it was meant to do: correct for state dependent reporting errors.

One way would be to generate cleansed health measures. The application of those measures is not straightforward as the imputation of cleansed measures will lead to errors in variables biases. It would therefore be interesting to investigate whether the model of reporting behaviour can be estimated simultaneously with a model of retirement or labour supply decisions.

ACKNOWLEDGEMENTS

We wish to thank Philip de Jong and the participants of the workshop on Health Econometrics in Antwerp, September 1994, for their helpful suggests and comments. The authors are members of CERRA (Center for Economic Research on Retirement and Aging) at Leiden University. The research in this paper was financed by a grant from NESTOR (the Dutch Stimulation Program for Aging Research) and from the Leiden University Speerpunten Program.

APPENDIX

Definition of variables

Age	Age of the respondent (January 1993)
Female	Gender dummy, equals 1 if female
Education	1 Lower general
	2 Lower vocational
	3 Medium general
	4 Medium vocational
	5 Higher general
	6 Higher vocational
	7 Academic
Married	Dummy for marital status equals 1 if married or living together
Religious	Dummy, equals 1 if respondent attends the church at least once a week
H^s	Responses to question 'How good would you rate your health?'
	1 Very good
	2 Good
	3 Fair
	4 Sometimes good sometimes bad
	5 Bad

Table A3.1 Cross-tabulations of the health measures controlling for labour-market state

Employed

	H^s				
H^o	1	2	3	4	5
1	225	305	21	2	1
2	167	335	47	9	3
3	116	305	71	29	4
4	25	97	48	10	3
5	6	37	13	9	0
6	6	32	17	12	3
7	0	8	11	4	5
Total	545	1119	228	75	19

Early retired

	H^s				
H^o	1	2	3	4	5
1	82	132	7	2	0
2	57	123	15	4	0
3	31	124	19	4	1
4	9	26	11	1	0
5	3	12	2	2	0
6	1	6	5	1	0
7	0	2	2	2	1
Total	183	425	61	16	2

Unemployed

	H^s				
H^o	1	2	3	4	5
1	44	49	4	2	0
2	25	70	14	4	0
3	25	68	28	5	4
4	8	50	15	11	1
5	2	12	7	3	1
6	2	9	9	11	1
7	1	4	12	10	3
Total	107	262	89	46	10

Disabled

	H^s				
H^o	1	2	3	4	5
1	7	30	8	4	1
2	5	27	28	14	4
3	4	60	63	32	8
4	4	28	39	36	11
5	0	12	18	13	6
6	1	27	35	43	15
7	1	8	16	36	28
Total	22	192	207	178	73

H^o Hopkins symptom Checklist (HSCL) score

1 Very good
2 Good
3 Above average
4 Average
5 Below average
6 Bad
7 Very bad

REFERENCES

1. Lambrinos, J. Health: A source of bias in labour supply models. *Review of Economics and Statistics* 1981; **63**: 206–212.
2. Parsons, D.O. Male labour force participation decision: health, reported health and economic incentives. *Economica* 1982; **49**: 81–91.
3. Anderson, K.H. and Burkhauser, R.V. The retirement-health nexus: a new measure of an old puzzle. *Journal of Human Resources* 1985; **20**: 315–330.
4. Bazzoli, G. The early retirement decision: New empirical evidence on the influence of health. *Journal of Human Resources* 1985; **20**: 214–234.
5. Butler, J.S., Burkhauser, R.V., Mitchell, J.M. and Pincus, T.P. Measurement error in self-reported health variables. *Review of Economics and Statistics* 1987; **69**: 644–650.
6. Stern, S. Measuring the effect of disability on labour force participation. *Journal of Human Resources* 1989; **24**: 361–395.
7. Bound, J. Self-reported versus objective measures of health in retirement models. *Journal of Human Resources* 1991; **26**: 107–137.
8. Bartel, A. and Taubman, P. Health and labour market success: the role of various diseases. *Review of Economics and Statistics* 1979; **61**: 1–8.
9. Lee, L.F. Health and wage: A simultaneous equation model with multiple discrete indicators. *International Economic Review* 1982; **20**: 199–221.
10. Chirikos, T.N. and Nestel, G. Further evidence on the economic effects of poor health. *Review of Economics and Statistics* 1985; **67**: 61–9.
11. Fuchs, V.R. Time preference and health: An exploratory Study. In: V.R. Fuchs (ed.), *Economic Aspects of Health.* Chicago: University of Chicago Press, 1982.
12. Sickless, R. and Taubman, T. An analysis of the health and retirement status of the elderly. *Econometrica* 1986; **14**: 1339–1356.
13. Burkhauser, R.V. The pension acceptance decision of older workers. *Journal of Human Resources* 1979; **14**: 63–75.
14. Aarts, L.J.M. and de Jong, Ph.R. *Economic Aspects of Disability Behaviour.* Amsterdam: North Holland, 1991.
15. Wagstaff, A. and van Doorslaer, E. Measuring inequalities in health in the presence of multiple-category morbidity indicators. *Health Economics* 1994; **3**: 281–291.
16. McKelvey, R. and Zavoina, W. A statistical model for the analysis of ordinal level dependent variables. *Journal of Mathematical Sociology* 1975; **4**: 103–120.

4

The Effect of Smoking on Health Using a Sequential Self-selection Model

KAJAL LAHIRI AND JAE G. SONG

Department of Economics, State University of New York at Albany, USA

INTRODUCTION

Ever since a causal relationship between cigarette smoking and coronary heart disease was reported at the Mayo Clinic in 1940, the effect of cigarette smoking on health has been extensively studied by both epidemiologists and social scientists. Now cigarette smoking is considered to be the number one source of preventable morbidity and premature mortality in the United States (see [1]). Since the 1960s, various public policy efforts have been devoted to reducing the prevalence of cigarette smoking. Still over 25% of the population, or nearly 46.3 million adults in the US and many more around the world smoke on a regular basis [2].

There have been two approaches to reducing the prevalence of cigarette smoking: discouraging non-smokers from initiating, and encouraging smokers to quit. Even though smoking prevalence has steadily decreased since the 1960s, this decrease has been due to more people quitting but not due to fewer people initiating [2]. Hence, a comprehensive model of smoking participation that considers both initiation and cessation behaviour and their health effects is essential for developing an effective public policy approach to reducing the prevalence of smoking, and in estimating the proper human costs of cigarette smoking.

Unlike the consumption of a normal good, consumption of cigarettes increases not only the immediate satisfaction for smokers but also the probability of adverse health effects in the future, neither of which are directly observable. Hence, the subjective judgement on the costs and benefits of cigarette smoking plays a crucial role in smoking participation decisions. This subjective judgement depends largely on the assessment of the probability of the occurrence of side effects and the time preference between the immediate benefits and the future side effects of smoking.

An important factor affecting the initial smoking decision is an individual's prior belief on risks and benefits from smoking, which could depend on his demographic and other socio-economic characteristics. Those who decide to smoke gather additional information through their experience of smoking, and update their prior beliefs. Based on the updated belief, a decision of continuation or cessation is made. Therefore, individual risk assessment of cigarette smoking takes a critical role in each phase of the smoking cycle. Viscusi [3] studied individual risk perception and smoking decision by questioning whether smokers are risk cognizants, and whether the risk perception is reflected in smokers' behaviour. Viscusi [3] finds that the risk perception by the young is quite high, but it has no significant influence on their initiation behaviour.

Recently, the participation behaviours of smokers has been empirically examined by Jones [4,5] and Hsieh *et al.* [6]. In these studies, the role of health condition, health knowledge, social interaction, and other demographic characteristics are explored. There is another group of studies that examines the various human costs of smoking, such as health conditions, medical expenditures, and other economic consequences. Miller *et al.* [7] estimates medical care expenditures attributable to cigarette smoking. Mattson *et al.* [8] calculate the long-term risk of death contributed by individual smoking status for various age groups. The later group of studies, however, treat smoking status as exogenous, disregarding the dynamic interaction between individuals' health conditions and their smoking behaviour.

Econometric Analysis of Health Data. Edited by Andrew M. Jones and Owen O'Donnell
© 2002 John Wiley & Sons Ltd. Previously published in *Health Economics*, Vol. 9; pp. 491–511 (2000). © John Wiley & Sons Ltd

In this paper, we study the participation behaviour of smokers, both initiation and cessation, and integrate them into a model of health consequences of smoking. We examine the possibility of the presence of any un-measured heterogeneity bias in the probability distributions of smoking-related diseases for different smoking groups, and we study whether the observed proportions of smoking-related diseases in the sample correctly represent the risk factor associated with a particular smoking behaviour. The second issue we examine is whether the individual smoking choices are made in a way that is consistent with economic optimality. The rational addiction approach of cigarette smoking behaviour considers smoking choice as the outcome of individual utility maximization under uncertainty (see [9,10]). Even though there are several empirical studies on the rational addiction model, they tend to focus on the role of price on the demand for addictive goods without considering the role of implicit health cost.

This paper is organized as follows. In 'The Econometric Model' and 'Data and Empirical Specifications', we develop a sequential selection model of smoking behaviour based on a typical smoking cycle. 'Empirical Strategy' and 'Empirical Estimates' describe our data and the econometric strategy and presents and discusses empirical findings, respectively, and the paper ends with 'Conclusions'.

THE ECONOMETRIC MODEL

The smoking participation decisions, both initiation and cessation, are modelled as outcomes of utility maximization under uncertain occurrence of smoking-related diseases (SRDs) using a random utility model. Our model is based on the following fundamental premise: the baseline (autonomous) and induced risk factors of cigarette smoking are not always equal for all individuals, and that each individual possesses a subjective prior belief concerning the probability of occurrence of SRDs associated with each smoking choice, and this belief is updated using the information gained through the smoking experience and the realization of changes in his/her health condition.

Consider a simple two-period model with a time-separable indirect utility function. A rational individual lives two periods indexed by $t = 1, 2$. At the beginning of each period, individual i faces a decision to make a choice between two alternatives: to not smoke or to smoke, indexed by $j = 0, 1$ based on his own subjective judgement of the costs and the benefits of the alternatives. The length of each period varies across individuals. Let there be two discrete states of health condition, good and bad, indexed by $l = 1, 2$. The bad-health state indicates the presence of any undesirable health condition, caused by factors including smoking.

Individual i possesses a prior belief on the probability of the occurrence of each health state for a given smoking status. This probability is optimally updated each period. Let P_{jl} be the individual's subjective probability for lth health state when the smoking status is j. There are four possible states (S_{jl}) of the world an individual could be falling into. Further let U_{ijl}^t be an unobservable indirect utility of individual i choosing alternative j at period t when his/her health condition is l. Then the expected utility of each choice for each period t can be expressed as the sum of the utilities in each health state weighted by its probability:

$$EU_{ij}^t = \sum_{l=1}^{2} P_{ijl}^t U_{ijl}^t \tag{4.1}$$

At the beginning of each period, an individual chooses alternative j over j' if and only if $E_t U_{ij} > E_t U_{ij'}$. The discounted sum of expected utilities for the two periods realized at the beginning of period τ is:

$$E_\tau U_{ij} = \sum_{t=\tau}^{2} \theta_i^{t-1} \sum_{l=1}^{2} P_{ijl}^t U_{ijl}^t \tag{4.2}$$

where θ_i is an individual-specific time preference parameter.

The initiation decision rule at the beginning of period 1 is governed by the sign of $I_{1i}^* = E_1 U_{i1} - E_1 U_{i2}$. Once an individual starts to smoke then another subsequent decision rule can be defined in a similar way. The cessation decision rule for the second period is governed by the sign of $I_{2i}^* = E_2 U_{i1} - E_2 U_{i2}$. Thus, the selection criteria are:

Pr(choose to start smoking) = $\Pr(I_{1i}^* > 0)$

Pr(choose not to start) = $\Pr(I_{1i}^* \leq 0)$

Pr(choose to continue) = $\Pr(I_{2i}^* > 0, I_{1i}^* > 0)$

Pr(choose to quit) = $\Pr(I_{2i}^* \leq 0, I_{1i}^* > 0)$

I_{1i}^* and I_{2i}^* can be interpreted as present values of 'net' utilities at the time of initiation and cessation. They are not observable; we observe only their binary outcomes, I_{1i} and I_{2i}. There are three mutually exclusive outcomes of the selection process:

Group I (nonsmoker, I_{00}): $I_{1i} = 0$

Group II (ex-smoker, I_{10}): $I_{1i} = 1$ and $I_{2i} = 0$

Group III (current smoker, I_{11}):

$I_{1i} = 1$ and $I_{2i} = 1$

The two selection equations are parameterized as:

$$I_{1i}^* = Z_{1i}\eta_1 + W_{1ij}\delta_1 + \varepsilon_{1i}$$
$$I_{2i}^* = Z_{2i}\eta_2 + W_{2ij}\delta_2 + H_{2i}\zeta_2 + \varepsilon_{2i} \qquad (4.3)$$

where (Z_{1i}, Z_{2i}) are individual characteristics and (W_{1ij}, W_{2ij}) are the characteristics of the alternatives specific to the individual. The updated probability assessment at the beginning of the second period depends on the realization of a change in health conditions (H_{2i}) which may or may not be related to the smoking status in period 1, individual characteristics (Z_i), and characteristics of the alternatives specific to the individual (W_{ij}).

Finally, we specify an equation for the appropriate response variable for measuring the effect of the initiation and the cessation decisions. Since smoking participation decisions heavily influence the probability of SRDs such as lung diseases and various types of cancer, presence of any SRDs is the most appropriate and direct outcome variable for our purpose. Further, we will specify one equation for each smoking group in order to capture the full interactions among them (see [11]). The equations are:

$$Y_{ni}^* = X_{ni}\beta_n + \varepsilon_{ni}: \text{nonsmokers' disease equation}$$
$$Y_{xi}^* = X_{xi}\beta_x + \varepsilon_{xi}: \text{ex-smokers' disease equation}$$
$$Y_{ci}^* = X_{ci}\beta_c + \varepsilon_{ci}: \text{current smokers' disease equation} \qquad (4.4)$$

In Equations 4.3 and 4.4, Z_{1i} and W_{1ij} are $N \times K_1$ and $N \times K_2$ vectors of explanatory variables; η_1 and δ_1 are $K_1 \times 1$ and $K_2 \times 1$ vectors of unknown coefficients; Z_{2i}, W_{2ij} and H_{2i} are $N_1 \times K_3$, $N_1 \times K_4$ and $N_1 \times K_5$ vectors of explanatory variables; and η_2, δ_2 and ζ_2 are $K_3 \times 1$, $K_4 \times 1$ and $K_5 \times 1$ vectors of unknown coefficients; X_{ni}, X_{xi} and X_{ci} are $N_2 \times K_6$, $N_3 \times K_6$ and $N_4 \times K_6$ vectors of explanatory variables; β_n, β_x and β_c are $K_6 \times 1$ vector of unknown coefficients; $I_{1i}^*, I_{2i}^*, Y_{ni}^*, Y_{xi}^*$ and Y_{ci}^* are $N \times 1$, $N_1 \times 1$, $N_2 \times 1$, $N_3 \times 1$ and $N_4 \times 1$ unobservable latent indices; $N = N_2 + N_3 + N_4$ and $N_1 = N_3 + N_4$. We observe binary outcomes Y_{ni}, Y_{xi}, Y_{ci}, I_1 and I_2.

This completes our econometric model as a set of switching regressions with sequential self-selection rules. In the remainder of this paper, subscript i is omitted to avoid notational complexity. Also new variables C_1 and C_2 will represent the independent variables in the first and the second selection equations in Equation 4.3 with coefficients γ_1 and γ_2.

$$I_1^* = C_1\gamma_1 + \varepsilon_1: \text{initiation selection equation}$$

$$I_2^* = C_2\gamma_2 + \varepsilon_2: \text{cessation selection equation}$$

(observed, iff $I_1 = 1$)

$$Y_n^* = X\beta_n + \varepsilon_n: \text{nonsmoker's disease equation}$$
(observed, iff $I_1 = 0$)

$$Y_x^* = X\beta_x + \varepsilon_x: \text{ex-smoker's disease equation}$$
(observed, iff $I_1 = 1, I_2 = 0$)

$$Y_c^* = X\beta_c + \varepsilon_c: \text{current smoker's disease equation}$$
(observed, iff $I_1 = 1, I_2 = 1$)

The two sequential self-selection rules sort people into observed classes according to the expected present value of indirect utility. Hence, the presence of SRDs actually observed in each group are not random outcomes in the population, but instead are self-censored nonrandom samples. The initiation decision equation is defined over the entire population, but the cessation decision equation is defined only over the subset of observations for those who have started to smoke.

DATA AND EMPIRICAL SPECIFICATIONS

We use data from Health and Retirement Study (HRS) Wave I which was released in May 1995. The HRS is a national longitudinal study on health, retirement, and economic status focusing on individuals both between 1931 and 1941. A total of 12 652 individuals were interviewed during 1993, among these 2372 are single respondents and 5234 are paired (married or partnered) respondents. Their ages vary from 23 to 85 as of 1993. Mean age in the total sample is 55.6 and standard deviation is 5.66. Out of 12 652 individuals, 4626 are nonsmokers, 4588 are ex-smokers, and 3438 are current smokers.

The main advantage of this data set for our purpose is that the sample consists mainly of individuals in their 50s. The role of learning and regret throughout one's smoking cycle and the effects of smoking on health can be more fully observed in this data set because most smokers initiate smoking when they are relatively young. The HRS also provides complete classification of individuals' smoking status as nonsmoker, ex-smoker, and current smoker. Further, HRS has extraordinary information on current health conditions, health history, and various socio-economic factors. As a result, we are able to investigate the long-term health effects of 30–40 years of smoking.

To take full advantage of the data set for our purpose, we consider only individuals in the age group 52 and over.[a] We also drop those individuals who had quit smoking after they were diagnosed with various types of cancers and other smoking-related diseases to control for obvious endogeneity. As a result of these, our final sample for empirical analysis consists of 9109 individuals; among them 3287, 3368 and 2454 are nonsmokers, ex-smokers, and current smokers, respectively.[b]

The HRS data provides information that separate never smokers from ever smokers, and ever smokers are further subdivided into ex-smokers and current smokers. Technically, nonsmokers in HRS are defined as those individuals who smoked fewer than 100 cigarettes in his/her entire life time. Even though we observe complete outcomes of the two participation decisions, estimation of these equations based on a single cross-sectional data set requires careful thoughts. Fortunately, the data contain large amounts of information on current as well as historical health, socio-economic, and demographic factors. Our variables are categorized as pure demographic, social status, economic status, family life, current health condition and history, risk-taking behaviour, smoking related, and employment related variables. Some of these variables represent time invariant individual characteristics, such as sex, race, place of birth, and parents' education. We also include some other variables which are assumed to capture individuals' characteristics when they were young such as religion, tidiness, smoking status of the spouse, and occupation. This inclusion is particularly useful for our empirical model specification because our model contains two decisions that were possibly made many years ago.

We select the explanatory variables for each equation based on previous empirical specifications, theory, and data availability. From an economics standpoint, the individual's risk belief is assumed to have an important influence on the smoking behaviour. Barsky et al. [12] show that individual risk tolerance measured by HRS data is positively related to risk-taking behaviour in smoking and drinking. Their estimated preference parameters are related to the behaviour of individuals, and their risk tolerance estimates make prediction of smoking behaviour at least qualitatively correct. Viscusi [13,14] found some evidence that an individual's smoking decision responds to his/her risk perception. Differences in smoking behaviour among different demographic groups are reported in various studies. The Surgeon Generals' report of 1985 noted differences in smoking behaviour, both initiation and cessation, between white-collar and blue-collar workers. Breslau and Peterson [15,16] reported that smoking cessation varies by sex, race, education, and number of cigarettes smoked daily. They also found that smoking and drinking habits are correlated. The prevalence of alcohol abuse or dependence was significantly higher in smokers than nonsmokers. For the three SRD equations, we include occupation, smoking, nutrition, demographic, socio-economic, and general health-related variables. To control further for individual

heterogeneity, we include variables related to occupation, occupational hazards, fundamental health condition indicators, socioeconomic status, life-styles, and insurance status.

Our key dependent variable is the presence of one of the SRDs, which include various lung diseases and types of cancers that are directly related to smoking such as cancer of the abdomen, mouth, bladder, neck, nose, pancreas, brain, bronchia, cervix, oesophagus, stomach, throat, tongue, kidney, liver, and lung. Selection of such cancers is based on reports of the Surgeon General in 1982, 1983, and 1984 on the health consequences of smoking and on various medical and public health literature such as Bartecchi et al. [1], Mattson et al. [8], Yuan et al. [17] and Fielding [18]. Thus, our definition of SRD is very broad, giving us a reasonable sample size of people having SRDs. Detailed definitions of variables are shown in Appendix A and descriptive statistics by smoking status for some key variables are summarized in Table 4.1.

EMPIRICAL STRATEGY

Our empirical strategy is to estimate the model first by a two-step probit method using the Heckman–Lee two-step method and to use the two-step estimates as starting values for full information maximum likelihood (FIML) estimation. The conditional expectations of the dependent variables using the properties of truncated normal density functions are:

$$E(I_1^*) = G_1$$

$$E(I_2^* | I_1 = 1) = G_2 + E(\varepsilon_2 | - G_1 < \varepsilon_1)$$

$$= G_2 + \sigma_{12} \frac{\phi_1(G_1)}{\Phi_1(G_1)}$$

$$E(Y_n^* | I_1 = 0) = X_n \beta_n + E(\varepsilon_n | - G_1 \geq \varepsilon_1)$$

$$= X_n \beta_n + \sigma_{1n} \frac{-\phi_1(G_1)}{1 - \Phi_1(G_1)}$$

$$E(Y_x^* | I_1 = 1, I_2 = 0)$$

$$= X_x \beta_x + E(\varepsilon_x | - G_1 < \varepsilon_1, - G_2 \geq \varepsilon_2)$$

$$= X_x \beta_x + \sigma_{1x} \frac{\phi_1(G_1) \Phi_1(- G_2^*)}{\Phi_2(G_1, - G_2; - \sigma_{12})}$$

$$+ \sigma_{2x} \frac{- \phi_1(G_2) \Phi_1(G_1^*)}{\Phi_2(G_1, - G_2; - \sigma_{12})}$$

$$E(Y_c^* | I_1 = 1, I_2 = 1)$$

$$= X_c \beta_c + E(\varepsilon_c | - G_1 < \varepsilon_1, - G_2 < \varepsilon_2)$$

Table 4.1 Descriptive statistics for selected variables

Variables	Whole sample mean	Nonsmoker mean	Ex-smoker mean	Current smoker mean
AGE	1.0000	0.9967	1.0088	0.9922
ALCHOLIC	0.0543	0.0179	0.0537	0.1039
ARTHRTS	0.3974	0.3836	0.4041	0.4067
BADFIN	0.2244	0.1926	0.1900	0.3142
BLOODPRS	0.4062	0.4061	0.4353	0.3663
BMI	1.0000	1.0116	1.0189	0.9586
CATHOLIC	0.2734	0.2616	0.2892	0.2673
CHOLSTRL	0.2401	0.2443	0.2553	0.2135
DIABTS	0.1123	0.1071	0.1232	0.1043
DISEASE	0.0974	0.0542	0.0941	0.1597
EVDRINK	0.6078	0.5196	0.6660	0.6459
EXDRINK	0.2031	0.0904	0.2524	0.2865
EXER	0.2098	0.2212	0.2432	0.1487
FEDINS	0.1671	0.1263	0.1859	0.1960
FINJOB	0.0520	0.0593	0.0454	0.0513
FORNBORN	0.0973	0.1238	0.0900	0.0717
GOODFAM	0.2211	0.2379	0.2396	0.1732
HAZWORK	0.2040	0.1552	0.2224	0.2441
HELTHINS	0.8572	0.8598	0.8893	0.8097
INVEST	0.6253	0.6660	0.6758	0.5016
IRA	0.4197	0.4551	0.4822	0.2865
JOGAMILE	0.1447	0.1618	0.1571	0.1047
LIFEINS	0.7098	0.6988	0.7527	0.6659
MALE	0.5003	0.3614	0.6161	0.5273
MARIDIST	0.5405	0.6109	0.5621	0.4165
MARIED	0.7508	0.7682	0.7975	0.6634
MILIT	0.2956	0.1935	0.3833	0.3121
MYOPIC	0.1829	0.1682	0.1609	0.2327
NETWORTH	1.0000	1.1744	1.0607	0.6834
NEVERW	0.0349	0.0554	0.0187	0.0297
PAREDU	0.2999	0.2823	0.3141	0.3040
RACEB	0.1634	0.1667	0.1443	0.1850
RACEW	0.7254	0.7037	0.7548	0.7143
RELIGS	0.5256	0.6413	0.5220	0.3757
RISKAVER	0.8717	0.8862	0.8735	0.8496
SALESJOB	0.1547	0.1363	0.1485	0.1879
SCHLYRS	1.0000	1.0202	1.0171	0.9494
SERVJOB	0.0924	0.0931	0.0852	0.1015
SPOSENSM	0.5117	0.5634	0.4840	0.4804
SPOSEXSM	0.2855	0.2778	0.3480	0.1968
TECHJOB	0.1277	0.1451	0.1455	0.0799
WESTB	0.0784	0.0803	0.0808	0.0725

$$= X_c \beta_c + \sigma_{1c} \frac{\phi_1(G_1)\Phi_1(G_2^*)}{\Phi_2(G_1, G_2; \sigma_{12})} + \sigma_{2c} \frac{\phi_1(G_2)\Phi_1(G_1)}{\Phi_2(G_1, G_2; \sigma_{12})}$$

$$G_1^* = \frac{G_1 - \sigma_{12}G_2}{(1 - \sigma_{12}^2)^{1/2}},$$

$$G_2^* = \frac{G_2 - \sigma_{12}G_1}{(1 - \sigma_{12}^2)^{1/2}}.$$

where

$$G_1 = C_1\gamma_1,$$

$$G_2 = C_2\gamma_2,$$

$\Phi_g(\cdot)$ and $\phi_g(\cdot)$ are the standard g-variate normal distribution and density function, respectively.

Thus, we can rewrite the equations with new error terms which have zero conditional means:

$$I_1 = G_1 + \varepsilon_1$$

$$I_2 = G_2 + \sigma_{12}\lambda_{12} + e_2$$

$$Y_n = X_n\beta_n + \sigma_{1n}\lambda_{1n} + e_n$$

$$Y_x = X_x\beta_x + \sigma_{1x}\lambda_{1x} + \sigma_{2x}\lambda_{2x} + e_x$$

$$Y_c = X_c\beta_c + \sigma_{1c}\lambda_{1c} + \sigma_{2c}\lambda_{2c} + e_c \qquad (4.5)$$

where

$$\lambda_{12} = \frac{\phi_1(G_1)}{\Phi_1(G_1)},$$

$$\lambda_{1n} = \frac{-\phi_1(G_1)}{1 - \Phi_1(G_1)},$$

$$\lambda_{1x} = \frac{\phi_1(G_1)\Phi_1(-G_2^*)}{\Phi_2(G_1, -G_2; -\sigma_{12})},$$

$$\lambda_{1c} = \frac{\phi_1(G_1)\Phi_1(G_2^*)}{\Phi_2(G_1, G_2; \sigma_{12})},$$

$$\lambda_{2x} = \frac{-\phi_1(G_2)\Phi_1(\tilde{G}_1^*)}{\Phi_2(G_1, -G_2; -\sigma_{12})}$$

and

$$\lambda_{2c} = \frac{\phi_1(G_2)\Phi_1(G_1^*)}{\Phi_2(G_1, G_2; \sigma_{12})}.$$

Under the normality assumption, each of the above equations can be estimated sequentially by five separate probit regressions with the appropriate Heckman–Lee corrections as specified in Equation 4.5. Note that the error terms e_2, e_n, e_x and e_c are heteroskedastic by construction, and if there are overlapping variables in the selection and disease equations, the problem of significant multicollinearity may result in the structural equations.

ENDOGENEITY OF SOME HEALTH VARIABLE

A recent debate between Jones [4,5], and Shmueli [19] deals with the issue of endogeneity of health variables in the cessation decision equation. The health variables included in our equations are based more objectively on physical activity limitations and health history, which are expected to develop independent of smoking.

Blundell and Smith [20] provide a simple way to test for endogeneity by a two-stage approach. The first stage is to regress the suspicious variables on exogenous variables. The second step is to estimate the original probit equation with the residuals from stage 1 as additional regressors and to jointly test the hypothesis that coeffi-

cients of the residuals are zeros. Since our suspicious health variables are binary, we generated probit generalized residuals (see [21,22]). The probit generalized residuals for a model $Y_i^* = X_i\beta_i + \varepsilon_i$ are given by:

$$\hat{\varepsilon} = Y_i - \Phi_1(X_i\hat{\beta}_i)\phi_1(X_i\hat{\beta}_i)$$
$$\times ((1 - \Phi_1(X_i\hat{\beta}_i))^{-1}\Phi_1(X_i\hat{\beta}_i)^{-1} \qquad (4.6)$$

We tested the endogeneity of EXER (exercises regularly), JOGAMILE (can jog a mile with no difficulty), BLOODPRS (blood pressure), CHOLSTRL (cholesterol), ARTHRTS (arthritis), and DIABTS (diabetes) in the cessation decision and BLOODPRS, CHOLSTRL, ARTHRTS, and DIABTS in the switching disease equations.[c] The χ^2 statistics for the null hypotheses that these additional coefficients are zero for cessation, non-smokers', ex-smokers' and current smokers' equations are obtained as 6.585 (df = 6), 3.474 (df = 4), 3.232 (df = 4) and 3.123 (df = 4), respectively. These are not statistically significant at the 5% level of significance. Our specifications originally included a few other health variables, but we dropped them because they did not pass the endogeneity test.[d] These variables were replaced by the instruments used to test for their endogeneity, whenever they were statistically significant. Thus, we interpret our disease equations as purely reduced form specifications.

HETEROSKEDASTICITY

We examine the presence of heteroskedasticity using the following formulation [23]:

$$\mathrm{Var}(\varepsilon_i) = \sigma_i^2 = [\exp(V_i\omega)]^2$$
$$Y_i^* = X_i\beta + \varepsilon_i \qquad (4.7)$$

where V_i is $1 \times p$ vector of observations on a subset of variables, and ω is a vector of corresponding parameters. Then log of likelihood function is:

$$\ln 1 = \sum_i Y_i \ln \Phi_1\left(\frac{X_i\beta}{\exp(V_i\omega)}\right)$$
$$+ (1 - Y_i)\ln\left[1 - \Phi_1\left(\frac{X_i\beta}{\exp(V_i\omega)}\right)\right] \qquad (4.8)$$

Once this likelihood function is maximized, we can easily check for heteroskedasticity by the likelihood ratio test because $\omega = 0$ implies homoskedasticity. Further, we can identify the special structure of heteroskedasticity and are able to correct it by feasible GLS [24]. The results indicated that significant heteroskedasticity exists in all our equations at the 5% level. As a result, we specified our equations after allowing for heteroskedasticity:

$$I_1^* = D_1 + \varepsilon_1$$
$$I_2^* = D_2 + \sigma_{12}\lambda_{12}^* + \varepsilon_2$$
$$Y_n^* = D_n + \sigma_{1n}\lambda_{1n}^* + e_n$$
$$Y_x^* = D_x + \sigma_{1x}\lambda_{1x}^* + \sigma_{2x}\lambda_{2x}^* + e_x$$
$$Y_c^* = D_c + \sigma_{1c}\lambda_{1c}^* + \sigma_{2c}\lambda_{2c}^* + e_c \qquad (4.9)$$

where

$$D_1 = \frac{(C_1\gamma_1)}{\exp(V_1\omega_1)},$$

$$D_2 = \frac{(C_2\gamma_2)}{\exp(V_2\omega_2)},$$

$$D_n = \frac{X_n\beta_n}{\exp(V_n\omega_n)},$$

$$D_x = \frac{(X_x\beta_x)}{\exp(V_x\omega_x)},$$

$$D_c = \frac{(X_c\beta_c)}{\exp(V_c\omega_c)}$$

and Vs are the variables which condition heteroskedasticity for each equation. λ^*s are defined in the same way as in Equation (5) with Gs replaced by Ds.

NORMALITY TESTS

Pagan and Vella [25] derived a normality test for the tobit model with selectivity that can be directly applied to our probit model with selectivity. Since our cessation and nonsmokers' disease equations involve a single selection, we can apply the test developed by Pagan and Vella with minor modifications. However, we want to estimate our structural model by FIML, which requires evaluation of trivariate CDFs. As a result, we use the normality test based on Edgeworth expansion of CDF suggested by Lee [26], generalized to the trivariate case by Lahiri and Song [27]. Here we test for the bivariate normality of $(\varepsilon_1, \varepsilon_n)$ and the trivariate normality of $(\varepsilon_1, \varepsilon_2, \varepsilon_c)$ and $(\varepsilon_1, \varepsilon_2, \varepsilon_x)$. The χ^2 statistics were calculated as 12.97 (df = 9), 27.42 (df = 25), 31.64 (df = 25), respectively. Since these values are less than the critical χ^2 values at the 5% level of significance, we did not reject the multivariate normality assumption in our context. We should point out that without the heteroskedasticity correction, the normality assumption would have been resoundingly rejected in our sample (see [27]).

FULL INFORMATION MAXIMUM LIKELIHOOD ESTIMATION

The inefficiency of the two-step method relative to maximum likelihood has been critically examined by Nelson [28], who suggested the more difficult MLE. The poor performance of Heckman–Lee two-step method is also reported in Nawata and Nagase [29] and Stolzenberg and Relles [30]. Their results, based on Monte Carlo and empirical examples, suggest that the two-step method may not be a dependable estimator when there is strong multicollinearity between independent variables (X) and selectivity correction terms (λs). If there are no overlapping variables in the selection and the outcome regression equations, then the multicollinearity may not be very high. Since we have overlapping variables, especially in the second selection equation, we can not rule out the possibility of significant multicollinearity. As a result, it is advisable to estimate the model by FIML for correct inferences (see [31] for further discussion).

The log of likelihood function for the model Equation 4.9 is:

$$\ln L(\gamma_1, \omega_1, \gamma_2, \omega_2, \beta_n, \beta_x, \omega_x, \beta_c, \omega_c,$$
$$\sigma_{12}, \sigma_{1n}, \sigma_{1x}, \sigma_{1c}, \sigma_{2x}, \sigma_{2c})$$

$$= \sum_{i=1}^{m} \{(1 - I_1)Y \ln \Phi_2(-D_1, D_n; -\sigma_{1n})$$
$$+ (1 - I_1)(1 - Y)\ln \Phi_2(-D_1, -D_n; \sigma_{1n})$$
$$+ I_1(1 - I_2)Y \ln \Phi_3(D_1, -D_2, D_x;$$
$$- \sigma_{12}, -\sigma_{2x}, \sigma_{1x}) + I_1(1 - I_2)(1 - Y)$$
$$\times \ln \Phi_3(D_1, -D_2, -D_x; -\sigma_{12}, \sigma_{2x}, -\sigma_{1x})$$
$$+ I_1 I_2 Y \ln \Phi_3(D_1, D_2, D_c; \sigma_{12}, \sigma_{2c}, \sigma_{1c})$$
$$+ I_1 I_2(1 - Y)\ln \Phi_3(D_1, D_2, -D_c; \sigma_{12}, -\sigma_{2c}, -\sigma_{1c})$$
$$(4.10)$$

where $\Phi_2(.,.,;.)$ and $\Phi_3(.,.,.,;.,.,.)$ are the standard bivariate and trivariate densities, respectively. The parameters are $\gamma_1, \gamma_2, \gamma_3, \beta_n, \beta_x, \beta_c$, and 5×5 covariance matrix of disturbances, Σ:

$$\Sigma = \begin{bmatrix} 1 & \sigma_{12} & \sigma_{1n} & \sigma_{1x} & \sigma_{1c} \\ \sigma_{12} & 1 & \sigma_{2n} & \sigma_{2x} & \sigma_{2c} \\ \sigma_{1n} & \sigma_{2n} & 1 & \sigma_{nx} & \sigma_{nc} \\ \sigma_{1x} & \sigma_{2x} & \sigma_{nx} & 1 & \sigma_{xc} \\ \sigma_{1c} & \sigma_{2c} & \sigma_{nc} & \sigma_{xc} & 1 \end{bmatrix}$$

Note that $\sigma_{2n}, \sigma_{nx}, \sigma_{nc}$ and σ_{xc} do not explicitly appear in the likelihood function. It is well known that σ_{nx}, σ_{nc} and

σ_{xc} are not identified because the likelihood function does not depend on these parameters (for further discussion on this issue see [32]). Another parameter, σ_{2n}, is also not identified because the second selection equation is irrelevant for the nonsmoker group, and, hence, it is not in the likelihood function. This is because our two selection equations classify the sample not into four categories but into three categories. Hence, an additional restriction ($\sigma_{2n} = 0$) on the variance covariance matrix is required for identification. The rest of the parameters – $(K_1 + K_2) + 6 + (K_3 + K_4 + K_5) + 7 + 3K_6$ elements of regression coefficients γ_1, w_1, γ_2, w_2, β_n, β_x, ω_x, β_c and ω_c, plus six elements of the covariance matrix σ_{12}, σ_{1n}, σ_{1x}, σ_{1c}, σ_{2x} and σ_{2c} – are identifiable. It is well known that the likelihood function of the multivariate probit model is not globally concave, unlike that of the univariate probit model. The complexity of the likelihood function makes the FIML estimation difficult, and there is no ready-made guarantee that one has reached the global maximum.

We estimate the model by FIML with starting values from the Heckman–Lee two-step method with pre-tested forms of heteroskedasticity using GAUSS (version 3.2.4). FIML has seldom been used to estimate switching regression models with double selection because of computational difficulty. One useful tip to save a significant amount of computing time is to arrange the data by each of the six non-overlapping groups and maximize a form of the log of likelihood function given in Equation 4.11 rather than Equation 4.10:

$$
\begin{aligned}
\ln L(&\gamma_1, \omega_1, \gamma_2, \omega_2, \beta_n, \beta_x, \omega_x, \beta_c, \omega_c, \\
&\sigma_{12}, \sigma_{1n}, \sigma_{1x}, \sigma_{1c}, \sigma_{2x}, \sigma_{2c})
\end{aligned}
$$

$$
\begin{aligned}
= &\sum_{I_1=0, Y=1} \ln \Phi_2(-D_1, D_n; -\sigma_{1n}) \\
&+ \sum_{I_1=0, Y=0} \ln \Phi_2(-D_1, -D_n; \sigma_{1n}) \\
&+ \sum_{I_1=1, I_2=0, Y=1} \ln \Phi_3(D_1, -D_2, D_x; -\sigma_{12}, \\
&\quad -\sigma_{2x}, \sigma_{1x}) + \sum_{I_1=1, I_2=0, Y=0} \\
&\times \ln \Phi_3(D_1, -D_2, -D_x; -\sigma_{12}, \sigma_{2x}, -\sigma_{1x}) \\
&+ \sum_{I_1=1, I_2=1, Y=1} \ln \Phi_3(D_1, D_2, D_c; \sigma_{12}, \sigma_{2c}, \sigma_{1c}) \\
&+ \sum_{I_1=1, I_2=1, Y=0} \ln \Phi_3(D_1, D_2, -D_c; \\
&\quad \sigma_{12}, -\sigma_{2c}, -\sigma_{1c}) \qquad (4.11)
\end{aligned}
$$

If one wishes to maximize the likelihood function as written in Equation 4.11, GAUSS will evaluate two bivariate normal CDFs and four trivariate normal CDFs for each observation. In our estimation, we have saved more than three quarters of the computing time by maximizing (4.7). We also found that a 'good' starting value is critical to achieving smooth convergence. Further, we normalized all continuous variables by their means to prevent any possible interruption during the maximization of the likelihood function. We use the Berndt–Hall–Hall–Hausman (BHHH) algorithm for the FIML estimation and it took 29 iterations (with running time approximately 673 minutes in a 400 Hertz (Htz) PC) to converge with a pre-set tolerance level of 0.00001.[e] The variance–covariance matrix of the estimated structural parameters is obtained from the final information matrix on convergence. Interestingly, the estimates from the two-stage method and the FIML were very close except for the selectivity correction terms.[f]

EMPIRICAL ESTIMATES

SELECTION EQUATIONS

Table 4.2 presents heteroskedasticity corrected two-step and FIML estimates of the first selection equation together with marginal effects and odd ratios associated with different explanatory variables. To check for goodness-of-fit we compute various measures of pseudo R^2. Among those McKelvey and Zavonia's R^2 is 0.23, and the correct prediction rate is about 70%.

The initiation decision varies by different demographic characteristics; males tends to initiate more often than females. Participation in regular religious services (RELIGS), having a stable marriage life (MARIDIST), and having a nonsmoking spouse (SPOUSNSM) have high negative correlation with initiation. Individual drinking behaviour (EVDRINK, EXDRINK) has a significant positive effect. We also find that the propensity to initiate varies across different ethnic groups and education levels. SCHLYRS (school years) has a significant nonlinear effect on the initiation decision.

The variables RISKAVER, MYOPIC, and INVEST represent individuals' attitudes toward risk and play a major role in initiation. The variable RISKAVER represents individual risk aversion and MYOPIC represents an aspect of individual's time preference. For example, the individual with MYOPIC = 1 may be considered as a short-sighted individual who tends to prefer the immediate benefits of smoking over the future costs of health deterioration. These risk variables, which we can take to be largely time-invariant, turned out to have substantive impact on the initiation decision; odd ratios and marginal

Table 4.2 Estimates for the initiation equation

Variable	Two-step	FIML	SE (FIML)	Odds ratio	Marginal effect
Constant	0.8821	0.8964	0.1599	2.4508	0.3091
MALE	0.4142	0.4173	0.0451	1.5179	0.1452
RACEW	0.0871	0.0835	0.0559	1.0871	0.0305
RACEB	0.1053	0.1101	0.0754	1.1164	0.0369
FORNBORN	−0.2378	−0.2483	0.0591	0.7801	−0.0833
WESTB	−0.1118	−0.1104	0.0554	0.8955	−0.0392
SOUTHB	0.0189	0.0145	0.0339	1.1046	0.0066
SCHLYRS	0.5224	0.5205	0.2507	1.6829	0.1831
SCHLYRS2	−0.5048	−0.5071	0.1397	0.6022	−0.1769
PAREDU	0.0740	0.0784	0.0308	1.0816	0.0259
CATHOLIC	0.1495	0.1520	0.0362	1.1642	0.0524
RELGIS	−0.2729	−0.2764	0.0341	0.7585	−0.0956
MILIT	0.1477	0.1487	0.0424	1.1603	0.0518
MARIDIST	−0.3707	−0.3710	0.0354	0.6900	−0.1299
EVDRINK	0.2950	0.2996	0.0423	1.3493	0.1034
EXDRINK	0.8802	0.8823	0.1904	2.4165	0.3085
SPOUSNSM	−0.3499	−0.3488	0.0343	0.7055	−0.1226
NETWORTH	−0.0155	−0.0156	0.0057	0.9845	−0.0054
INVEST	−0.1482	−0.1489	0.0354	0.8617	−0.0519
SALESJOB	0.1236	0.1270	0.0397	0.1354	0.0433
FINJOB	−0.0698	−0.0691	0.0607	0.9332	−0.0245
TECHJOB	0.0787	0.0798	0.0477	1.0831	0.0276
SERVJOB	0.0408	0.0401	0.0469	1.0409	0.0143
NVRWORKD	−0.2655	−0.2677	0.0778	0.7651	−0.0931
RISKAVER	−0.0817	−0.0826	0.0428	0.9207	−0.0286
MYOPIC	0.0650	0.0678	0.0384	1.0702	0.0228
CLEAN	−0.0763	−0.0773	0.0292	0.9256	−0.0267
BMI	−0.3763	−0.3834	0.0820	0.6815	−0.1319
RACEB	0.3005	0.3088	0.0826		
MARIDIST	−0.2341	−0.2302	0.0602		
EVDRINK	0.1838	0.1862	0.0586	*Heteroskedasticity*	
EXDRINK	0.3354	0.3348	0.1334	*Specification*	
SPOUSNSM	−0.1738	−0.1677	0.0561		

effects of RISKAVER, MYOPIC, and INVEST are (0.92, 1.07. 0.86) and (−0.029, 0.022, −0.05), respectively. This evidence indicates that risk-average individuals tend not to initiate and that individuals with higher time preferences for the immediate tend to initiate more often. Other socio-economic status variables have significant explanatory power to explain individuals' initiation decisions. The direction of contributions from these variables are consistent with previous studies.

Table 4.3 presents estimates from heteroskedasticity-corrected two-step estimator of the second selection equation (continuation decision) by FGLS and FIML procedures together with the marginal effects and odd ratios. McKelvey–Zavonia's R^2 is 0.31 and the correct prediction rate is again about 70%. In terms of the R^2 measure, the fit of the second selection equation is slightly better than that of the first selection equation. As one would expect, spouse's cessation decision (SPOSEXSM)

has very strong effect on individual's cessation decision. Spouse's health status and the number of children in the household were not significant.

An interesting finding is that the presence of current good health conditions (EXER, JOGAMILE) and also bad health conditions (BLOODPRS, CHOLSTRL, DIABTS) have strong positive effects on the propensity for cessation. When people realize that they have developed some bad health conditions which might be aggravated by smoking, they tend to quit (see [4,19]). Current smokers who still enjoy good health sometimes quit in order to maintain the good health. This evidence simply implies that there are two groups of ex-smokers in our sample – one group quits in order to restore better health (curative), and the other group quite in order to maintain good health (preventive).

Risk variables in the cessation decision equation also have very interesting implications. RISKAVER, MY-

Table 4.3 Estimates for the continuation equation

Variable	Two-step	FIML	SE (FIML)	Odds ratio	Marginal effect
Constant	0.9862	1.0069	0.2036	2.7371	0.3900
MALE	−0.1056	−0.1202	0.0346	0.8867	−0.0417
RACEB	0.1491	0.1619	0.0701	1.1757	0.0590
RACEW	0.0917	0.1343	0.0662	1.1437	0.0363
FORNBORN	−0.1211	−0.1094	0.0534	0.8964	−0.0479
CATHOLIC	0.0556	0.0489	0.0264	1.0501	0.0220
RELIGS	−0.1972	−0.1968	0.0351	0.8214	−0.0779
MARRIED	−0.1635	−0.1633	0.0451	0.8493	−0.0646
NOMARAGS	0.0450	0.0443	0.0197	1.0453	0.0178
HOUSE	−0.0533	−0.0497	0.0250	0.9515	−0.0211
EXER	−0.1408	−0.1485	0.0341	0.8620	−0.0557
ALCHOLIC	0.1896	0.1858	0.0495	1.2042	0.0749
CLEAN	−0.1100	−0.1156	0.0267	0.8908	−0.0435
BADFIN	0.0799	0.0814	0.0287	1.0848	0.0316
SPOUSNSM	−0.2940	−0.2873	0.0574	0.7428	−0.1163
SPOUSXSM	−0.4094	−0.4209	0.0600	0.6565	−0.1619
OWNRV	−0.1512	−0.1566	0.0654	0.8550	−0.0598
IRA	−0.1353	−0.1465	0.0309	0.8637	−0.0535
LIFEINS	−0.0373	−0.0408	0.0260	0.9600	−0.0148
RISKAVER	−0.0498	−0.0486	0.0319	0.9526	−0.0197
HELTHINS	−0.0872	−0.0827	0.0339	0.9206	−0.0345
SCHLYRS	0.5217	0.5413	0.2149	1.7182	0.2063
SCHLYRS2	−0.3956	−0.4102	0.1186	0.6635	−0.1564
JOGAMILE	−0.1466	0.1696	0.0417	1.1848	−0.0580
BLOODPRS	−0.0946	−0.0983	0.0266	0.9064	−0.0374
CHOLSTRL	−0.0421	−0.0443	0.0254	0.9567	−0.0166
DIABTS	−0.0356	−0.0383	0.0355	0.9522	−0.0141
ARTHRTS	−0.0260	−0.0280	0.0226	0.9724	−0.0103
SALESJOB	0.0745	0.0725	0.0294	1.0752	0.0295
FINJOB	0.0946	0.0978	0.0492	1.1027	0.0374
MYOPIC	0.0691	0.0700	0.0296	1.0725	0.0273
ADDICTION	0.0595	0.0593	0.0142	1.0611	0.0235
BMI	−0.7590	−0.8134	0.1165	0.4433	−0.3001
R12	0.1137	0.1590	0.1227		
MALE	0.1671	0.1516	0.0671		
RACEW	−0.5697	−0.5365	0.0904		
MARRIED	−0.1372	−0.1209	0.0951	*Heteroskedasticity*	
SPOUSNEM	−0.2414	−0.2112	0.0832	*Specification*	
OWNRV	0.2249	0.1994	0.1233		

OPIC, IRA, LIFEINS, and HELTHINS are the variables that can capture individual risk behaviour. Our results show that those individuals who have higher time preferences for the current time continue to smoke. The variables LIFEINS and HELTHINS represent individuals' attitudes towards health risk, and these variables also have a meaningful interpretation. Individuals who have individual retirement accounts (IRA) can be considered to be more financially well planned, and the variable IRA has a positive contribution to the cessation decision. Schooling (SCHLYRS, SCHLYRS2) and Body Mass Index (BMI) variables have significant non-linear effects on the cessation decision. Another interesting variable is the cigarette addiction variable (ADDICTION) which is designed to capture the approximate strength of smokers' cigarette addictions. As one would expect, our result indicates that the stronger the addiction, the harder it is to quit. Also a stable married life (MARRIED, NOMARAGS) and drinking habit (ALCHOLIC) have significant effects on the cessation decision. We also observe variations in cessation propensity by different demographic, occupational, and economic classes, and they are consistent with prior findings.

Table 4.4 Estimates for the nonsmoker's disease equation

Variable	Two-step	FIML	SE (FIML)	Odds ratio	Marginal effect
Constant	−2.7242	−2.6669	0.9493	0.0695	−0.3230
MALE	−0.0873	−0.0747	0.1033	0.9280	−0.0104
RACEB	0.2413	0.2329	0.1699	1.2623	0.0286
FORNBORN	0.4258	0.4149	0.1692	1.5142	0.0505
WESTB	0.6618	0.6488	0.2103	1.9132	0.0785
MARIDIST	−0.0532	−0.0605	0.0898	0.9413	−0.0063
BLOODPRS	0.4400	0.4388	0.1589	1.5508	0.0522
CHOLSTRL	0.1947	0.1931	0.0760	1.2130	0.0231
DIABTS	−1.0859	−0.0799	0.5215	0.3396	−0.1287
ARTHRTS	0.2126	0.2132	0.0787	1.2376	0.0252
EXDRINK	−0.1684	−0.1548	0.1285	0.8566	−0.0200
BADFIN	0.2037	0.2042	0.0832	1.2265	0.0242
GOODFAM	0.0344	0.0324	0.1030	1.0329	0.0041
HAZWORK	0.3111	0.3122	0.0871	1.3664	0.0369
AGRIJOB	0.1120	0.1108	0.1879	1.1172	0.0133
SALESMAN	−0.0824	−0.0806	0.1495	0.9226	−0.0098
SERVJOB	−0.0907	−0.0885	0.1188	0.9153	−0.0108
NVRWORKD	0.5355	0.5319	0.1786	1.7022	0.0635
FEDINS	0.2415	0.2406	0.0933	1.2720	0.0286
LIFEINS	0.0312	0.0306	0.0808	1.0311	0.0037
RISKAVER	−0.0051	−0.0081	0.1106	0.9919	−0.0006
MYOPIC	−0.2119	−0.2067	0.1512	0.8133	−0.0251
SPOUSNSM	0.1722	0.1634	0.1291	1.1775	0.0204
SPOUSXSM	0.1780	0.1773	0.1281	1.1940	0.0211
NOJOBS	−0.0264	−0.0256	0.0641	0.9747	−0.0031
NOMARAGS	0.1876	0.1884	0.0863	1.2073	0.0222
AGE	0.3834	0.3763	0.4647	1.4569	0.0455
SCHOLYRS	−0.0697	−0.0741	0.1334	0.9286	−0.0083
NETWORTH	−0.0426	−0.0433	0.0344	0.9576	−0.0051
BMI	0.1914	0.1863	1.2774	1.2048	0.0227
BMI2	0.0138	0.0144	0.5548	1.0145	0.0016
Rln	−0.0247	0.0130	0.1791		
RACEB	−0.3961	−0.3923	0.1701		
FORNBORN	−0.5785	−0.5774	0.1665		
WESTB	−0.6623	−0.6529	0.2747		
BLOODPRS	−0.3126	−0.3127	0.1420	*Heteroskedasticity*	
DIABTS	0.9055	0.9067	0.2777	*Specification*	
NVRWORKD	−0.7137	−0.7206	0.2851		
MYOPIC	0.4190	0.4189	0.1356		

SWITCHING DISEASE EQUATIONS

Tables 4.4–4.6 present estimates of the disease equations by two-step and FIML methods for the three smoking status groups. We specify our switching disease equations using a number of demographic, occupational, economic, and fundamental health condition variables. An interesting variable is HAZWORK, which represents occupational exposure to hazards. In some sense, HAZWORK also represents individual risk-taking behaviour as well. The occupational exposure to hazards has significant effect on the probability of the occurrence of the SRDs for all three smoking groups. There are direct and indirect

effects of this variable. The direct effect in the contribution from the exposure. Some workers work in hazardous occupations not because they prefer them, but because they have no other choices. The indirect effect comes because individuals who work in hazardous occupations are often risk-takers (see [33]), and such attitudes can have positive effects on the probability of SRDs. A part of the indirect effect is expected to manifest itself through the selectivity correction terms.

The variable FEDINS, which indicates health insurance coverage by federal health insurance programs such as Medicaid and VA, has a positive effect on the probability of having SRDs for all three smoking groups. The

Table 4.5   Estimates for the ex-smoker's disease equation

Variable	Two-step	FIML	SE (FIML)	Odds ratio	Marginal effect
Constant	−0.8954	−1.1841	0.8318	0.3060	−0.1379
MALE	−0.1548	−0.1390	0.0948	0.8702	−0.0238
RACEB	−0.1923	−0.1884	0.1025	0.8283	−0.0296
FORNBORN	−0.5729	−0.5346	0.2005	0.5859	−0.0882
WESTB	−0.0830	−0.0777	0.1117	0.9252	−0.0128
MARIDIST	0.0794	0.0886	0.0911	1.0926	0.0122
BLOODPRS	−0.2342	−0.3002	0.1871	0.7407	−0.0361
CHOLSTRL	0.0018	0.0083	0.0692	1.0083	0.0003
DIABTS	0.1398	0.1355	0.0886	1.1451	0.0215
ARTHRTS	0.1581	0.1585	0.0647	1.1718	0.0244
EXDRINK	0.1066	0.0986	0.0784	1.1036	0.0164
BADFIN	0.0811	0.0602	0.0777	1.0620	0.0125
GOODFAM	0.2763	0.3265	0.1623	1.3861	0.0425
HAZWORK	0.4941	0.5138	0.1582	1.6716	0.0761
AGRIJOB	−0.0056	−0.0026	0.1825	0.9974	−0.0009
SALESMAN	−0.9838	−0.3988	1.3063	0.2469	−0.1515
SERVJOB	−0.0651	−0.0654	0.0962	0.9367	−0.0100
NVRWORKD	−0.2946	−0.2985	0.2684	0.7419	−0.0454
FEDINS	0.2136	0.2146	0.0838	1.2394	0.0329
LIFEINS	−0.0581	−0.0461	0.0698	0.9549	−0.0090
RISKAVER	−0.1243	−0.1189	0.0910	0.8879	−0.0191
MYOPIC	0.2735	0.3380	0.1666	1.4021	0.0421
SPOUSNSM	0.0467	0.0650	0.1030	1.0672	0.0072
SPOUSXSM	0.1109	0.1459	0.1039	1.1571	0.0171
NOJOBS	−0.0631	−0.0683	0.0455	0.9340	−0.0097
NOMARAGS	0.1436	0.1392	0.0681	1.1494	0.0221
AGE	0.3400	0.3822	0.4096	1.4655	0.0524
SCHOLYRS	−0.3158	−0.2746	0.1272	0.7599	−0.0486
NETWORTH	−0.0209	−0.0196	0.0217	0.9806	−0.0032
BMI	−1.8797	−1.6930	1.2346	0.1840	−0.2895
BMI2	0.8676	0.8014	0.5460	2.2287	0.1336
CIGARETS	0.2299	0.2219	0.0448	1.2484	0.0354
R1x	0.2359	0.2230	0.2485		
R2x	−0.2189	−0.3908	0.1743		
BLOODPRS	0.2710	0.2659	0.1206		
GOODFAM	−0.4824	−0.4197	0.1386		
HAZWORK	−0.3551	−0.2886	0.1475	*Heteroskedasticity*	
SALESMAN	0.6186	0.6660	0.4368	*Specification*	
MYOPIC	−0.3588	−0.3315	0.1439		

marginal effect of FEDINS for nonsmokers, ex-smokers, and current smokers are 0.03, 0.03, and 0.08, respectively, implying that the interaction of smoking status and FEDINS is a significant factor in the health production function (see [11]). Since FEDINS captures mostly people with low socio-economic status, these estimates suggest that smoking by individuals has a considerable social cost as well. Unstable married life (NOMARAGS) also has a significant impact on the presence of the diseases for all three groups of smokers. We also find demographic variations in the incidence of SRDs.

One of the most significant findings of this study is the presence of significant selectivity coefficients in previous smokers' and current smokers' disease equations. Some of the selectivity coefficients in FIML estimation turned out to be substantially different from those in two-step estimations – underscoring the importance of FIML approach in these kinds of models. The selectivity coefficient in the nonsmokers' equation turned out to be insignificant. The statistically significant selectivity coefficients in the last two disease equations imply the endogenous nature of switching in our structural model. We should emphasize that we took utmost care to fully specify our five equations such that the significance of the selectivity terms is not due to the omission of observable explanatory variables. For instance, interaction of a number of

Table 4.6   Estimates for current smoker's disease equation

Variable	Two-step	FIML	SE (FIML)	Odds ratio	Marginal effect
Constant	−0.9730	−0.8839	0.8575	0.4132	−0.1590
MALE	0.0275	−0.0065	0.1638	0.9935	0.0045
RACEB	−0.5621	−0.5266	0.1262	0.5906	−0.0919
FORNBORN	−0.6234	−0.6189	0.1976	0.5385	−0.1019
WESTB	−0.2598	−0.2481	0.1523	0.7803	−0.0425
MARIDIST	0.0584	0.0569	0.0976	1.0585	0.0095
BLOODPRS	0.1616	0.1477	0.0811	1.1592	0.0264
CHOLSTRL	0.1864	0.1697	0.0915	1.1849	0.0305
DIABTS	−0.1212	−0.0644	0.2057	0.9376	−0.0198
ARTHRTS	0.3358	0.3250	0.0798	1.3840	0.0549
EXDRINK	0.0223	0.0043	0.1047	1.0043	0.0036
BADFIN	0.2615	0.2610	0.0951	1.2982	0.0427
GOODFAM	−0.2212	−0.2172	0.1306	0.8048	−0.0361
HAZWORK	0.2300	0.2224	0.0935	1.2491	0.0376
AGRIJOB	0.5055	0.4835	0.2286	1.6217	0.0826
SALESMAN	−0.3303	−0.3215	0.1484	0.7251	−0.0540
SERVJOB	−0.1556	−0.1485	0.1196	0.8620	−0.0254
NVRWORKD	0.5811	0.5481	0.1791	1.7300	0.0950
FEDINS	0.4773	0.4648	0.1025	1.5917	0.0780
LIFEINS	−0.2028	−0.1435	0.1442	0.8663	−0.0331
RISKAVER	−0.0055	−0.0086	0.1035	0.9914	−0.0009
MYOPIC	0.0855	0.0894	0.0869	1.0935	0.0140
SPOUSNSM	0.1659	0.1583	0.1065	1.1715	0.0271
SPOUSXSM	0.2418	0.2105	0.1355	1.2343	0.0395
NOJOB	0.0061	0.0026	0.0586	1.0026	0.0010
NOMARAGS	0.1321	0.1352	0.0590	1.1448	0.0216
AGE	1.0138	0.9496	0.5889	2.5847	0.1657
SCHOLYRS	−0.2571	−0.2513	0.1692	0.7778	−0.0420
NETWORTH	−0.0249	−0.0237	0.0414	0.9766	−0.0041
BMI	−2.2286	−2.2623	1.0911	0.1041	−0.3642
BMI2	0.6494	0.6637	0.5072	1.9420	0.1061
CIGARETS	0.1854	0.1875	0.0682	1.2062	0.0303
R1c	0.1777	0.0931	0.3218		
R2c	−0.3443	−0.2373	0.1452		
MALE	−0.1564	−0.1497	0.1336		
DIABTS	0.3646	0.3744	0.2216		*Heteroskedasticity*
NVRWORKD	−0.8484	−0.9518	0.3737		*Specification*
LIFEINS	0.3288	0.3080	0.1316		

statistically significant explanatory variables were not found to be important in the specifications.

FURTHER IMPLICATIONS OF OUR FINDINGS

The model estimated in this paper provides a way to identify the true risk of smoking by correcting the self-selection problem in the observed proportions of SRDs in different smoking groups. The evidence on the presence of unobserved heterogeneity in ex-smokers' and current smokers' disease equations suggests that the risk factor for smokers may be different from that of nonsmokers, even if smokers had never smoked. The coefficients $(\sigma_{1x}, \sigma_{1c})$ from the initiation equation are both positive, but they are not significant at the 5% level. On the other hand, the coefficients $(\sigma_{2x}, \sigma_{2c})$ from the cessation equation are both negative and statistically significant at the 5% level. The significance of these terms suggests that the observed relative frequencies of SRDs in the sample are biased estimates of the true risk factors for the ex-smokers and the current smokers. The observed proportions based on our sample indicate that the probability of getting SRDs for ex-smokers and current smokers are 9.41% and 15.97%, respectively. The signs of the coefficients $(\sigma_{2x}, \sigma_{2c})$ indicate the direction of the selection bias.

The observed risk factors have two components: risk factor due to smoking and selectivity. The estimated negative values of σ_{2x} and σ_{2c} capture an unobservable negative correlation between the propensity of getting SRDs and the propensity of continuing to smoke. Ignoring this correlation, which manifests through the cessation selection, would yield an upward bias for ex-smokers' and downward bias for current smokers' risk factors. Since the signs of the selectivity coefficients allow us to make other interesting inferences, we devote the rest of this section to interpreting the results.

Our prediction shows that the true mean risk factor for ex-smokers is about 6%, which is slightly more than that for nonsmokers and much less than the observed risk factor (9.41%). The risk factor for current smokers is about 20%, which is much higher than the observed risk factor for current smokers (15.9%).[g] This finding has significant implications for previous empirical studies on the costs of cigarette smoking. For example, Miller et al. [7] estimated medical care expenditures attributed to cigarette smoking based on observed frequencies of SRDs, without considering the unobserved heterogeneity in the baseline risk factors of smokers. In order to estimate the actual effect of cigarette smoking on health, this unobserved heterogeneity first has to be controlled for.

Further, our model is useful for investigating whether individual smoking participation decisions are consistent with economic rationality or forward looking behaviour. The counter-factual conditional mean risk factor predictions are useful for this purpose (see [34]). Table 4.7 presents the probabilities for getting SDRs for nonsmokers, if they had chosen to be ex-smokers ($P[\hat{Y}_x = 1 | X_n, I_1 = 0]$), and chosen to be current smokers ($P[\hat{Y}_c = 1 | X_n, I_1 = 0]$); the probabilities for ex-smokers, if they had chosen not to start smoking ($P[\hat{Y}_n = 1 | X_x, I_1 = 1, I_2 = 0]$), and had chosen not to quit smoking ($P[\hat{Y}_c = 1 | X_x, I_1 = 1, I_2 = 0]$); and finally the probabilities for current smokers, if they had chosen not to start smoking ($P[\hat{Y}_n = 1 | X_c, I_1 = 1, I_2 = 1]$), and if they had chosen to quit smoking ($P[\hat{Y}_x = 1 | X_c, I_1 = 1, I_2 = 1]$).[h] However, $P[\hat{Y}_n = 1 | X_c, I_1 = 1, I_2 = 1]$ and $P[\hat{Y}_n = 1 | X_x, I_1 = 1, I_2 = 0]$ are

not identifiable because our model can not identify σ_{2n}.

We find from Table 4.7 that the risk factor for an ex-smoker had he/she not chosen to quit ($P[\hat{Y}_c = 1 | X_x, I_1 = 1, I_2 = 0]$) is even higher than that of a current smoker ($P[\hat{Y}_c = 1 | X_c, I_1 = 1, I_2 = 1]$). This evidence indicates that ex-smokers incorporate the hazards of smoking into their beliefs based on private information, and that they reverse their smoking behaviour because they could foresee health deterioration. Current smokers may not fully realize the hazards of smoking because they have not yet run down their health stock below the individual-specific critical threshold, are ignoring the signs of health deterioration, or are unable to quit simply because of addiction. This implies either that there is an information failure that prevents current smokers from smoking or that current smokers may not readily accept the foreseeable adverse health effects due to addition. This apparent market failure requires different types of policy interventions that are specifically targeted on current smokers who continue to smoke for various different reasons.

Our empirical model can also examine the presence and direction of comparative advantage (or more appropriately, 'comparative risk' in our context) in the initiation and cessation decisions. Our empirical evidence has indicated that self-selection has a non-ignorable effect on the observed risk factors for both ex-smokers and current smokers. Under self-selection, individuals will choose an alternative for which they have a comparative advantage (see [35–37]). The existence of comparative risk will suggest a lack of forward looking behaviour in that choice.

First, we examine the presence of comparative risk in the cessation decision by looking at the counter-factual conditional mean risk predictions, $P[\hat{Y}_n = 1 | X_x, I_1 = 1, I_2 = 0]$ and $P[\hat{Y}_x = 1 | X_c, I_1 = 1, I_2 = 1]$. In the absence of comparative risk in the cessation decision, we expect:

$$\frac{P[Y_x = 1 | X_x, I_1 = 1, I_2 = 0]}{P[Y_x = 1 | X_c, I_1 = 1, I_2 = 1]}$$

$$< \frac{P[\hat{Y}_c = 1 | X_x, I_1 = 1, I_2 = 0]}{P[Y_c = 1 | X_c, I_1 = 1, I_2 = 1]}.$$

The left hand side of the inequality indicates the mean relative risk taken by observed quitters, whereas the right hand side of the inequality indicates the relative risk foregone by them. Based on the predictions presented in Table 4.7, we see that the inequality holds, which suggests rational risk-taking in the cessation decision.[i] Second, in order to examine the existence of comparative risk at the initiation stage, we obtain the following counter-factual mean risks: $P[\hat{Y}_n = 1 | X_x, I_1 = 1]$, $P[\hat{Y}_x = 1 | X_n, I_1 = 0]$, $P[\hat{Y}_x = 1 | X_x, I_1 = 1]$, $P[\hat{Y}_n = 1 | X_c, I_1 = 1]$,

Table 4.7 Counter-factual risk factor predictions

Observed smoking status	Counter-factual smoking status		
	$E[Y_n | .]$ (None)	$E[Y_X | .]$ (Ex.)	$E[Y_C | .]$ (Current)
None ($I_1 = 0$)	0.054	0.056	0.111
Ex ($I_1 = 1, I_2 = 0$)	*	0.094	0.214
Current ($I_1 = 1, I_2 = 1$)	*	0.082	0.159

$P[\hat{Y}_c = 1 \mid X_n, I_1 = 0]$ and $P[\hat{Y}_c \mid X_c, I_1 = 1]$. Since we want to compare nonsmokers with ex-smokers and current smokers in the initiation decision, the mean prediction here excludes the effect of the second selection. If the rational risk-taking behaviour is valid on the average at the initiation stage, we expect the follow-up inequalities to hold:

$$\frac{P[Y_n = 1 \mid X_n, I_1 = 0]}{P[\hat{Y}_n = 1 \mid X_x, I_1 = 1]} < \frac{P[\hat{Y}_x = 1 \mid X_n, I_1 = 0]}{P[\hat{Y}_x = 1 \mid X_x, I_1 = 1]},$$

and

$$\frac{P[Y_n = 1 \mid X_n, I_1 = 0]}{P[\hat{Y}_n = 1 \mid X_c, I_1 = 1]} < \frac{P[\hat{Y}_c = 1 \mid X_n, I_1 = 0]}{P[\hat{Y}_c = 1 \mid X_c, I_1 = 1]}.$$

Each side of the inequalities has similar interpretations as before. Our predictions show little evidence of forward-looking behaviour in the initiation decision.[j]

These results are broadly consistent with those of Viscusi [14] who found that young people have a high risk perception but that this risk perception does not influence their smoking behaviour. Most at the initiation stage are too young to think about the hazard of smoking, which may or may not happen until many years in the future. At this age, they tend to experiment with various alternative life styles. The lack of rationality in the initiation behaviour could be more transparent in our analysis because the hazards of cigarette smoking were not very well known to the public a few decades ago, and cigarette smoking was a more acceptable social behaviour during the period in which the smokers in our sample initiated. Unlike the initiation decision, the rationality in the cessation decision is observed because individuals get first-hand information on the risk and utility of smoking from their past smoking experiences.

CONCLUSIONS

Almost all previous empirical studies on cigarette smoking estimated a particular part of our structural model and focused on the interpretation of the estimated coefficients. Thus, a particular association between a dependent variable (smoking behaviour or the presumed effect of smoking) and the covariates is the main issue in these studies. They uncover many interesting empirical regularities such as the demographic variations in smoking behaviour, and the correlation of smoking with drinking habits. The estimation of our initiation and cessation equations corroborates results which are consistent with previous studies. However our objective is not to confirm these previous findings using new data, but to go beyond the mere interpretation of estimated regression coefficients. Fundamentally, our two selection equations explore individual attitudes towards risk, and how these risk attitudes lead to different health outcomes that are represented by the prevalence of SRDs. By combining smoking motivation and its outcomes, our model reveals many useful aspects of how individuals incorporate their risk beliefs into smoking choices, and further it provides a clear direction for future public policy.

We find significant evidence of self-selection effects on both previous and current smokers' probabilities for getting SRDs. This indicates that previous studies on the effects of smoking on health or medical expenditures should be revisited after considering self-selection behaviour of smokers. We find that the true mean risk factor for ex-smokers is about 6%, which is slightly more than that of never-smokers and is much less than their observed risk factor (9.4%) in the sample. The true mean risk factor for the current smokers is about 20% which is much higher than their observed risk factor (16%). Based on counterfactual conditional mean risk factor predictions, we find that the risk factor for an ex-smoker, had he not chosen to quit, is even higher than that of a current smoker. Our evidence also suggests that self-selection in the cessation decision is consistent with economic rationality, but the same is not found in the initiation decision. This finding underscores the importance of public policy initiatives on teenage initiation. In addition, our analysis suggests a direction for anti-smoking campaigns; it should target those groups of individuals who tend to initiate more easily, because those who tend to initiate have higher risk factors for the diseases as well.

ACKNOWLEDGEMENTS

Earlier versions of the paper were presented at the 1998 Econometric Society Meetings at Chicago and at the Triangle Health Economics Workshop. We are grateful to Andrew Jones, Terrence Kinal, Hamp Lankford, Maarten Lindeboom, Angel Lopez-Nicolas, Edward Norton, Ilde Rizzo, Michael Sattinger, Frank Sloan, Insan Tunali, and Michelle White and two anonymous referees for many helpful comments. We thank Deb Dwyer for first suggesting to us the possible use of HRS data in the present context.

APPENDIX

Variable names and definitions

Variable	Definition

Unless otherwise noted, all variables denoted below are (0 1) dummies

Initiation Equation

Variable	Definition
Dependent variable	Ever-smoker = 1, never smoker = 0.
BMI	Body Mass Index (weight/height^2) normalized by sample mean (not a dummy).
CATHOLIC	Religious preference, Catholic.
CLEAN	Interior of the dwelling units is clean.
EVDRINK	Ever drink any alcoholic beverages such as beer, wine, or liquor.
EVRSMOKD	Ever smoked cigarette.
EXDRINK	Excessive drinking habits.
FINJOB	Worked in the business of finance, insurance, or real estate. (US Census Code: 700-712.)
FORNBORN	Not born in the US.
INVEST	Invests in stock, bond, real estate, or t-bill.
MALE	Male.
MARIDIST	First marriage and currently married.
MILIT	Ever been in military service.
MYOPIC	The most important financial planning horizon for the individual is the next few months.
NETWORTH	Total net worth normalized by sample mean (not a dummy).
NVRWORKD	Never worked for pay.
PAREDU	Either mother or father has more than 12 years of schooling.
RACEB	Black.
RACEW	White/Caucasian.
RELIGS	Attends religious services more than two or three times a month.
RISKAVER	Would not take new job with a 50–50 chance of doubling income and 50–50 chance of cutting income by half.
SERVJOB	Service related job (US Census Code: 403-407, 413-427, 433-469).
SALESJOB	Worked in the business of retail or whole sale.
SCHLYRS	Years of schooling normalized by sample mean (not a dummy).
SCHLYRS2	SCHLYRS^2
SOUTHB	Born in southern states.
SPOUSNSM	Individual's spouse is nonsmoker.
TECHJOB	Professional specialty operation and technical support job (US Census Code: 043-235).
WESTB	Born in western states.

Continuation Equation

Variable	Definition
Dependent variable	Current smoker = 1, ex-smoker = 0.
BMI2	BMI^2
ADDICTION	Years of smoking times number of cigarettes smoked, normalized by sample mean (not a dummy).
ALCHOLIC	Drinks more than 3 or 4 a day.
ARTHRTS	Ever had arthritis.
BADFIN	Dissatisfied with his/her financial condition.
BLOODPRS	Ever had high blood pressure problem.
CHOLSTRL	Ever had high cholesterol problem.
DIABTS	Ever had diabetes.
EXER	Does both light and heavy exercise more than three times a week.
FINJOB	Worked in the business of fiance, insurance, and real estate (UK Census Code: 700-712).
HELTHINS	Individual has health insurance policy, either federally funded, privately funded, or employer provided.
HOUSE	Living in a detached single family house.
IRA	Individual has an IRA account.
JOGAMILE	Individual has no difficulty at all in running or jogging a mile.
LIFEINS	Individual has one or more life insurance policies.
MARRIED	Currently married.
NOMARAGS	Number of marriages including current one normalized by sample. Mean (not a dummy).
OWNRV	Owns a recreational vehicle (RV).
RACEB	Race dummy for Black.
SPOSEXSM	Individual's spouse is ex-smoker.
R12(σ_{12})	Inverse of Mill's ratio for the first selection equation (initiation).

BMI, CATHOLIC, CLEAN, FINJOB, FORNBORN, MALE, MYOPIC, RELIGS, RISKAVER, SALESJOB, SCHLYRS, SCHLYRS2, SPOUSNSM have already been defined above.

Disease equations

Dependent variable	Ever had smoking related diseases = 1. Never had the disease = 0.
	Smoking related diseases (SRDs): lung disease (not including asthma) such as chronic bronchitis or emphysema, or any following type of the cancers of the abdomen, mouth, bladder, neck, nose, pancreas, bronchia, cervix, esophagus, stomach, throat, tongue, kidney, liver, and lung.
AGE	Age normalized by sample mean (not a dummy).
AGRIGJOB	Work in the area of agriculture, forestry, and fishing (US Census Code: 010-031).
CIGARETS	Number of cigarettes smoked per day normalized by sample mean.
SALESMAN	Sales job (US Census Code: 243-285).
FEDINS	Federally funded health insurance, such as Medicaid, CHAMPUS, VA, or other military programs.
GOODFAM	Satisfied with family life.
HAZWORK	Ever exposed and continuously exposed more than 1 year to dangerous chemicals or other hazards at work.
NOJOBS	Number of jobs including current one normalized by sample mean (not a dummy).
$R12(\sigma_{12})$	Inverse of Mill's ratio for the first selection equation (initiate), ever-smoker.
$R1n(\sigma_{1n})$	Inverse of Mill's ratio for the first selection equation (not initiate), nonsmoker.
$R1x(\sigma_{1x})$	Inverse of Mill's ratio for the first selection equation (initiate), ex-smoker.
$R2x(\sigma_{2x})$	Inverse of Mill's ratio for the first selection equation (quit), ex-smoker.
$R1c(\sigma_{1c})$	Inverse of Mill's ratio for the first selection equation (initiate), current smoker.
$R2c(\sigma_{2c})$	Inverse of Mill's ratio for the first selection equation (continue), current smoker.

ARTHRITS, BADFIN, BLOODPRS, BMI, BMI2, CATHOLIC, CHOLESTRL, DIABTS, EXDRINK, FORNBORN, LIFEINS, MARIDIST, MYOPIC, NETWORTH, NEVERW, NOMARAGS, RISKAVER, RACEB, SCHLYRS, SERVJOB, SPOSEXSM and SPOSENSM have already been defined above.

NOTES

a. Thus, we will be estimating the effect of smoking on a more homogenous group of individuals, for whom the effect of aging will be similar.

b. We drop a total of 3543 individuals from our final sample: 2407 individuals whose ages are less than 52, 269 individuals who quit smoking after they were diagnosed with various diseases, 96 individuals whose household-level information is not available, and the rest who have missing information in any one of our variables. Of the 269 individuals who quit after they were diagnosed with various diseases, only 54 had developed SRDs as defined later in the paper. Arguably, the 54 smokers who quit after being diagnosed as having SRDs should be treated as current smokers and the remaining 215 should be included in the ex-smokers group for calculating the risk factors. This would result in a slightly higher risk factor for current smokers and a slightly lower risk factor for the ex-smokers than the one reported later in the paper. Following a suggestion of a referee, when we estimated our model with this reclassification, the basic conclusions of this paper remained unchanged.

c. We use following variables as exogenous regressors for the first stage probit regression: MALE, FORN-BORN, WESTB, RACEW, RACEB, RACEA, SCHLYRS, SCHLYTS2, PAREDU, CATHOLIC, MILIT, MARIDIST, HOUSE, NOMARAGS, RIS-KAVER, RELIGS, AGE and a few other obvious exogenous variables like the regional dummies.

d. The variables were: self-reported current health status, change in health condition during last year, presence of various limitations on daily activities, presence of asthma disease, and heart attack.

e. We found that the BHHH algorithm tends to converge much faster than other Quasi-Newton methods, such as Broyden–Fletcher–Goldfarb–Shanno (BFGS) or Davidon–Fletch–Powell (DFP). In our experiments, BHHH took nearly 30 iterations, whereas BFGS and DFP took more than 150 iterations to converge at the tolerance level 0.00001 with the starting values from the Heckman–Lee two-stage method.

f. In order to make sure that our estimates maximize the likelihood function globally, we experimented with different starting values and also with the method of simulated annealing (see [38]). Since this estimation can take a very long time, we use FIML estimates as starting values for the simulated annealing method.

g. Note that the risk factors for the ever smokers will be slightly higher than that of the non-smokers if we consider the differential sample attrition rates due to deaths for the three smoking groups. During the 2-year period between waves 1 and 2, the annual mortality rates in our sample for the non-smokers, ex-smokers, and current smokers with SRDs (aged 52 and more) were calculated to be approximately 0.40%, 0.50%, and 1.50%, respectively.

h. Our conditional mean risk factor predictions are computed in the following way:

$$P[\hat{Y}_i = 1 | X_j, I_1 = 1, I_2 = 1]$$

$$= \frac{\Phi_3(X_j\beta_i, I_1^*, I_2^*, \sigma_{1i}, \sigma_{12}, \sigma_{2i})}{\Phi_2(I_1^*, I_2^*, \sigma_{12})}$$

and similarly

$$P[\hat{Y}_i = 1 | X_j, I_1 = 1] = \frac{\Phi_2(X_j\beta_i, I_1^*, \sigma_{1i})}{\Phi_1(I_1^*)},$$

where $i = n, x, c$ and $j = n, x, c$.

i. The results from our predictions are:

$$\frac{P[Y_x = 1 | X_x, I_1 = 1, I_2 = 0]}{P[\hat{Y}_x = 1 | X_c, I_1 = 1, I_2 = 1]} = \frac{0.094}{0.082} = 1.146,$$

and

$$\frac{P[\hat{Y}_c = 1 | X_x, I_1 = 1, I_2 = 0]}{P[Y_c = 1 | X_c, I_1 = 1, I_2 = 1]} = \frac{0.214}{0.160} = 1.33.$$

j. The results of our predictions are:

$$\frac{P[Y_n = 1 | X_n, I_1 = 0]}{P[\hat{Y}_n = 1 | X_x, I_1 = 1]} = \frac{0.054}{0.088} = 0.614,$$

$$\frac{P[\hat{Y}_x = 1 | X_n, I_1 = 0]}{P[Y_x = 1 | X_x, I_1 = 1]} = \frac{0.039}{0.067} = 0.582,$$

$$\frac{P[Y_n = 1 | X_n, I_1 = 0]}{P[\hat{Y}_n = 1 | X_c, I_1 = 1]} = \frac{0.054}{0.111} = 0.486$$

and

$$\frac{P[\hat{Y}_c = 1 | X_n, I_1 = 0]}{P[\hat{Y}_c = 1 | X_c, I_1 = 1]} = \frac{0.099}{0.205} = 0.483.$$

Since we are not conducting any statistical tests on the validity of these inequalities, our results on comparative risk are only suggestive.

REFERENCES

1. Bartecchi, C.E., MacKenzie, T.D. and Schrier, R.W. The human cost of tobacco use (first of two parts). *New Engl. J. Med.* 1994; **330**: 907–921.
2. National Center for Health Statistics. *Health, United States, 1995.* Public Health Service: Hyattsville, Maryland, 1996.
3. Viscusi, W.K. *Smoking: Making the Risky Decision.* Oxford University Press: New York, 1992.
4. Jones, A.M. Smoking cessation and health: a response. *J. Health Econ.* 1996; **15**: 755–759.
5. Jones, AM. Health, addiction, social interaction and the decision to quit smoking. *J. Health Econ.* 1994; **13**: 93–110.
6. Hsieh, C.-R., Yean, L.-L., Liu, J.-T. and Lin, C.J. Smoking health knowledge, and anti-smoking campaign: An empirical study in Taiwan. *J. Health Econ.* 1996; **15**: 87–104.
7. Miller, L.S., Bartlett, J.C., Rice, D.P., Max, W.B. and Novotny T. *Medical-care expenditures attributable to cigarette smoking, 1993: Methodology, descriptive statistics, parameter, and expenditure estimates.* Center for Disease Control and Prevention, August 1994, 1994.
8. Mattson, M.E., Pollack, E. and Cullen, J.W. What are the odds that smoking will kill you? *Am. J. Public Health* 1987; **77**: 425–431.
9. Becker, G.S. and Murphy, K. A theory of rational addiction. *J. Polit. Econ.*, 1988; **96**: 675–701.
10. Orphanides, A. and Zervos, D. Rational addiction with learning and regret. *J. Polit. Econ.* 1995: **103**: 739–758.
11. Cantoyannis, P. and Forster, M. The distribution of health and income: a theoretical framework. *J. Health Econ.* 1999; **18**: 605–622.
12. Barsky, R.B., Juster, F.T., Kimball, M.S. and Shapiro, M.D. Preference parameters and behavioral heterogeneity: an experimental approach in the health and retirement study. *Quart. J. Econ.* 1997; **112**: 537–579.
13. Viscusi, W.K. Age variations in risk perceptions and smoking decisions. *Rev. Econ. Stats.* 1991; **73**: 577–589.
14. Viscusi, W.K. Do smokers underestimate risks? *J. Polit. Econ.* 1990; **98**: 1253–1269.
15. Breslau, N. and Peterson, E. Smoking cessation in young adults: Age at initiation of cigarette smoking and other suspected influences. *Am. J. Public Health* 1996; **86**: 214–220.
16. Breslau, N., Peterson, E., Schultz, L., Andreski, P. and Chilcoat, H. Are smokers with alcohol disorders less likely to quit? *Am. J. Public Health* 1996; **86**: 985–990.
17. Yuan, J.-M., Ross, R.K., Wang, X.L., Gao, Y.T., Henderson, B.E. and Yu, M.C. Morbidity and Mortality in relation to cigarette smoking in Shanghai, China. *J. Am. Med. Assoc.* 1996; **275**: 1646–1650.
18. Fielding, J.E. Smoking: Health effects and control. *New Engl. J. Med.* 1985; **313**: 491–497.
19. Shmueli, A. Smoking cessation and health: A comment. *J. Health Econ.* 1996; **15**: 751–754.
20. Blundell, R. and Smith, R. An exogeneity test for a simultaneous equation Tobit model with application to labor supply. *Econometrica* 1986; **54**: 679–685.
21. Gourieroux, C., Monfort, A., Renault, E. and Trognon, A. Generalized residuals. *J. Econom.* 1987; **34**: 5–32.
22. Vella, F. A simple estimator for simultaneous models with censored endogenous regressors. *Int. Econ. Rev.* 1993; **34**: 441–457.
23. Greene, W.H. *Econometric Analysis.* Macmillan: New York, 1993.

24. Yatchew, A. and Criliches, Z. Specification error in probit models. *Rev. Econ. Stats.* 1984; **66**: 134–139.

25. Pagan, A. and Vella, F. Diagnostic tests for models based on individual data: A survey. *J. Appl. Econom.* 1989; **4**; s29–s59.

26. Lee, L.-F. Tests for the bivariate normal distribution assumption in econometric models with selectivity. *Econometrica* 1984; **52**: 843–863.

27. Lahiri, K. and Song, J.G. Testing for normality in a probit model with double selection. *Econ. Lett.* 1999; **65**: 33–39.

28. Nelson, F.D. Efficiency of the two-step estimator for models with endogenous sample selection. *J. Econom.* 1984; **24**: 181–196.

29. Nawata, K. and Nagase, N. Estimation of sample selection bias models. *Econom. Rev.* 1996; **8**: 387–400.

30. Stolzenberg, R.M. and Relles, D.A. Tools for intuition about sample selection bias and its correlation. *Am. Sociol. Rev.* 1997; **65**: 494–507.

31. Leung, S.F. and Yu, S. On the choice between sample selection and two-part models. *J. Econom.* 1996; **72**: 197–229.

32. Koop, G. and Poirier, D.J. Learning about the across-regime correlation in switching regression models. *J. Econom.* 1997; **78**: 217–227.

33. Burtless, G. Occupational effects on the health and work capacity of older men. In *Work, Health, and Income Among the Elderly*, Burtless G. (ed.). The Brookings Institution: Washington, DC, 1987; 103–142.

34. Vella, F. Generating conditional expectations from models with selectivity bias. *Econ. Lett.* 1988; **28**: 97–103.

35. Sattinger, M. Comparative advantage in individuals. *Rev. Econ. Stats.* 1978; **60**: 259–267.

36. Maddala, G.S. *Limited Dependent and Qualitative Variables in Econometrics*. Cambridge University Press, Cambridge, 1983.

37. Fishe, R.P.H., Trost, R.P. and Lurie, P.M. Labor force earnings and college choice of young women: An examination of selectivity bias and comparative advantage. *Econ. Educ. Rev.* 1981; **1**: 169–191.

38. Goffe, W.L., Ferrier, G. and Rogers, J. Global optimization of statistical functions with simulated annealing. *J. Econom.* 1994; **60**: 65–99.

Section II

Count Data and Survival Analysis

5

A Comparison of Alternative Models of Prescription Drug Utilization

PAUL V. GROOTENDORST

St Joseph's Hospital, Hamilton, Ontario, Canada

In Canada, public spending on prescription medicines is one of the fastest rising components of overall health care expenditures [1]. Nominal expenditures on the government-funded Ontario Drug Benefit (ODB) program – which provides 100% reimbursement on a formulary of selected prescription medicines for seniors (aged 65 or older) and those on welfare assistance – rose from $212.2m in 1985 to $645.6m in 1992 [2]. Such expenditure growth on government-funded drug plans has caused a number of Canadian provinces, such as Ontario, British Columbia, New Brunswick and Saskatchewan to actively consider or implement some form of patient copayment for prescription drugs among groups previously eligible for subsidy. There is evidence from econometric time-series studies in the UK [3–5] that increased charges are associated with decreased utilization; this has also been found in similar studies of US Medicaid programs [6,7], US studies of managed care settings [8,9] and analysis of data from the US RAND Health Insurance Experiment [10]. The evidential base for policy on public drug insurance coverage is, however, incomplete. While knowledge of the fiscal impact of patient charges on program expenditures is important, little is known about the health and/or distributional consequences of prescription drug copayments. Evidence from both Medicaid populations [6,11] and enrolees in managed care organizations [8] indicate that potentially needed medications are relinquished after the imposition of drug copayments. There is no evidence, however, on the differential effect of copayments on individuals with differing levels of health status. Moreover, little is known about the effects of copayments on drug utilization of older adults, who are by far the largest consumers of medicines.

Universal health insurance in Canada provides first dollar coverage for all citizens for medical services such as hospital care and physician consultations. But universal public insurance does not extend to out-of-hospital prescription medicines. The 'natural experiment' analysed in this study is the 65th birthday of Ontario residents, the age at which they become eligible for zero copayment medicines on the publicly-funded Ontario Drug Benefit plan. Prior to this age of eligibility many Ontarians will be paying some out-of-pocket amount for prescription medicines, typically as copayments on employment-related plans, or in some cases 100% copayment for persons without any insurance coverage for medicines [12]. After their 65th birthday Ontarians become relatively homogeneous with respect to the financial cost to them of using medicines because they are all eligible for the government plan with zero copayment.

Data from the 1990 Ontario Health Survey (OHS) on self-reported use of medicines in the past 4 weeks are used to address how eligibility for ODB benefits by virtue of turning 65 affects the expected number of different medicines used per respondent. In order to assess the distributional effects of copayment, attention is paid to the effect of eligibility for ODB benefits across individuals who are heterogeneous in their levels of self-reported health status.

The distribution of the dependent variable – the number of different medicines used per respondent – has characteristics which may have implications for the choice of estimation technique. The distribution is discrete, contains a rather large number of zeroes, and has a long right tail. The answers to the study questions appear to depend on the estimation technique chosen. Several estimation techniques suitable for estimation using data with these characteristics are considered and are evalu-

Econometric Analysis of Health Data. Edited by Andrew M. Jones and Owen O'Donnell
© 2002 John Wiley & Sons Ltd. Previously published in *Health Economics*, Vol. 4; pp. 183–198 (1995). © John Wiley & Sons Ltd

ated on the basis of within-sample forecasting performance and model selection tests. Candidate models include the Poisson, negative binomial, zero altered negative binomial, and the two-part models. These are described below.

METHODS

THE POISSON MODEL

One approach to dealing with the analysis of data involving counts of events per time interval is to use the Poisson regression. Ordinary Least Squares (OLS) regression admits negative predictions which are inconsistent with non-negative data. Moreover, the disturbance terms associated with OLS regression models of count data are typically left-skewed, non-normal and heteroskedastic. As counts must be integers as well as non-negative, maximum likelihood techniques based on discrete distributions are potentially more efficient, produce positive predictions, and may produce more powerful inference on the estimated parameters than OLS or ad-hoc corrections to OLS.

The contribution to the likelihood of the ith observation of a Poisson-distributed random variable Y is:

$$f(y_i) = \Pr(Y_i = y_i) = \frac{\lambda_i^{y_i} \exp(-\lambda_i)}{y_i!}, \quad y_i = 0, 1, 2, \ldots \quad (5.1)$$

The density of Y_i is made conditional on the explanatory variables x_i by parameterizing the mean λ_i, as:

$$\ln \lambda_i = x_i'\beta \quad (5.2)$$

This particular transformation ensures that the estimated mean is positive. The Poisson model has the possibly unattractive restriction that the first and second conditional moments of the Poisson-distributed variable are both equal to λ_i. Hence:

$$E[y_i | x_i] = Var[y_i | x_i] = \lambda_i = \exp(x_i'\beta) \quad (5.2a)$$

THE NEGATIVE BINOMIAL MODEL

Many types of count data are characterized by 'overdispersion' meaning that the (conditional) variance exceeds the (conditional) mean. In these cases, the assumptions of the Poisson model are not satisfied and a more general specification should be adopted. Over-dispersion may be due to unobservable individual heterogeneity in drug consumption. The negative binomial regression model

arises if this heterogeneity is modelled using the gamma probability distribution. The density of the negative binomial is derived by adding an error term to the conditional mean of the Poisson (Equation 5.2):

$$\ln \lambda_i = x_i'\beta + \varepsilon \quad (5.3)$$

where $\exp(\varepsilon)$ follows a gamma distribution with mean one and variance α. Substituting Equation 5.3 into Equation 5.1 and integrating ε out of the expression yields the negative binomial density:

$$f(y_i) = \Pr(Y_i = y_i) = \frac{\Gamma(\theta + y_i)}{\Gamma(\theta)y_i!} u_i^{\theta}(1 - u_i)^{y_i},$$

$$y_i = 0, 1, 2, \ldots \quad (5.4)$$

where:

$$u_i = \frac{\theta}{\theta + \lambda_i}, \theta = \frac{1}{\alpha}, \Gamma(\cdot) = \text{gamma function}$$

The variance of the negative binomial distributed random variable y_i is:

$$Var[y_i] = E[y_i](1 + \alpha E[y_i]) \quad (5.5)$$

The introduction of the extra parameter, α, permits the mean to differ from the variance. The Poisson model is a special case of the negative binomial in which the variance parameter α is equal to zero (in which case the variance and mean of y_i are identical). A test for overdispersion in the context of the Poisson model conveniently reduces to a t-test on the significance of the estimated value of α.

A TWO-PART MODEL

According to simulation results reported by Duan et al. [13], the 'two-part model' is well suited to model individual level health care utilization data characterized by a large proportion of individuals who do not consume drugs and skewness in the distribution of consumption among user. The essence of the two-part model is to decompose the number of different drugs taken (y_i) into two observed random components: '$y_i > 0$' and '$y_i | y_i > 0$' and specify a probability model appropriate for each part. Predictions from these two models, the probability of any consumption: $\Pr(y_i > 0 | x_i)$, and expected number of drugs conditional upon any use: $E(y_i | y_i > 0, x_i)$ are used to predict the mean number of drugs used, $E(y_i | x_i)$, conditional on the vector of covariates, x_i, using the decomposition:

$$E(y_i \mid \mathbf{x}_i) = \Pr(y_i > 0 \mid \mathbf{x}_i) E(y_i \mid y_i > 0, \mathbf{x}_i). \tag{5.6}$$

To implement the model, the sample of n observations is partitioned so that the first N observations have positive expenses, and the last $(n - N)$ observations have no drug expenditures. The likelihood of the N users is:

$$L = \Pr(y_i > 0 \mid \mathbf{x}_i) \times density(y_i \mid y_i > 0, \mathbf{x}_i), i = 1, \ldots, N \tag{5.7}$$

The likelihood of the $(n - N)$ individuals who do not consume drugs is:

$$L_i(\delta_1) = \Pr(y_i = 0 \mid \mathbf{x}_i), \quad i = N + 1, \ldots, n \tag{5.7a}$$

The likelihood of the entire sample is therefore:

$$L = \prod_{i=1}^{N} \Pr(y_i > 0 \mid \mathbf{x}_i) \times density(y_i \mid y_i > 0, \mathbf{x}_i)$$

$$\times \prod_{i=1}^{N} \Pr(y_i = 0 \mid \mathbf{x}_i) \tag{5.7b}$$

A convenient feature of the likelihood function is that it factors into two multiplicative terms:

$$L1 = \prod_{i=1}^{N} \Pr(y_i > 0 \mid \mathbf{x}_i) \times \prod_{i=N+1}^{N} \Pr(y_i = 0 \mid \mathbf{x}_i) \tag{5.7c}$$

$$L2 = \prod_{i=1}^{N} density(y_i \mid y_i > 0, \mathbf{x}_i) \tag{5.7d}$$

As Duan et al. [13] note, the first term depends exclusively on parameters in the model of the binary outcome equation: '$y_i > 0$'; the second term depends exclusively on parameters in the equation explaining expenditures of the users. Because of this separability, maximizing the likelihood is equivalent to maximizing the likelihood functions Equations 5.7c and 5.7d separately. The two part model has been used by Leibowitz and colleagues [10] to analyse drug expenditures data from the RAND study. In that study, the probit model was used to model the probability of any use (Equation 5.7c), and OLS was used to predict the log of expenditures (Equation 5.7d). For the present model, the probit will be used to model the probability of any use. Because the consumption variable is discrete, however, the negative binomial is used to model the number of different drugs taken by users.

THE ZERO ALTERED MODEL

There is sometimes substantial heterogeneity between individuals reporting zero levels of consumption. Non-smokers, for example, will not smoke at any level of price or income. For 'potential smokers' nonconsumption might be a strictly economic decision. Similar heterogeneity might apply to those reporting no drug consumption. Many people who are healthy would not consume drugs at any price. Indeed, for otherwise healthy individuals, drug consumption may even be hazardous. People with a medical need, on the other hand, could experience a health status improvement from prescription drug use. Zero consumption could still arise, however, due to economic factors such as financial barriers to care.

If the process describing consumption behaviour of healthy individuals differs from those who are 'potential' drug users, it makes sense to let the parameters differ between the two sets of observations. If it were possible to discern between these individuals on the basis of values of observable variables, then standard methods (such as estimating separate models) could be used. When this information is not available, however, some other mechanism must be used to discern between these groups. One approach is to estimate conditional probabilities that individuals are one of these two types. Models using mixtures of discrete distributions proposed by Greene [14], the *zero altered Poisson* and *zero altered negative binomial* models, appears well suited for the estimation of these models. The model consists of two behavioural processes depicted in the schematic below:

- a *splitting model* which estimates a conditional probability that an individual is one of the two types discussed above: nondrug users and potential drug users, and

- a *Poisson or negative binomial model* of the drug consumption of the potential drug users.

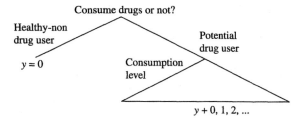

Zero consumption may arise in both regimes. For otherwise healthy individuals, however, non-consumption is automatic. Drug consumption would not be optimal even at a zero price. Potential and actual drug users, on the other hand, respond to prices and income in their consumption decision. Zero consumption is but one possible outcome at this stage. Formally, the probability q_i of being a non drug user is made conditional on a vector of covariants z_i:

$$q_i = prob(nondruguser) = F(\mathbf{z}_i'\delta) \qquad (5.8)$$

where $F(\mathbf{z}_i'\delta)$ is a cumulative distribution function. The Poisson or negative binomial density could be used to model the consumption for potential drug users. For either model, the mean of the distribution λ_i is made conditional on another set of covariants, $\mathbf{x}_i$ using the transformation $\lambda_i = \exp(\mathbf{x}_i'\beta)$.

Defining $f(.)$ as either the Poisson or negative binomial density function, the sample densities for drug consumption (y_i) are as follows:

$$prob(yi = 0) = q_i + (1 - q_i)f(y_i = 0) \qquad (5.9a)$$

$$prob(yi = j > 0) = (1 - q_i)f(y_i = j) \qquad (5.9b)$$

If the observed frequency of zeroes in the data exceeds that predicted by the simple Poisson model, there are at least two possible reasons. First, there could be unobservable heterogeneity in drug use which causes zero to be observed more frequently than expected. This could be accommodated by employing the negative binomial model. Alternatively, the additional zeroes could be generated by the presence of individuals for whom zero consumption is automatic. In this case, the zero altered Poisson model could be employed. Notice from Equation 5.9a that the zero altered model has the effect of adding a probability mass to observations on zero consumption. If both unobservable heterogeneity and a splitting mechanism are operational, then the zero altered negative binomial may be preferred.

MODEL SELECTION CRITERIA

With several plausible competing statistical models, some mechanism must be established to choose among them. In principle, it is possible to devise 'goodness of fit' measures that are comparable across the models. These performance measures, however, favour more complicated models that could over-fit the data [13]. The additional complications in the models might be simply fitting artefacts of the particular sample and hence may not generalize to other samples. Instead the 'split sample analysis' was conducted to devise performance measures.

The set of observations was randomly partitioned into estimation and forecast subsamples. All the models were fitted to this estimation subsample, which consisted of approximately 70% of all observations. Observations from the forecast subsample were then used to calculate predictions that could be compared to the actual values of the dependent variable. The differences between the predicted and actual number of different drugs form the basis of the mean squared error (MSE) performance measure.

The statistic is defined as:

$$MSE_j = \frac{1}{n} \sum_{i=1}^{n} (\hat{y}_{ij} - y_i)^2 \qquad (5.10)$$

where the summation extends over the n individuals in the forecast subsample, $\hat{y}_{ij}$ is the predicted number of different drugs of the ith individual using the jth estimator and y_i is the actual number of different drugs consumed. MSE takes on values from zero (indicating no forecast error) to positive infinity (indicating a rather poor fit).

The performance of the alternative models was assessed using a second method, the Vuong [15] non-nested test. To test two competing probability models, f_1 and f_2, the statistic V is computed:

$$V = \frac{N^{1/2}\tilde{m}}{s_m}, \text{ where } m_i = \log\left[\frac{f_1(y_i)}{f_2(y_i)}\right] \qquad (5.11)$$

This statistic (which is asymptotically normal) tests the null that $E[m_i] = 0$. An attractive feature of this test is in its ability to discriminate between the different models; a large positive value (e.g. greater than 1.96) favours model 1, whereas a large negative value favours model 2.

As Greene [14] notes, testing the zero altered negative binomial against the negative binomial using this statistic allows us to make statements as to whether any excess zeroes are a consequence of the splitting mechanism or are due to unobserved heterogeneity. If the zero altered model is rejected in favour of the negative binomial, then the splitting model is rejected. If, in addition, the estimate of the 'heterogeneity' parameter α in the negative binomial is found to be significant, then individual level heterogeneity may be at work. A finding that the negative binomial is rejected in favour of the zero altered model coupled with a finding that the estimate of α in the zero altered model is significant would indicate that both the splitting mechanism and individual heterogeneity in drug consumption are operational.

THE ONTARIO HEALTH SURVEY

The Ontario Health Survey was a comprehensive survey of Ontarians to assess population health status, disease risk factors and use of health services. The target population of the Ontario Health Survey was all residents of private dwellings in Ontario over the survey period January through December 1990 [16]. Residents of Indian reserves, inmates of institutions, foreign service personnel and residents of remote areas were excluded. For the purposes of sampling, the population of Ontario was stratified by geographic regions known as Public Health

Units (PHUs). Respondents were selected using a two-stage stratified cluster sampling frame designed to obtain 1000 completed responses per PHU.

Once a household was selected for inclusion into the survey, the questionnaire was administered in two stages. The first stage was an in-person interview with one respondent (referred to as the index respondent) in which the health status, health care utilization and socio-demographic information of all household members was collected. The index respondent responded both on behalf of himself or herself (self-report) and on behalf of other household members (acting as a proxy respondent). Supplementary information was then collected through self-completed written questionnaires left for each member of the household (aged 12 and older). The response rate for the interview part of the survey was 87% and the response rate for the self-completed questionnaire was also high (77%).

OHS VARIABLES ON MEDICINES USE

The OHS asked each subject how many different drugs they had taken in the past four weeks. An advantage of this measure is that it probably suffers from a lower degree of recall bias on the part of survey respondents, than say nominal drug expenditures [17]. In addition, this measure records actual consumption rates. Expenditures, on the other hand, record the purchase of drugs, which may not necessarily coincide with consumption.

The modelling approach used here is quite simple. No behavioural model of medicines use is posited; instead a reduced form equation is estimated relating the number of drugs taken to insurance prices, health status and demographic variables. Being reduced form, the estimates are consistent with a number of structural models of patient and physician behaviour. Given that a patient's access to prescription medicines is via a physician, an association between changes in prescription copayment and number of different drugs taken must work via changes in patient-initiated factors, such as physician consultations or compliance with prescription, via physician-initiated factors such as changes in the number or type of prescriptions written or both of these factors. Unfortunately, these cross-sectional data are not informative enough to distinguish between these alternative structures. Moreover, attempts to model supply effects on utilization by including, say, physician visits as an explanatory variable introduces the statistical problems associated with regressor endogeneity.

SAMPLE AND INDEPENDENT VARIABLE SELECTION

The aim of the analysis was to isolate the effect of becoming eligible for zero copayment medicines on ODB by virtue of age; it was therefore necessary to identify other groups eligible for ODB coverage in selecting the sample of survey data and regression covariates. Individuals are eligible for ODB by virtue of age (age 65 or older); income (social assistance recipients); specific diseases (e.g., cancer, diabetes); specific drugs (e.g., AZT, cyclosporin) or residency in a long-term care facility or recipient of home care. To sharpen the focus on the effect of turning age 65 on drug use we dropped respondents from the OHS sample if they had received social assistance in the past year (and hence would have been eligible for ODB). Within the OHS data it was not possible to identify precisely respondents with particular drugs or diseases that would have made them eligible for ODB at the time of the survey. However, persons in long-term care institutions and eligible for ODB were not surveyed in the OHS.

Individuals were restricted to be between 55 and 75 years, inclusive. This avoided the problem of modelling substantial age-related variation in drug use before age 55, especially among females of reproductive age. After the age of 75, it appears that drug use declines slightly with age. This may be an artefact of the sampling process: to be eligible for inclusion, individuals must be healthy enough to avoid institutionalization or death. Finally, given the marked gender differences in health care utilization, a likelihood ratio test for parameter homogeneity between males and females was conducted using the negative binomial estimator. The null was decisively rejected (LR = 82.09, $P < 0.001$); separate models for males and females were therefore estimated. Dependent and independent variables, for males and females, are detailed in Table 5.1 and described below.

Age and ODB Eligibility

Non-parametric analysis suggested that the effect of age on medicines use, controlling for other covariates, was approximately linear over the age range 55–75 years. This analysis consisted of plotting the coefficients associated with age-specific dummy variables estimated from an OLS regression in which the health status and demographic variables were also used as covariates. (The use of age-specific dummy variables is a useful exploratory device since it does not impose any functional form restrictions on age, while at the same time controlling for the effects of variables correlated with age.)

Table 5.1 Descriptive statistics: Ontario health survey, males and females, age 55–75

Variable	Definition	Females (n = 3099)				Males (n = 2644)			
		Mean	Std. Dev.	Min.	Max.	Mean	Std. Dev.	Min.	Max.
QTYDRUG1	Number of different drugs taken over the last 4 weeks	2.11	2.33	0	30	2.02	2.71	0	30
QTYDRUG2	Number of different drugs taken over the last 4 weeks in the sub-sample of users	2.62	2.32	1	30	2.73	2.82	1	30
DRUGUSER	=1 if prescription drugs were taken over the last 4 weeks	0.81	0.40	0	1	0.74	0.44	0	1
AGE65	=1 if eligible for ODB benefits (age 65 or older)	0.47	0.50	0	1	0.46	0.50	0	1
DRUGINS	=1 if covered by other drug insurance	0.69	0.46	0	1	0.74	0.44	0	1
AGE65* DRUGINS	Interaction between AGE65 and other drug insurance	0.34	0.47	0	1	0.34	0.47	0	1
WORKING	=1 if main activity over past year was working at a job	0.20	0.40	0	1	0.37	0.48	0	1
EXCLHLTH	=1 if self-assessed health, relative to others same age: excellent	0.11	0.32	0	1	0.12	0.32	0	1
VGHLTH	=1 if self-assessed health, relative to others same age: very good	0.34	0.47	0	1	0.31	0.46	0	1
GOODHLTH	=1 if self-assessed health, relative to others same age: good	0.36	0.48	0	1	0.34	0.47	0	1
FAIRHLTH	=1 if self-assessed health, relative to others same age: fair	0.16	0.36	0	1	0.18	0.38	0	1
POORHLTH	=1 if self-assessed health, relative to others same age: poor	0.03	0.18	0	1	0.05	0.22	0	1
NPROB	Number of chronic health problems	2.52	1.84	0	8	2.27	1.69	0	8
AGE65*NPROB	Interaction between AGE65 and number of chronic health problems	1.33	1.93	0	8	1.16	1.71	0	8
LHSIZE	Log household size	0.64	0.40	0	2	0.76	0.35	0	2
INC1	=1 if household income: $0–11 999	0.11	0.31	0	1	0.05	0.23	0	1
INC2	=1 if household income: $12 000–29 999	0.43	0.49	0	1	0.38	0.48	0	1
INC3	=1 if household income: $30 000–59 999	0.34	0.47	0	1	0.38	0.49	0	1
INC4	=1 if household income: $60 000 and over	0.12	0.33	0	1	0.19	0.39	0	1
PRIMARY	=1 if highest level of education completed: primary, or lower	0.23	0.42	0	1	0.29	0.45	0	1
SOMEHIGH	=1 if highest level of education completed: some highschool	0.29	0.46	0	1	0.26	0.44	0	1
CPMPHIGH	=1 if highest level of education completed: highschool	0.25	0.43	0	1	0.21	0.40	0	1
SOMEPOST	=1 if highest level of education completed: some college, or some university	0.18	0.39	0	1	0.13	0.34	0	1
UNDEGREE	=1 if highest level of education completed: university degree	0.05	0.21	0	1	0.11	0.31	0	1
AGE	Age in completed years	64.06	5.72	55	75	64.02	5.68	55	75

Note: This is a subsample of/with persons removed if they received social assistance payments in the previous year (i.e. would have been eligible for zero copayment medicines through ODB due to low income).

Insurance Status

To identify the effect of eligibility for zero copayment medicines on ODB by virtue of age, the binary indicator variable *AGE65* was constructed which was set equal to one if the respondent's age at the time of the survey was 65 or older and equal to zero otherwise. To allow the effect of eligibility for ODB to vary by health status level, interaction terms were added, as described below. Data on respondents' birthdates and date of the survey were not available. It was therefore not possible to determine if individuals who were 65 years at the time of the survey were eligible for zero copayment medicines during the entire 4 week period prior to the survey. It was also not possible to control for seasonal effects on drug use.

A possible source of confounding on the association between public insurance for medicines at age 65 and utilization is whether the respondent has private insurance for prescription drugs from occupational or other plans. The OHS did contain a question on private health insurance coverage for 'medicines and other health services'. For persons responding positively to this question we have defined a variable *DRUGINS* to take the value one if they had such coverage and zero otherwise. Because this question is non-specific to drug insurance it may introduce measurement error, but insurance industry sources suggest around 90% of persons who respond positively to this item will have some form of private prescription drug coverage [12]. This indicator variable will also fail to capture any heterogeneity in the terms of private drug insurance coverage.

It is possible that any drug utilization response observed at age 65 for individuals who have additional prescription drug insurance coverage is different from the response by those with no such coverage. For example, persons with no insurance coverage prior to age 65 will be faced with the greatest reduction in out-of-pocket expense; persons with prior private coverage with zero copayment face no change in the out-of-pocket cost of medicines when they become eligible for ODB. To allow the effect of eligibility for ODB to vary by insurance coverage status, an interaction term between *DRUGINS* and the *AGE65* dummy variables was created.

Labour Force Participation

The financial cost of drugs is only one dimension of the cost to patients of seeking care; another cost is the opportunity cost of time. Individuals who are employed, for example, may incur a larger 'time price' of going to the physician than non-employed [18,19]. Our models are potentially confounded because, for many persons, the typical age of retirement from work will also be age 65. In other words, a reduction in the opportunity cost of time is coincident with the removal of the prescription copayment. This reduction in time price would be predicted to increase the number of physician consultations and therefore the likelihood of medicines use. Fortunately not all retirement from work in Ontario appears to be coincident with the 65th birthday; for example, 8% of our male respondents and 6% females were still in paid employment at age 67. To explore this effect we have created a variable called *WORKING* which takes the value one if the main activity reported over the past year was working at a job. To the extent that some persons do not retire at age 65 this will enable us to disentangle, to some extent, the impact of time price versus copayment on use of medicines.

Health Status

Health status is typically an important predictor in empirical models of health care utilization. As Manning *et al.* [20] note in their review of the literature, health status often explains most of the variance in regression models of medical care utilization. More importantly, controlling for it can affect the magnitude of other estimated coefficients because of the correlations between health status and other regressors such as education, income and age. The level of self-assessed health status was ascertained in the OHS with the following survey question: 'In general, compared to other persons your age, would you say your health is: excellent, very good, good, fair or poor'. The five-point health status scale has been used successfully in many other health care utilization studies [21] and this type of measure has been shown to correlate well with physician ratings of health [22–24] and other measures of functional status [21,23]. The number of current chronic health problems (*NPROB*) experienced by individuals has also been used in a variety of empirical models of health care utilization [25,26].

To allow the effect of eligibility on use to vary by health status level, an interaction term between the number of health problems and the age 65 variable (*AGE65*NPROB*) was created. A positive coefficient on this interaction term indicates larger increases in medicines use at age 65 among persons with a greater number of chronic health problems.

Other Demographic Effects

Covariates on income and education were also used as conditioning variables. These variables were included primarily to avoid confounding with the variable of primary

Table 5.2 Mean squared error statistics of alternative estimators: males and females

Model	Mean squared error – male models	Mean squared error – female models
Poisson regression	6.983	4.821
Negative binomial regression	6.593	4.433
Zero altered – Probit and negative binomial	7.657	5.975
Two-part model – probit and negative binomial	6.168	4.375

interest *AGE65* and to improve model fit. Given that the model is a reduced form, it is difficult to interpret the coefficients associated with these variables. For example, income might have a positive association with drug use via ability to pay, but a negative association with drug use because income and health status are positively correlated. Ths OHS questions on household income have been grouped into four categories (see Table 5.1). Log household size was also included to deflate income to per person levels. Covariates on education are included with highest level of education completed by the respondent in five groups from 'primary or lower' through to 'completed university degree'.

RESULTS

The results of the MSE estimator selection exercise appear in Table 5.2. A total of 1857 observations on males (from 2644) were used for estimation; 2174 observations on females (from a total of 3099) were used for estimation. For both the male and female models, the two-part model consisting of a probit model for the binary outcome (use vs. no use) and a negative binomial model for the drug use on the subsample of drug users outperformed the other candidates. Prediction errors were uniformly lower in the models estimated using females data.

The zero altered model failed to converge when the splitting model was a function of all of the regressors. To remedy this, zero restrictions were placed on all but the health status variables in the splitting model. The model still predicted number of different drugs in the forecast subsample substantially worse than the others. The zero altered negative binomial model was also rejected when tested against the negative binomial model using the Vuong test statistic ($V = -2.24$ for males and $V = -5.64$ for females; 5% critical value $= -1.96$). This suggests that the conceptual distinction between 'non drug users' and 'potential users' may not be necessary for estimation purposes, at least for individuals between 55–75. It does appear to be the case, however, that there is substantial unobserved heterogeneity in drug utilization. The Poisson models were found to substantially under-predict the proportion of zeroes in the data (approximately 30%

underprediction for females and 20% for males). The findings that the estimate of the parameter α in the negative binomial model was highly significant on the basis of its *t*-ratio ($t = 10.82$ for males and $t = 10.77$ for females; 5% critical value $= 2.01$), together with the earlier rejection of the splitting function provide some support for this view.

These tests appear to reject the zero altered negative binomial and Poisson specifications in favour of the negative binomial model. It remained to be seen whether the rankings from the mean squared error exercise are consistent with the Vuong test. The negative binomial model was therefore tested against the two-part model using the Vuong test. The test provided unambiguous support for the two-part specification ($V = -8.39$ for males and $V = -6.24$ for females; 5% critical value $= -1.96$).

DIAGNOSTIC TESTS

A variety of diagnostic tests were performed on the two-part models to ensure that the parameter estimates and inferences drawn on them were reasonably robust to potential misspecifications. Specifically, assumptions regarding the form of the variance in all of the models were tested.

The first set of tests concern the probit models of drug use-non use. The model generating the binary outcome I, which equals one if any drugs are consumed, and zero otherwise, can be thought of as arising from an underlying latent model of drug utilization (p_i), where $\mathbf{z}_i$ is the vector of conditioning variables and δ is the vector of associated parameters:

$$p_i = \mathbf{z}_i'\delta + \varepsilon_i$$

$$I_i = 1 \text{ if } p_i > 0 \text{ and } I_i = 0 \text{ if } q_i \leqslant 0$$

$$\varepsilon_i \sim N(0, 1) \tag{5.12}$$

An assumption implicit in the estimation of the probit models of prescription drug utilization is that the disturbances in the underlying latent model of drug utilization has constant (unit) variance. The assumption that the variance is constant across all observations ('homoskedasticity') may not, however, be realistic. Individuals with lower levels of health status may have higher variability in the latent level of drug utilization (p_i) than those with higher levels of health status. Heteroskedasticity affects the consistency properties of both the covariance matrix *and* the vector of slope coefficients in the probit and negative binomial models. It is therefore important to test for its existence. These results contrast with both nonlinear and linear regression models, in which heteroskedasticity does not affect the consistency of the estimated (slope) coefficients.

To accommodate heteroskedastic errors in the context of the probit model, the variance of the disturbances in the underlying model was generalized as follows (where w_i is the vector of covariates in the variance or 'skedastic' function):

$$\varepsilon_i \sim N(0, [\exp(w_i'\gamma)]^2) \quad (5.12a)$$

The sample density for observations on users corresponding to this model is:

$$\text{Prob}(I_i = 1 \mid \Omega_i = E(I_i \mid \Omega_i) = \Phi\left(\frac{z_i'\delta}{[\exp(w_i'\gamma)]^2}\right) \quad (5.12b)$$

When $\gamma = 0$, Equation 5.12b reduces to the homoskedastic probit model:

$$\text{Prob}(I_i = 1 \mid \Omega_i) = E(I_i \mid \Omega_i) = \Phi(z_i'\delta) \quad (5.12c)$$

The null hypothesis of homoskedasticity is easily tested using the likelihood ratio test. The vector of covariates in the skedastic function, w_i, was initially set equal to those in the mean function z_i. Significant variables in the skedastic function were, however, limited to the four self assessed health status dummies and the number of health problems. In the interests of parsimony, these five variables were therefore used exclusively in all subsequent skedastic function specifications. The negative binomial model can be generalized in a similar manner.

The variance of the random variable y_i in the standard model is:

$$Var[y_i] = E[y_i](1 + \alpha E[y_i])$$
$$= \lambda_i(1 + \alpha\lambda_i) \quad (5.13)$$

As it stands now, the variance is not constant across observations, but is increasing in λ_i. This variance process may be further generalized by parameterizing $\alpha_i = \exp(\gamma_0 + z_i'\gamma)$. In essence the standard negative binomial model restricts the pattern of heterogeneity in the occurrence rate λ_i to be constant across individuals. This gener-

Table 5.3 Likelihood ratio tests for heteroskedasticity

Model	Female subsample	Male subsample
Probit model of prescription drug use	LR = 79.6	LR = 77.3
Negative binomial model of prescription drug use by users	LR = 105.6	LR = 65.2

Note: the five percent critical value: $\chi^2(5) = 11.07$.

alization allows the heterogeneity in λ_i to depend on the vector of health status covariates unique to the individual. Again, when $\gamma = 0$, the generalized model reduces to the usual negative binomial model.

The results of the tests on assumptions concerning the variances (i.e. $\gamma = 0$) for both probit and negative binomial models for prescription drug use are reported in Table 5.3. The null hypotheses are soundly rejected in each case, which lend some support for the more general specifications.

PARAMETER ESTIMATES – TWO-PART MODEL

Empirical results of the heteroskedasticity-adjusted two-part models, estimated over both the females and male subsamples are reported in Table 5.4. Pseudo R^2 measures of model fit based on the sample size, n, the maximized values of the log likelihood functions evaluated at the unrestricted estimates (LU) and estimates restricted to be zero (LR) were calculated using the formula outlined in Magee [27]:

$$R^2 = 1 - \exp\left(\frac{-2*(LU - LR)}{n}\right). \quad (5.14)$$

Pseudo R-squared measures were in the range 0.22–0.27, which is typical goodness of fit for cross-sectional models of health care utilization.

Estimates of the effect of publicly funded prescription drug insurance on the number of prescription drugs taken depends on both health status (*NPROB*: the number of chronic health problems) and on whether or not the individual has additional drug insurance coverage (*DRUGINS*). Technically, if the estimated model is $QRX = a_0 + a_1 AGE65 + a_2 AGE65*NPROB + a_3 AGE65 *DRUGINS +$ other regressors, then the increase in utilization at age 65 is approximated by: $\partial QRX/ \partial AGE65 = a_1 + a_2 NPROB + a_3 DRUGINS$. Testing the hypothesis that there is no overall effect ($\partial QRX/ \partial AGE65 = a_1 + a_2 NPROB + a_3 DRUGINS = 0$) there-

Table 5.4   Two-part model estimates of prescription drug utilization

Covariate	Females				Males			
	Probit		Negative binomial		Probit		Negative binomial	
	Coef.	t-ratio	Coef.	t-ratio	Coef.	t-ratio	Coef.	t-ratio
Constant	−0.841	−0.82	−0.074	−0.25	−2.631	−2.79	−0.127	−0.34
AGE65	0.133	0.55	0.097	1.24	−0.215	−0.91	−0.086	−0.85
AGE	0.006	0.36	0.006	1.36	0.024	1.66	0.007	1.24
DRUGINS	0.133	1.05	0.127	2.83	0.036	0.28	−0.058	−1.02
AGE65* DRUGINS	−0.160	−0.78	−0.183	−3.09	0.086	0.45	0.085	1.12
WORKING	−0.143	−1.25	−0.045	−1.03	−0.073	−0.71	−0.059	−1.30
EXCLHLTH	—	—	—	—	—	—	—	—
VGHLTH	0.607	4.11	0.065	0.99	0.314	2.45	0.180	2.41
GOODHLTH	0.984	5.01	0.249	3.85	0.566	3.97	0.374	5.12
FAIRHLTH	1.459	4.11	0.441	6.52	0.935	3.91	0.692	8.79
POORHLTH	1.905	0.71	0.779	9.23	1.400	1.22	0.899	9.52
NPROB	0.929	8.35	0.065	5.76	0.857	7.63	0.079	5.51
AGE65* NPROB	0.255	2.78	0.037	2.70	0.249	2.67	0.033	1.80
LHSIZE	−0.038	−0.28	0.101	2.57	0.213	1.71	0.013	0.25
INC1	0.131	0.55	0.100	1.45	−0.281	−1.21	0.282	3.32
INC2	−0.084	−0.52	0.075	1.42	−0.168	−1.22	−0.058	−1.00
INC3	−0.145	−1.02	0.001	0.01	−0.064	−0.54	−0.036	−0.67
INC4	—	—	—	—	—	—	—	—
PRIMARY	−0.665	−2.88	−0.047	−0.64	0.031	0.19	0.067	1.01
SOMEHIGH	−0.573	−2.67	−0.045	−0.63	0.090	0.57	0.019	0.29
COMPHIGH	−0.381	−1.83	−0.070	−0.97	0.032	0.20	0.007	0.10
SOMEPOST	0.528	−2.43	−0.115	−1.54	0.179	1.03	−0.023	−0.32
UDEGREE	—	—	—	—	—	—	—	—
Skedastic function								
Constant	—	—	−0.709	−2.16	—	—	−17.959	−5.13
VGHLTH	0.118	0.97	−0.627	−1.70	0.012	0.09	15.739	4.49
GOODHLTH	0.133	1.05	0.063	0.19	−0.111	−0.78	16.300	4.66
FAIRHLTH	0.005	0.03	−1.887	−1.18	−0.309	−1.82	17.293	4.94
POORHLTH	−0.245	−0.23	1.349	3.10	−0.279	−0.65	17.376	4.96
NPROB	0.206	8.55	0.752	5.80	0.239	8.68	−0.226	−3.55
Loglikelihood	−1152.30		−4479.01		−1125.10		−3644.69	
R Squared	0.22		0.23		0.25		0.27	
n	3099		2495		2644		1959	

fore depends on the estimated coefficients (a_1, a_2 and a_3) and on specific values for the two covariates.

Likelihood ratio (LR) tests of the hypothesis that there is no overall effect after the onset of eligibility for ODB coverage were conducted on both parts of the two-part models (Table 5.5). Six different restrictions were imposed, each with a different combination of number of chronic health problems ($NPROB = 0, 2, 4$) and indicator of other drug insurance coverage ($DRUGINS = 0, 1$). The tests revealed that the statistical significance of the effect of ODB coverage on the probability of using any medicines increased, the greater the number of chronic health

conditions. Males and females reporting a total of four chronic health conditions, for example, were found to have positive, significant increases in the probability of utilization, irrespective of their additional insurance coverage ($P < 0.01$ in all tests). Individuals with no chronic health conditions, on the other hand, had negligible increases in probability of use after becoming eligible for ODB. The results for the level of use equations were mixed. Female drug users with no prior insurance coverage ($DRUGINS = 0$) but suffering from 2 or more health problems had significant increases in utilization ($P \leqslant 0.01$). Female drug users with prior insurance cover-

Table 5.5 Likelihood ratio tests for zero increased use of drugs after eligibility for ODB, by level of health status, prior drug insurance coverage and sex

Restriction	Probability of any prescription drug use		Number of drugs taken by users	
	Females	Males	Females	Males
$DRUGINS = 0$,	0.2	1.0	1.5	0.7
$NPROBS = 0$	$(P = 0.65)$	$(P = 0.32)$	$(P = 0.21)$	$(P = 0.40)$
$DRUGINS = 0$,	8.0	1.8	6.7	0.1
$NPROBS = 2$	$(P < 0.01)$	$(P = 0.18)$	$(P = 0.01)$	$(P = 0.81)$
$DRUGINS = 0$,	12.8	6.4	14.7	0.3
$NPROBS = 4$	$(P < 0.01)$	$(P < 0.01)$	$(P < 0.01)$	$(P = 0.61)$
$DRUGINS = 1$,	0.01	0.4	1.4	0.0
$NPROBS = 0$	$(P = 0.98)$	$(P = 0.53)$	$(P = 0.24)$	$(P = 0.99)$
$DRUGINS = 1$,	5.8	4.4	0.0	0.8
$NPROBS = 2$	$(P = 0.02)$	$(P = 0.04)$	$(P = 0.84)$	$(P = 0.36)$
$DRUGINS = 1$,	10.8	9.6	1.2	3.6
$NPROBS = 4$	$(P < 0.01)$	$(P < 0.01)$	$(P = 0.28)$	$(P = 0.06)$

age ($DRUGINS = 1$), on the other hand, did not significantly increase the number of drugs taken, irrespective of the number of health problems ($P > 0.24$ in all tests). The effects of ODB eligibility on the level of use by male drug users was found to approach conventional levels of significance only for individuals with four or more health conditions and with additional insurance coverage ($P = 0.06$).

PARAMETER ESTIMATES – POISSON, NEGATIVE BINOMIAL AND ZERO ALTERED MODELS

Parameters estimated using the Poisson, negative binomial and zero altered negative binomial models are reported in Tables 5.6A (females) and 5.6B (males). The results obtained using the two-part specification do not appear to be robust to the choice of estimator. For females, $AGE65$ was statistically significant on the basis of its t-ratios in all models. The $AGE65*NPROB$ interaction was statistically insignificant and had the anticipated positive sign in only the zero altered model. Likelihood ratio tests of the hypothesis that the onset of ODB eligibility has no effect on utilization could only be rejected for an individual with 4 health problems and no additional drug insurance when estimated using the zero altered negative binomial ($P = 0.031$). For males, tests of this hypothesis were not rejected in any of the models ($P > 0.137$).

DISCUSSION

The efficiency and predictive ability of models of individual-level health care utilization data can often be improved by using estimation techniques which take into account the special characteristics of the data. The distribution of the utilization measure considered here – the number of different drugs consumed – is typical of other health care utilization data such as physician visits or length of hospital stay. Specifically, the distribution is discrete, contains a large proportion of zeroes (is left-skewed) and has a long right tail. This distribution mirrors the stylized fact that a large proportion of individuals do not consume any health care services; a small proportion of individuals, on the other hand, use a large number of services. An estimation technique advocated for modelling individual-level data with these characteristics – the two-part model [13] – was one of several candidate estimators and was found to perform well according to model selection tests. The model consists of a probit model of the use vs. non-use of prescription medicines and a negative binomial model of the number of different drugs taken in the subsample of drug users. This two-part model dominated the Poisson, negative binomial and the 'zero altered' negative binomial model on both the mean squared error (MSE) and Vuong non-nested model selection criterion. Duan *et al.* [13] report success of this technique in estimating models of continuous individual-level medical care expenditure data.

One of the candidate estimation techniques – the zero altered model – is useful when there exists a large proportion of zeroes and there is some evidence that there is heterogeneity between individuals reporting no drug consumption over the survey period. This was thought to be the case with the number of different drugs taken, in so far as some of the zeroes might represent individuals with no medical need, who had no intention of seeking health care, and others were individuals who may very well have had medical need, but did not seek care because of lack of insurance, or other reasons. The zero altered model is

Table 5.6A Poisson, negative binomial, and zero altered negative binomial estimates of prescription drug utilization: females

Covariate	Poisson		Negative binomial		Zero altered negative binomial	
	Coef.	t-ratio	Coef.	t-ratio	Coef.	t-ratio
Constant	−0.845	−3.06	−0.917	−2.58	−0.566	−1.45
AGE65	0.282	4.00	0.296	3.80	0.239	2.82
DRUGINS	0.154	3.70	0.151	3.24	0.174	3.37
AGE65* DRUGINS	−0.212	−3.84	−0.207	−3.53	−0.214	−3.39
WORKING	−0.090	−2.20	−0.076	−1.47	−0.045	−0.75
VGHLTH	0.306	5.16	0.302	4.74	0.240	3.13
GOODHLTH	0.574	9.83	0.571	9.03	0.455	6.02
FAIRHLTH	0.810	12.98	0.811	11.43	0.671	8.23
POORHLTH	1.151	15.63	1.159	14.62	1.022	11.48
NUMBPRB	0.132	13.47	0.147	10.76	0.119	7.75
AGE65* NPROBS	−0.003	−0.22	−0.012	−0.72	0.029	1.56
LHSIZE	0.086	2.33	0.086	2.07	0.090	1.98
INC1	0.120	1.87	0.126	1.51	0.138	1.52
INC2	0.055	1.12	0.069	1.10	0.085	1.23
INC3	−0.041	−0.86	−0.036	−0.58	−0.026	−0.37
PRIMARY	−0.157	−2.32	−0.187	−2.54	−0.101	−1.23
SOMEHIGH	−0.154	−2.34	−0.193	−2.63	−0.114	−1.39
COMPHIGH	−0.143	−2.16	−0.172	−2.29	−0.122	−1.45
SOMEPOST	−0.219	−3.20	−0.258	−3.25	−0.230	−2.59
AGE	0.009	2.17	0.010	1.85	0.007	1.14
log alpha			0.187	17.89	0.165	13.54
Splitting function						
NPROBS					−0.688	−12.59

novel in that it models two separate processes which are assumed to have produced the observed distribution of drug utilization. First, a latent variable – the probability that an individual is in need of health care – is made conditional on a vector of covariates. Second, the mean utilization by those who are in need of health care (that is conditional on another set of covariates) is estimated.

Estimates from the zero altered model were consistent with prior hypotheses. For example, a regressor which appeared in both parts of the model, the number of health problems afflicting the individual, was associated with a lower probability that the individual was not in need of prescription drugs and also associated with an increased level of drug utilization by those deemed in need of prescription drugs. This model was explicitly rejected, however, indicating that either the splitting function was misspecified or the conceptual distinction between nonusers and potential users is not important, at least for older adults.

The way in which health status was modelled in the estimating models proved to be important. Specifically,

the standard homoskedastic probit models of prescription drug use was found to be rejected in favour of probit models in which the variance (of the disturbances of the underlying latent variable) was a function of self assessed health status and the number of health problems. This adjustment resulted in modest changes to the estimated parameters of the standard probit model. This generalized model also indicates that both the conditional mean and dispersion in the underlying latent level of drug use are increasing in the number of health problems. One reason is that those reporting lower levels of health status might have either untreatable conditions (and report consuming only a few drugs) or be treatable with a large number of different drugs. This latter effect could be explained by the fact that therapeutic drugs may generate side effects that induce additional prescriptions to ameliorate the side effects.

The empirical model examined the effects on drug utilization of eligibility for zero copayment medicines under the Ontario Drug Benefit programme. This exogenous change in the effective price of prescription drugs was

Table 5.6B Poisson, negative binomial, and zero altered negative binomial estimates of prescription drug utilization: males

Covariate	Poisson		Negative binomial		Zero altered negative binomial	
	Coef.	t-ratio	Coef.	t-ratio	Coef.	t-ratio
Constant	−1.493	−4.85	−1.567	−3.70	−1.421	−3.19
AGE65	0.082	1.00	0.036	0.41	−0.176	−1.86
DRUGINS	−0.015	−0.33	−0.041	−0.93	−0.107	−2.37
AGE65* DRUGINS	0.056	0.90	0.107	1.48	0.204	2.78
WORKING	−0.092	−2.37	−0.077	−1.74	−0.067	−1.44
VGHLTH	0.422	5.71	0.415	4.74	0.364	3.57
GOODHLTH	0.761	10.57	0.736	8.64	0.644	6.53
FAIRHLTH	1.174	15.77	1.169	13.23	1.071	10.54
POORHLTH	1.328	15.84	1.328	12.36	1.271	10.67
NUMBPRB	0.163	14.50	0.183	12.44	0.106	6.87
AGE65* NPROBS	−0.008	−0.57	−0.003	−0.15	0.010	0.48
LHSIZE	0.112	2.61	0.088	1.59	0.092	1.60
INC1	0.269	3.93	0.214	3.01	0.296	3.98
INC2	−0.096	−1.92	−0.108	−2.06	−0.088	−1.60
INC3	−0.022	−0.49	−0.032	−0.57	−0.017	−0.28
PRIMARY	0.058	1.01	0.087	1.06	0.092	1.07
SOMEHIGH	0.013	0.22	0.030	0.37	0.028	0.32
COMPHIGH	0.000	−0.01	0.005	0.06	0.007	0.08
SOMEPOST	0.008	0.13	0.015	0.16	0.002	0.02
AGE	0.014	2.96	0.015	2.37	0.020	3.00
log alpha			0.309	18.25	0.268	14.64
Splitting function						
VGHLTH					−0.253	−1.00
GOODHLTH					−0.618	−2.11
FAIRHLTH					−0.597	−1.25
POORHLTH					−0.595	−0.47
NPROBS					−1.262	−5.48

exploited to investigate aspects of the drug utilization by individuals aged 55–75. Consistent with the existing evidence, the onset of full insurance was associated with an increase in drug utilization. The focus of the analysis was, however, on the incidence of the subsidy. Are the increases in utilization observed concentrated among those with lower health status? If the additional health services are provided to seniors with lower health, then a policy of subsidizing prescription drugs may be satisfying distributional criteria.

Estimates from the two-part model indicated that the provision of public insurance favours individuals with lower levels of health status. Increases in utilization after the onset of public insurance were found to be higher among individuals with lower levels of health status. It should be noted, however, that these results were somewhat sensitive to the choice of estimator. Specifically, other models did not predict this distributive effect.

ACKNOWLEDGEMENTS

Funding for this research was provided by a doctoral fellowship from the Social Sciences and Humanities Research Council of Canada. I would like to thank Andrew Jones, an anonymous referee, Martin Browning, David Feeny, Lonnie Magee, Michael Veall, seminar participants at McMaster University and participants at the Third European Workshop on Econometrics and Health Economics for useful comments. All errors are my own.

REFERENCES

1. Anderson, G., Kerluke, K.J., Pulcrins, I.R., Hertzman, C. and Barer, M.L. Trends and determinants of prescription drug expenditures in the elderly: Evidence from the British Columbia Pharmacare Program. *Inquiry* 1993; **30**: 199–207.
2. Institute for Clinical Evaluative Sciences. *Patterns of Health*

Care in Ontario. Toronto: Sunnybrook Hospital, 1994.

3. O'Brien, B.J. The effect of patient charges on the utilisation of prescription medicines. *Journal of Health Economics* 1989; **8**: 109–132.

4. Ryan, M. and Birch, S. Charging for health care: evidence on the utilisation of NHS prescribed drugs. *Social Science and Medicine* 1991; **33**: 681–687.

5. Lavers, R.J. Prescription charges, the demand for prescriptions and morbidity. *Applied Economics* 1989; **21**: 1043–1052.

6. Soumerai, S.B., Ross-Degnan, D., Gortmaker, S. and Avorn, J. Payment restrictions for prescription drugs under Medicaid: effects on therapy, cost and equity. *New England Journal of Medicine* 1987; **317**: 550–556.

7. Nelson, A.A., Reeder, C.E. and Dickson, W.M. The effect of a Medicaid drug co-payment on the utilization and cost of prescription services. *Medical Care* 1984; **22**: 724–735.

8. Harris, B.L., Stergachis, A. and Ried, L.D. The effect of drug co-payments on utilization and cost of pharmaceuticals in a Health Maintenance Organization. *Medical Care* 1990; **28**: 907–917.

9. Smith, D.G. The effects of co-payments and generic substitution on the use and costs of prescription drugs. *Inquiry* 1993; **30**: 189–198.

10. Leibowitz, A., Manning, W.G. and Newhouse, J.P. The demand for prescription drugs as a function of cost-sharing. *Social Science and Medicine* 1985; **21**: 1063–1069.

11. Reeder, C.E. and Nelson, A.A. The differential impact of co-payment on drug use in a Medicaid population. *Inquiry* 1985; **22**: 396–403.

12. Canadian Life and Health Insurance Association Inc. *Survey of health insurance benefits in Canada – 1992*. Toronto, 1994.

13. Duan, N., Manning, W.G., Morris, C.N. and Newhouse, J.P. A comparison of alternative models for the demand for medical care. *Journal of Business and Economic Statistics* 1983; **1**: 115–126.

14. Greene, W.H. *Accounting for excess zeroes and sample selection in Poisson and negative binomial regression models*. Department of Economics Working Paper EC-94-10, Stern School of Business, New York University, 1994.

15. Vuong, Q. Likelihood ratio tests for model selection and non-tested hypotheses. *Econometrica* 1989; **57**: 307–334.

16. Ontario Ministry of Health. *Ontario Health Survey, 1990, User's Guide. Vol. 1: Documentation*. Toronto: Ontario Ministry of Health, 1990.

17. Berk, M.L., Schur, C.L. and Mohr, P. Using survey data to estimate prescription drug costs. *Health Affairs* 1990; **9**: 147–156.

18. Phelps, C.E. and Newhouse, J.P. Coinsurance, the price of time, and the demand for medical services. *The Review of Economics and Statistics* 1974; **56**: 334–342.

19. Cauley, S.D. The time price of medical care. *The Review of Economics and Statistics* 1987; **13**: 59–66.

20. Manning, W.G., Newhouse, J.P. and Ware, J.E. The status of health in demand estimation. In: Fuchs, V.R. (ed.), *Economic Aspects of Health*. Chicago: The University of Chicago Press, 1982.

21. Davies, A.R. and Ware, J.E. *Measuring Health Perceptions in the Health Insurance Experiment*. Santa Monica: The Rand Corporation, 1981.

22. Linn, L.S., Hunter, K.I. and Linn, B.S. Physicians' orientation toward the legitimacy of drug use and their preferred source of new drug information. *Medical Care* 1980; **18**: 282–288.

23. Linn, B.S. and Linn, M.W. Objective and self-assessed health in the old and very old. *Social Science and Medicine* 1980; **14A**: 311–315.

24. LaRue, A.L., Bank, L., Jarvik, L. and Hetland, M. Health in old age: how do physician ratings and self ratings compare? *Journal of Gerontology* 1979; **14**: 687–691.

25. Acton, J.P. Demand for health care among the urban poor, with special emphasis on the role of time. In: Rosett, R.N. (ed.), *The role of health insurance in the health services sector*. National Bureau Conference Series No. 27. New York: National Bureau of Economic Research, 1976.

26. Davis, K. and Reynolds, R. The impact of medicare and medicaid on access to medical care. In: Rosett, R.N. (ed.), *The role of health insurance in the health services sector*. National Bureau Conference Series No. 27. New York: National Bureau of Economic Research, 1976.

27. Magee, L. R^2 measures based on Wald and likelihood ratio joint significance tests. *The American Statistician* 1990; **44**: 250–253.

6

Estimates of Use and Costs of Behavioural Health Care: a Comparison of Standard and Finite Mixture Models

PARTHA DEB[1] AND ANN M. HOLMES[2]

[1]*Department of Economics and* [2]*School of Public and Environmental Affairs, Indiana University – Purdue University Indianapolis, Indianapolis, USA*

INTRODUCTION

Estimates of health care demand (and policy recommendations based on such estimates) have been shown to depend on the empirical specification used in the analysis. If such specifications do not reflect the underlying behavioural structures that drive health care utilization, estimates will not accurately reflect actual use, and suggested policies may have unintended consequences. In this paper, we evaluate an innovative specification, the finite mixture model (FMM), to estimate utilization and expenditure relationships in behavioural health care.

The FMM has the ability to distinguish between distinct classes of users of behavioural health care (for instance, the severely mentally ill, who typically are high intensity users, and persons without severe mental illness, who are typically more moderate users of care). Mental illness has been classified by diagnosis, severity of symptoms, aetiology and clinical course. Although adequate for some purposes, for resource allocation purposes, it may be preferable to group patients on the basis of utilization. In applications where data exist in subgroups, FMMs offer a number of advantages over standard specifications, including more accurate predictions of average use and expenditure for each subgroup.

Mental health care is increasingly financed on a capitated basis in the USA. Payment rates are usually set according to some function of the mean cost of providing treatment for a particular patient type, sometimes with an adjustment for financial risk. While some jurisdictions set rates through a competitive bid process (e.g. Medicaid in Massachusetts and New York, although the latter had to adjust such rates in 1996 to bring the rates into line with provider costs), more commonly, rates are set through some process of risk assessment and risk adjustment [1]. Multivariate techniques are usually used in the first stage of this process to identify the relative importance of different risk factors. For instance, the Medicare programme uses model fit between historic costs and potential risk stratifiers as one criterion for choosing risk adjusters [2]. Some states 'carve-out' mental health care from Medicaid, and carve-out providers may or may not be paid on a capitated basis. When they are paid on such a basis, the rates are often set to reflect some measure of projected or historical costs [3]. Because the FMM is more flexible than standard specifications, fitted means, variances and predicted distributions based on such estimates may more accurately reflect the true distributions of costs. These advantages could result in more rational allocations of health care resources that are necessary to ensure persons with severe mental illness are able to receive adequate care.

The main objective of this paper is to determine if the FMM does indeed provide a better fit of behavioural health care data than the standard models currently used in practice. We are particularly interested in the ability of the FMM to predict the use and expenditures of care for high intensity users. Standard models consistently fail to accurately estimate the resource consumption needs of this group [4].

We demonstrate the practical importance of correctly specifying health care utilization relationships in the con-

Econometric Analysis of Health Data. Edited by Andrew M. Jones and Owen O'Donnell

text of setting appropriate reimbursement rates in capitated environments. Should capitation rates not reflect the true average costs of treating certain patient groups, providers will have an incentive to cream-skim – denying care to patient groups whose costs of treatment systematically exceed the reimbursement rate and recruiting patient groups whose costs of treatment are below the reimbursement rate. Furthermore, if providers cannot adequately pool risks across a sufficiently large client base, care may also be denied to patients whose treatment costs are highly variable unless reimbursement strategies are also adjusted for financial risk. Thus, to ensure that vulnerable populations are adequately served in such financial environments (e.g. rural settings), payors need to be able not only to predict accurately mean costs of care for various patient populations, but also to predict the distribution of these costs.

It is well documented that a minority of patients consumes the larger share of outpatient behavioural health care. In a review of the literature, Kent et al. [5] reported most studies found 10–20% of patients could be classified as 'heavy users', consuming between 50–80% of all mental health services. For instance, Taube et al. [6] found fewer than 10% of persons who used any outpatient mental health care made more than 25 visits, and used 50% of all services. At the other extreme of the care distribution, Howard et al. [7] found two-thirds of their patients used less than one-quarter of all services. Such distributions are endemic in a variety of behavioural health care settings and insurance environments [8,9].

While economists have usually represented such phenomena using a continuous distribution with extreme skew, epidemiological analyses have found that behavioural health care users empirically tend to fall into discrete groupings. Ford et al. [10] determined depressives could be classified into two groups (those patients with major depression and those patients with depressed mood) by use of health services. Perry et al. [11], in a study of persons suffering from personality and affective disorders, determined these patients fell into one of three clusters of users. Smith and Loftus-Rueckheim [12] identified four distinct groupings among mental health care users in general, with degree of disability acting as a critical stratifying variable. Unfortunately, such analyses have tended to be exploratory in nature, and are of limited use when predicting economically-relevant behaviours. These findings suggest, however, that users of mental health care may indeed fall into distinct groups, and that utilization behaviours may differ across user groups.

Most economic analyses of health care utilization have adopted the two-part empirical specification. Two-part models represent the utilization decision with two equations: one to identify which factors affect the decision to seek any care, and the second to determine how much care is demanded among the subgroup of users. Such specifications were developed and evaluated in general health care applications by Duan et al. [13]. The model has been recently adapted to accommodate count data, appropriate when use is measured by number of contacts rather than total cost of all contacts [14]. Two-part models are also the standard specification in the analysis of behavioural health care demand [15–19].

The performance of the two-part model is potentially superior to single-equation models because it can accommodate possible heterogeneity between users and non-users of (behavioural) health care. Statistical comparisons of these two models suggests differences between users and non-users are meaningful [15,16,18,20]. Because its authors recognized that users and non-users of health care might behave differently, they were able to predict much more accurately the cost of care and responses to various demand stimuli than could be obtained from single equation models. However, behavioural health care tends to be characterized by extreme distributions that this model is unable to completely accommodate. Other researchers have had to resort to truncating data at some arbitrary amount in order to achieve satisfactory statistical performance with standard models [4,21,22]. The FMM may be better able to predict the tail of the distribution if that tail represents a unique group of users.

The two-part model forces a sharp dichotomy between users and non-users of care. This is intuitively appealing when examining episodes of care since the decision to seek care is usually determined unilaterally by the patient, whereas patient and provider jointly determine subsequent use. Such arguments do not apply when estimating annual patterns of use, since multiple episodes of care may occur in any given year. Thus, the structural appeal of the standard two-part model is less obvious when the goal is to predict annual costs as required for rate-setting exercises. Furthermore, because all users of care are represented by one equation in the two-part model, it does not allow for heterogeneity in behaviours between subgroups of users. If users of behavioural health care are drawn from distinct groups (e.g. high, medium, and low intensity users), the two-part model will not be able to adequately represent demand for behavioural health care services.

In this paper, we employ an innovative specification, the FMM, to estimate the utilization of and expenditures on behavioural health care. The FMM offers a number of potential advantages over standard specifications: two-part count models for visits and the log repression as the second part of the two-part model for expenditures. Not only does the FMM accommodate heterogeneity between types of users of behavioural health care, but the model can serve as an approximation to any true, but unknown, probability density [23,24]. Its growing popularity is reflected in an increase in the number of recent regression-based applications in economics that employ the method [25–30]. To our knowledge, however, the only published application of the FMM in health care utilization analysis is the study by Deb and Trivedi on the use of outpatient visits by the elderly [31].

ECONOMETRIC MODELS

Consider demand measured in terms of expenditures on care (c) or utilization of specific services (e.g. number of visits, v). Utilization and expenditures are assumed to depend on a set of observable explanatory variables, which is denoted by the vector, x.

COUNT DATA (VISITS)

The two-count models we wish to consider for visits are the two-part model and the FMM. We choose the negative binomial density as the base-line density for both classes of models. Of the densities available in the statistical literature for econometric models of count data, the family of negative binomial densities is the most general and flexible.

The negative binomial density is given by:

$$f(v_i \mid x_i) = \frac{\Gamma(v_i + \psi_i)}{\Gamma(v_i + 1)\Gamma(\psi_i)} \left[\frac{\psi_i}{\psi_i + \lambda_i}\right]^{\psi_i} \left[\frac{\lambda_i}{\lambda_i + \psi_i}\right]^{v_i}, \quad (6.1)$$

where $\lambda_i = \exp(x_i\beta)$ and $\psi_i = (1/\alpha)\lambda_i^k$. The parameter α measures the degree of overdispersion relative to the Poisson density (which is a special case obtained when $\alpha = 0$). Most health utilization data are strongly overdispersed and cannot be adequately represented by the Poisson model. While α measures the degree of overdispersion, the choice of k dictates the functional relationship between the mean and the variance of the random variable. We choose $k = 1$ because of the evidence in its favour demonstrated in previous studies [14,31]. While, in general, it is possible to estimate k among with α, it is not desirable for identification reasons.

We use the hurdle model [14] as the standard specification for comparison purposes. The hurdle model belongs to the class of two-part models in that it consists of a first stage, that identifies factors that distinguish between users and non-users of care, and a second stage, that determines which factors affect the level of health care chosen by users. The first equation of such models esti-

mates the dichotomous event of having zero or positive health care use. For a model based on negative binomial densities. (Equation 6.1), the first equation is defined by:

$$\text{Prob}_1(v_i = 0 \mid x_i) = (\psi_{1,i}/(\lambda_{1,i} + \psi_{1,i}))^{\psi_{1,i}} \quad (6.2)$$

and

$$\text{Prob}_1(v_i > 0 \mid x_i) = 1 - (\psi_{1,i}/(\lambda_{1,i} + \psi_{1,i}))^{\psi_{1,i}}. \quad (6.3)$$

A second equation is used to determine how much care is demanded conditional on utilization being positive. Hence, once the 'hurdle' of positive use is crossed, the data are assumed to follow the density for a truncated binomial distribution given by:

$$f(v_i \mid x_i, v_i > 0) = \frac{\Gamma(v_i + \psi_{2,i})}{\Gamma(v_i + 1)\Gamma(\psi_{2,i})}$$
$$\times \left[\left[\frac{\lambda_{2,i} + \psi_{2,i}}{\psi_{2,i}}\right]^{\psi_{2,i}} - 1\right]^{-1} \left[\frac{\lambda_{2,i}}{\lambda_{2,i} + \psi_{2,i}}\right]^{v_i}. \quad (6.4)$$

The second stage equation is estimated over the subsample of users of care. The coefficients of both stages, β_1 and β_2, can be estimated by maximum likelihood techniques.

In a FMM, the random variable, v_i, is postulated as a draw from a superpopulation which is an additive mixture of C distinct populations in proportions $\pi_1, \ldots, \pi_C$, where $\Sigma_{j=1}^{C}\pi_j = 1$, $\pi_j > 0$ $(j = 1, \ldots, C)$. The density is given by:

$$f(v \mid \Theta) = \pi_1 f_1(v \mid \theta_1) + \pi_2 f_2(v \mid \theta_2) + \cdots + \pi_C f_C(v \mid \theta_C) \quad (6.5)$$

where the mixing probabilities, π_j, are estimated along with all other parameters, denoted θ_j, and the $f_j(v \mid \theta_j)$ are defined by the density in Equation 6.1. Note that α and β are allowed to vary across components, i.e. both location and scale are freely estimated. In this paper, we consider models with only two points of support, i.e. $C = 2$. The results of Deb and Trivedi [31] suggest the two-point FMM is sufficiently flexible to explain health care counts quite well.

CONTINUOUS DATA (EXPENDITURES)

Most density functions for non-negative continuous random variables (e.g. lognormal, gamma, Weibull) exclude zero from their support. Moreover, continuous densities do not allow positive mass at any particular value in their supports. Thus, in the continuous case, there exists no density function that can represent the typical utilization pattern in which a large number of people consume no health care. Consequently, it is possible to devise a continuous version of the FMM, but only for positive expenditures. For this reason, we limit our comparisons in the continuous case to specifications that model only the behaviour of the subpopulation of users of any behavioural health care. We present a new approach to modelling the second part of standard two-part models.

For continuous variables such as expenditures, the second part of the two-part model is typically estimated using a linear regression with the logarithm of expenditures as the dependent variable. This approach provides the same parameter estimates for regression coefficients as a maximum likelihood approach that assumes expenditures follow a lognormal distribution, i.e.:

$$f(c_i \mid x_i) = \frac{1}{c_i \sigma (2\pi)^{0.5}} \exp[-(\log(c_i) - x_i \beta)^2 / 2\sigma^2]. \quad (6.6)$$

When the data are not lognormally distributed, linear regression (or lognormal maximum likelihood) provides consistent (but not efficient) coefficient estimates. Consistent estimates of $E(c_i \mid x_i)$ are typically obtained by the homoskedastic smearing retransformation of Duan et al. [13]. Such estimates of $E(c_i \mid x_i)$ can be significantly biased in the presence of heteroskedasticity so heteroskedastic smearing transformations may be preferable [32]. If the data can be stratified into groups such that the errors within each group are homoskedastic, then heteroskedastic smearing factors can be obtained by calculating a separate smearing factor for each group.

In the FMM for expenditures, the density of c_i is postulated as a draw from a superpopulation which is an additive mixture of C distinct populations in proportions $\pi_1, \ldots, \pi_C$, where $\Sigma_{j=1}^{C} \pi_j = 1$, $\pi_j > 0$ $(j = 1, \ldots, C)$. The density is given by:

$$f(c \mid \Theta) = \pi_1 f_1(c \mid \theta_1) + \pi_2 f_2(c \mid \theta_2) + \cdots + \pi_C f_C(c \mid \theta_C), \quad (6.7)$$

where $f_j(c \mid \theta_j)$ is the component lognormal density defined by Equation 6.6. Both σ and β are allowed to vary across components.

Maximum likelihood estimates for all models are obtained using the Broyden–Fletcher–Goldfarb–Shanno algorithm in SAS/IML [33]. Robust standard errors (sandwich-type) of parameter estimates are reported.

MODEL SELECTION STATISTICS

We use three criteria to compare models in-sample. These include two traditional model selection criteria based on the maximized log-likelihood values with penalties for the number of parameters. The Akaike information criteria (AIC) is given by:

$$\text{AIC} = -2 \operatorname{Log} L + 2K,$$

and the Bayesian information criteria (BIC) by:

$$\text{BIC} = -2 \log L + K \log(N),$$

where $\log L$ denotes the maximized log-likelihood value, K is the number of parameters in the model and N is the sample size. Models with smaller AIC or BIC values are preferred. These are valid even in the presence of misspecification [34]. In addition to the model selection criteria, we evaluate the goodness of fit (GoF) of each model using a chi-square test statistic that compares the difference between sample and fitted cell frequencies in general models with covariates [35]. The test is quite general and is applicable to discrete and continuous data. If a model adequately predicts the cell frequencies observed in the data, the GoF statistic fails to reject the null hypothesis of adequate fit. Smaller values of the test are associated with models with better fit. Note that the GoF test is based on the data density, hence requires no retransformation in the log ordinary least squares (OLS) case. We also evaluate the ability of the two models to estimate the conditional mean in the right tail of the distribution by comparing fitted values from the standard and FMMs for several upper-tail percentiles.

When highly non-linear models, such as the FMM, are estimated, there is always a risk of over fitting the model, i.e. in-sample comparisons may favour complex models even when there may be no gains in out-of-sample forecasting. Although the AIC and BIC are designed to guard against such possibilities, whenever possible, split-sample analysis is desirable to compare the performance of the competing models out of sample. Thus, we also estimate the models using 75% of the sample, holding back 25% of the observations for out-of-sample analysis to check the validity of our conclusions based on in-sample model selection criteria. The log-likelihood value is the most direct measure of out-of-sample fit of the model. Models with larger log-likelihood values are preferred. The negative of the log likelihood may be interpreted as the Kullback–Leibler information criterion (up to a constant), a powerful 'badness' criterion [36]. We also use a modified version of the Andrews' test as a heuristic with the expectation that models with better fit will have smaller values of the test statistic in the hold-out sample. In each case, we repeat the split-sample analysis 100 times to assess the robustness of our conclusions.

DATA

We base our analysis on data from the 1987 National Medical Expenditure Survey [37], a national probability sample of the civilian, non-institutionalized population, consisting of 38 000 individuals from 15 000 households. We restrict our analysis to respondents aged 18 and older. We believe the emotional disorders experienced by children, and their pathways to care, are distinct from those of adults with behavioural disorders. Data were collected on self-reported health status, use of health care, associated expenditures and respondent characteristics. Data on use and expenditures were verified with providers of these services. We base our analysis on a sub-sample of 1594 individuals who had any medical encounter, including prescription medications, with an associated ICD-9 code indicative of a behavioural disorder (i.e. ICD-9 codes 290–319, 331).

No standard definition of a mental health visit exists in the literature [38]. We identify office-based use of mental health care when the respondent reported that mental health was the main reason for seeking services. Since this definition is likely to truncate less rather than more intensive service users, it should minimize the observed differences between groups of users. Thus, any findings of distinct user groups should be robust to more liberal definitions. Use of care is measured by a count of the number of outpatient visits made in calendar year 1987.

Expenditures on care are measured as the total actual payments made from all sources (paid directly by patients, or through public or private insurers) for all outpatients modes of care and prescription drug expenditures for which a mental health condition was listed as the main reason for seeking care. Consequently, every individual in the sample has positive expenditures. However, only 51% of these individuals sought office-based treatment for a mental illness. Thus our visits variable includes zeros, although our expenditure variable does not.

We restrict our set of covariates to variables that are typically used to stratify expenditures for rate-setting purposes: patient age, gender and diagnosis [39]. These variables are commonly available in different data sets. We also include whether or not a patient resided in an urban setting. This variable serves as a proxy for differences in practice costs, which are usually higher in urban than rural areas. Such adjustments for geographic differences in practice costs are not uncommon in rate-setting exercises, and are mandated for the Medicare programme in the USA [40]. While a larger set of variables is often used in a full demand specification (including, notably, price and income), our purpose in this paper is not to study demand relationships *per se*, but to predict expenditures and utilization. Our decision to take the more limited approach stems from our desire to improve the methods by which expenditures and use are predicted for setting appropriate reimbursement rates under capitation. As a result, it is appropriate to limit our analysis to the set of variables commonly used in such exercises.

Respondents were asked to report both age and gender. Gender is represented by a dummy variable that assumes a value of 1 if the respondent reported being female, 0 otherwise. Respondents were also asked to provide diagnostic information, and their responses were converted to International Classification of Diseases 9th Revision (ICD-9) codes by trained transcribers. These data may be less reliable than diagnoses available in medical charts. To partially compensate for the imprecision with which respondents may have reported their diagnoses, we define our diagnostic categories very broadly, e.g. substance/alcohol abuse (ICD-9 codes 303–305), schizophrenia (code 295), major affective disorders (codes 291–292, 296–299) and all other mental disorders. Furthermore, such broad categorizations are typically used in rate-setting exercises. Location is a dummy variables that assumes a value of 1 if the respondent resided in an urban setting (metropolitan statistical area), 0 otherwise.

RESULTS

Table 6.1 provides summary statistics for the personal characteristics used in this analysis. The average age of respondents was 53 years, with a range of 18–99 years. Males made up 29% of the sample. The most common diagnosis was other mental disorder (92%), followed by substance and alcohol abuse disorders (5%), affective disorders (1.9%) and schizophrenia (1.8%). Table 6.2 reports summary statistics of the distribution of visits and expenditures. The number of annual visits averaged

Table 6.1 Summary statistics of patient characteristics

Variable	Mean or percentage
Age (years)	53.17
Gender (female = 1)	71.27
Diagnosis	
Substance/alcohol abuse	4.64
Schizophrenia	1.82
Major affective disorder	1.88
Other mental illness	91.66
Location (urban = 1)	24.91

N = 1594.

Table 6.2 Summary statistics of use

Statistic	No. visits	Expenditures ($)
Mean	3.88	401.77
S.D.	11.59	1171.40
Skewness	8.08	9.37
Minimum	0	1.00
5%	0	10.00
10%	0	15.00
25%	0	34.00
50%	1	99.78
75%	3	297.60
90%	9	861.80
95%	18	1860.00
Maximum	218	22 385.00

$N = 1594$.

slightly less than four, and the average utilization was $402. In both cases, however, a great deal of variability can be observed, and the data are very skewed.

Manning [32] has shown that the performance of the log regression model can be improved if any existing heteroskedasticity is taken into account. In our data, an analysis of the residuals from the log OLS regression using the White test for heteroskedasticity shows that age and urban status are strong sources of heteroskedasticity. Therefore, we split the data into four groups stratified by urban status and age (greater or less than 55). White tests for heteroskedasticity conducted on the residuals within each group show virtually no evidence of additional heteroskedasticity.

Tables 6.3 and 6.4 provide the parameter estimates and model selection criteria of the standard and FMMs based on the full sample for number of visits and positive expenditures, respectively. Based on the full sample analysis, both the BIC and AIC support the FMM specification over the standard specification, including the heteroskedastic specification of the log regression model in the case of expenditures. This result is further supported by the Andrews GoF test. Although not tested formally, it is also apparent that the impacts of some of the variables are very different for different sub-groups of users. For

Table 6.3 Parameter estimates and model selection criteria of models for visits

	Hurdle		Finite mixture	
	Binary choice	Positives	Component 1	Component 2
Constant	1.492*	0.269	1.258*	3.392*
	(0.127)	(0.643)	(0.254)	(0.316)
Schizophrenia	0.573*	3.626*	1.057*	1.247*
	(0.276)	(0.597)	(0.392)	(0.231)
Major affective disorder	1.181*	2.415*	1.237*	1.752*
	(0.362)	(0.548)	(0.306)	(0.262)
Drug or alcohol abuse	−0.159	0.303	−0.243	0.160
	(0.174)	(1.732)	(0.295)	(0.253)
Urban	0.253*	1.988*	0.045	0.824*
	(0.084)	(0.394)	(0.150)	(0.185)
Female	−0.031	−0.443	0.053	0.011
	(0.083)	(0.321)	(0.117)	(0.167)
Age	−2.967*	−4.214*	−2.600*	−3.362*
	(0.214)	(0.923)	(0.470)	(0.590)
σ		21.063*	1.896*	18.740*
		(2.177)	(1.208)	(4.514)
π			0.666*	
			(0.091)	
Log likelihood	−3108		−3096[†]	
AIC	6246		6226[†]	
BIC	6326		6317[†]	
GoF	75.8*		47.4*	

*Significant at the 5% level.
[†]Model preferred by the statistic.
$N = 1594$, df of GoF = 19.
GoF $= (f - F)'\Sigma^{-1}(f - F)$, where f is an $M \times 1$ vector denoting the empirical frequency of observations lying in M mutually exclusive partitions of the range of the outcome variable (with the $(M + 1)$th partition exhausting the range), F is the vector of associated predicted probabilities and Σ is the covariance matrix of the difference in frequencies. In the case of a count variable, each count value forms a natural partition. All count values greater than the 95th percentile are aggregated into one partition because the data are very thinly distributed across individual values in that range.

Table 6.4 Parameter estimates and model selection criteria of models for expenditures

	Lognormal	Finite mixture	
		Component 1	Component 2
Constant	5.144*	3.936*	6.731*
	(0.135)	(0.193)	(0.417)
Schizophrenia	1.877*	2.699*	0.875
	(0.209)	(0.435)	(0.601)
Major affective disorder	1.580*	1.684*	1.394*
	(0.267)	(0.495)	(0.305)
Drug or alcohol abuse	0.332	−0.168	0.716*
	(0.217)	(0.192)	(0.247)
Urban	0.355*	0.164	0.546*
	(0.091)	(0.116)	(0.148)
Female	−0.154	−0.183	−0.241
	(0.085)	(0.113)	(0.157)
Age	−1.005*	−0.187	−2.117*
	(0.198)	(0.268)	(0.427)
σ	1.486*	1.057*	1.241*
	(0.025)	(0.078)	(0.073)
π		0.535*	
		(0.090)	
Log likelihood	−10 333 [−10 321]	−10 299[†]	
AIC	20 682 [20 665]	20 631[†]	
BIC	20 725 [20 724]	20 722[†]	
GoF	89.8* [74.3*]	25.6	

*Significant at the 5% level.
[†]Model preferred by the statistic.
$N = 1594$, df of GoF = 19.
GoF $= (f - F)'\Sigma^{-1}(f - F)$, where f is an $M \times 1$ vector denoting the empirical frequency of observations lying in M mutually exclusive partitions of the range of the outcome variable (with the $(M + 1)$th partition exhausting the range), F is the vector of associated predicted probabilities and Σ is the covariance matrix of the difference in frequencies. In the continuous case, successive decile values of expenditures (in the full sample) are used as cutoff values to create the endpoints of each partition.
Values in square brackets are from the heteroskedastic log regression model.

instance, while an age gradient is apparent in the expenditure equation for high intensity users, age has no significant impact on expenditures for low intensity users. The standard model cannot uncover such a pattern because it assumes that all users come from the same population.

The ability of the two models to estimate the conditional mean (fitted values) in the upper tail is important for their use in the design of reimbursement strategies that adjust for financial risk. Without such strategies, small providers who cannot adequately pool risks across a sufficiently large client base may also deny care to patients whose treatment costs are highly variable. For visits, conditional means are calculated using the formulae implied by the distributions underlying each model. The conditional means for expenditures based on the FMM are also calculated using expectation formulae. In the case of the standard model for expenditures, retransformation from the log scale to the raw scale is conducted using homoskedastic and heteroskedastic smearing factors.

Figure 6.1 compares fitted values from the standard and FMMs for several upper-tail percentiles. Although fitted values from both models are much smaller than the corresponding percentile values of actual use (to be expected given the small proportions of variance explained by models with demographic covariates), the FMM does considerably better than the standard model with homoskedastic retransformation, especially as higher percentile values are considered. The standard model with heteroskedastic retransformation performs substantially better than the model with homoskedastic retransformation and compares favourably with the FMM except in the extreme upper tail of the distribution. If the objective of the statistical exercise is to estimate conditional means for 'typical' individuals (not the sickest), the standard model with heteroskedastic retransformation may be adequate. But overall, in spite of using the same set of covariates, the FMM has superior ability to predict the actual distributions of visits and costs, particularlly in the upper tail.

Table 6.5 reports statistics used to compare the per-

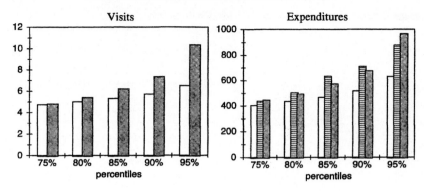

Figure 6.1. Upper tail of the distribution of fitted values. Light bars denote the standard model (for expenditures, homoskedastic retransformation is applied to the standard model). Striped bars denote the standard model for expenditures with heteroskedastic retransformation. Dark bars denote the FMM

Table 6.5   Model selection comparisons using split-sample replications

	Visits (% cases in favour of finite mixture versus hurdle)		Expenditures (% cases in favour of finite mixture versus lognormal)	
	In-sample	Out-of-sample	In-sample	Out-of-sample
Log likelihood	97	74	100 [100]	93 [88]
GoF	99	92	100 [100]	80 [73]

Values in square brackets are comparisons between the finite mixture and the heteroskedastic log regression model.

Table 6.6   Distribution of fitted means from finite mixture component densities

	Visits		Expenditures	
	Component 1	Component 2	Component 1	Component 2
Mean	1.1	9.5	102.5	750.1
S.D.	0.8	11.2	200.9	635.1
Min.	0.3	1.2	56.2	186.3
Max.	8.6	154.2	5378.4	8794.6

formance of the different specifications using split-sample analysis. As expected, the FMM does considerably better than the standard model (even with heteroskedastic retransformation) across the 100 in-sample replications. However, even based on out-of-sample results, the FMM dominates the standard model in the vast majority of cases, both in terms of improvement in log likelihood, and the smaller GoF statistic. The size of the advantage of the FMM over the standard specification can be represented by the difference in the log likelihood of the two models as observed in reeated split-sample analyses. In a Bayesian context with equally likely priors of either the FMM or the standard model being the true data generating process, the difference in the log-likelihood values of the two models is the log of the posterior odds ratio of the FMM

over the standard model given the data. The distribution of these log odds ratios across the split-sample replications is displayed in Figure 6.2. Positive values indicate the FMM fits the data better than the standard specification. Depicted graphically, it becomes obvious not only that the FMM dominates the standard model in the majority of cases, but also that the modal log odds ratio of the difference, even in the out-of-sample distribution, is approximately 5 for both visits and expenditures. Taken together, the in-sample and out-of-sample results provide strong evidence that the standard model does not adequately capture the hterogeneity amongst users of behavioural health care. Indeed, these results suggest that there are (at least) two distinct groups of users of behavioural health care.

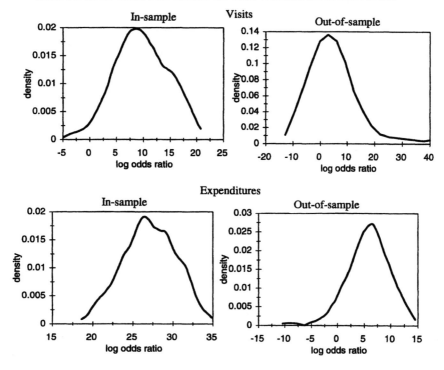

Figure 6.2. Log odds ratio of the likelihood of the data generating process being FMM relative to the standard model

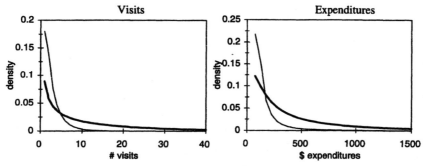

Figure 6.3. Component densities of the FMM. The bold curves correspond to the density associated with the high average-use, high variability group

Table 6.6 reports the distribution of fitted means from the component densities of the FMM. In the case of visits, low intensity users (about two-thirds of the sample) average 1.1 visits apiece, while high intensity users average 9.5 visits. Similarly, low intensity users average $102 in mental health care expenditures, while high intensity users average $750. Inspection reveals the group with distinctly higher average use also has higher variance. Differences in the higher moments are also apparent as can be seen in Figure 6.3 which displays the average component den-

sities (average of densities at each point for all individuals in the sample). In both cases, the right tail of the density associated with the high mean and variance component is considerably longer than the right tail of the density associated with low-mean component. This pattern of less predictable use in the high intensity group has significant implications for the feasibility of capitated financing of behavioural health care.

AN APPLICATION TO RATE-SETTING

To demonstrate the practical importance of the differences in model fit, we compare the relative performance of the two models in estimating risk-adjusted capitation rates (which we assume are set equal to the predicted use and costs for patients with particular diagnoses). Such rates should mimic the distribution of non-parametric estimates of group-specific averages over repeated samples taken from the same population. In order to limit potential cream-skimming of patients with certain diagnoses, the estimated rates should not systematically be above or below the non-parametric estimates. For this exercise, we use the median value of rates calculated for repeated samples as a (robust) measure of central tendency. It is also desirable for the estimated rates to be relatively precise: if a method generates sample means that are more variable than the non-parametric estimates, it increases the chance that the model-based estimate will result in a rate that will be considered too high or too low.

More precisely, let u_i denote mental health care use (as measured by visits and costs) for patient i. For each pair of samples (all individuals and specific sub-groups) in the split-sample analysis, we calculate rates using (i) the average of u_i, (ii) the average of $E(u_i | x_i)$ based on the FMM, and (iii) the average of $E(u_i | x_i)$ based on the standard model. In the case of expenditures, conditional means based on the standard model are calculated using homoskedastic and heteroskedastic smearing retransformations. Each of these three measures is calculated for all persons with any behavioural disorder diagnosis, as well as two subgroups (those with a diagnosis of schizophrenia and those with a diagnosis of a major affective disorder). Because (i) is a non-parametric estimate of the group averages, it serves as the benchmark rate for the comparison.

To measure the precision of our estimates, we calculate the 2.5th and 97.5th percentile values of the distribution of estimated costs based on 100 bootstrap replications. These may be somewhat imprecise, in general, given the number of replications. Although precise standard deviations (SDs) could be calculated using similar methods, the percentile approach accommodates asymmetry in confidence intervals. Since such asymmetry is likely in data of this nature, we chose to report percentile-based results rather than the more typical SDs. Note that while more replications are generally recommended, the statistics in this case are the percentiles of the distribution of sample means, not of the distribution of individual values. The former are considerably more stable than the latter and we found 100 replications to be adequate for our purpose.

Figure 6.4 displays the median values of the distributions of both the in-sample and out-of-sample non-parametric and parametric means of visits and expenditures, calculated for each of 100 replicated in-sample and out-of-sample estimates from the split-sample analysis. The dispersion of these means is represented by their 95% confidence intervals over the 100 replications. The figure shows that the FMM rates mimic the distribution of the non-parametric means much better than means based on the standard model for the severely ill, high-risk groups (although the difference between the two models is small for the overall sample). Median values of the means calculated using standard models sometimes differ substantially from the means based on non-parametric and FMM methods. Furthermore, the confidence intervals are considerably wider when the standard model rather than the FMM is used to generate means. For expenditures, there is little difference between rates set by homoskedastic and heteroskedastic retransformation methods. The superior performance of the heteroskedastic retransformation relative to the homoskedastic method in terms of individual predictions does not appear to translate into superior predictions of means across samples. This is likely because standard model estimates are based on an inferior distribution compared to FMM regardless of type of retransformation. It appears that the superior performance in terms of traditional measures of fit of the FMM translates into stabler estimates of subgroup average visits and costs, and this has important implications for rate-setting applications.

Reinterpreted in terms of rate-setting performance, the first four columns of Figure 6.4 reveal that, taken over all groups of patients, the average costs are about the same regardless of method of estimation. While the FMM generates predicted costs that are higher for high-intensity users than standard models, it also predicts lower costs for lower-intensity users (hence, the overall average cost is about the same). Given the FMM has better overall fit than the standard models, we conclude that standard models underestimate the resource requirements of this high-use sub-population, which typically includes the most severely and persistently mentally ill patients.

DISCUSSION

The objective of this paper was to compare the performance of the FMM to the standard two-part model used to represent health care utilization in the past. In the case of visits, the FMM is compared to the two-part count model. In the case of expenditures, the FMM for positive expenditures is compared to the second part of the standard two-part model, a log regression. One significant

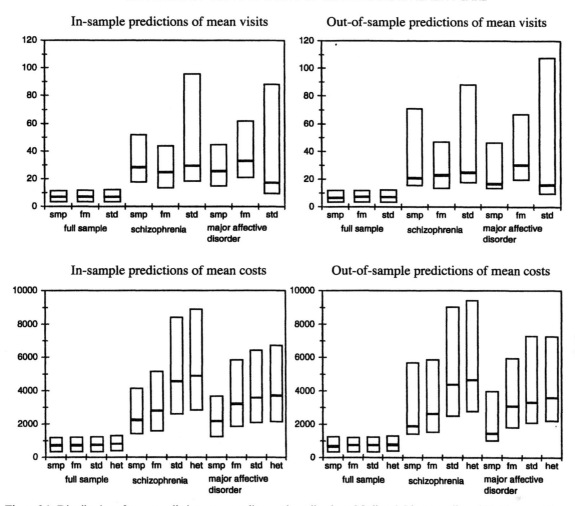

Figure 6.4. Distribution of mean predictions across split-sample replications. Median, 2.5th percentile and 97.5th percentile are shown. 'smp' denotes estimates based on the sample mean; 'fm' denotes mean predictions based on the FMM; 'std' denotes mean predictions based on the standard model (lognormal with homoscedastic smearing retransformation); 'het' denotes mean predictions based on the heteroscedastic standard model (lognormal with heteroscedastic smearing retransformation)

disadvantage of the two-part model is that it assumes that all users come from the same population. A number of descriptive studies in the behavioural health care arena suggest that users of behavioural health care may belong to distinct user classes stratified by illness severity. Because severity of illness is difficult to operationalize in a meaningful way, it becomes an important source of unobserved heterogeneity in health economic analyses. Unlike standard two-part models, FMMs can, theoretically, accommodate such latent differences in illness severity.

We evaluated the empirical performance of the FMM against the standard specification using data from the National Medical Expenditure Survey. Using a variety of model evaluation strategies, we conclude that the FMM does indeed provide a better fit of cost and use data than the standard model, particularly in the upper tail of the distribution.

Previous analyses have shown the inadequacy of established models for risk adjustment purposes. Newhouse [41] has argued that the future viability of capitated payment structures will require improvements in risk adjustment, either through expanding the set of stratifying variables or by changing the estimation methods used. Measurement issues limit the feasibility of the first solution. In contrast, it appears that the FMM constitutes a superior estimation strategy for setting capitation reimbursement rates because it can more accurately predict overall expenditures than standard estimation strategies.

Our results suggest there are (at least) two distinct

groups of users of behavioural health care. The high intensity user group exhibited not only higher expected expenditures, but less predictable expenditures as well. If the costs of caring for this group are less predictable than for the low intensity users, these patients may be at risk for cream-skimming by risk averse providers, and may be at higher risk of being denied care. Unlike standard models, the FMM generates superior estimates of variance that are necessary to make such adjustments. Furthermore, for variability that can be attributed to observable characteristics (e.g. diagnosis), the FMM generates superior estimates of subgroup average costs.

There are a number of caveats to these results. First, there are many possible sources of unobserved heterogeneity of which illness severity is only one. Regardless of the source of this heterogeneity, the FMM performs better than the standard specification in its presence. However, the source of the heterogeneity is important from a policy standpoint: if the high intensity user group is also the group of most severely ill patients, cream-skimming under capitation will effectively deny care to the group in greatest need.

Second, we restricted our analysis to a comparison of the two-component FMM and the standard specification. It may be that users of behavioural health care can be stratified into more than two groups. We felt it was inappropriate to consider a larger number of components with a sample of this size. Further analysis involving a larger number of observations is needed to determine whether users of behavioural health care belong to more than two groups. The results of this paper do support the position that there are at least two groups of users, and that the standard model that treats these two groups as being from the same population is mis-specified.

Third, we have not evaluated the FMM against other strategies for count [42] and continuous [43] data recently proposed in the literature. Although beyond the scope of this paper, these new approaches may also have desirable properties and deserve further study.

Fourth, these results are based on data taken from a period when behavioural health care was generally delivered on a fee-for-service basis. Further analysis is needed to determine to what extent our results may depend on institutional arrangements for the payment and delivery of care.

In conclusion, it appears that the FMM may offer a superior specification of behavioural health care use compared to the two-part model that has been the standard specification in the field for the past 15 years. The FMM provides more accurate estimates of the distribution of use and expenditures, particularly in the upper tail of the distribution. As a consequence, the FMM provides a more appropriate rate-setting method for capitated reimbursement. While our results are only preliminary, it would appear that the advantages of the FMM could result in a more rational allocation of health care resources that would ensure persons with severe mental illness are able to receive adequate care.

REFERENCES

1. Holahan, J., Rangarajan, S. and Schirmer M. Medicaid managed care payment methods and capitation rates: results of a national survey, 1999. Urban Institute Working Paper OP-26 1999.
2. Office of Strategic Planning. Report to Congress: Proposed method of incorporating health status risk adjusters into Medicare + choice payments, 1999. Health Care Financing Administration.
3. Mauch, D. Rhode Island: an early effort at managed care. In *Paying for Services: Promises and Pitfalls in Capitation*, Mechanic, D., Aiken, L.H. (eds). Jossey-Bass: San Francisco, CA, 1989; 55–64.
4. Fowles, J., Weiner, J., Knutson, D., Fowles, E, Tucker, A. and Ireland, M. Taking health status into account when setting capitation rates: a comparison of risk-adjustment methods. *J. Am. Med. Assoc.* 1996; **276**: 1316–1321.
5. Kent, S., Fogarty, M. and Yellowees, P. A review of studies of heavy users of psychiatric services. *Psychiatric Services* 1995; **46**: 1247–1253.
6. Taube, C., Goldman, H., Burns, B. and Kessler, L. High users of outpatient mental health services, I: Definition and characteristics. *Am. J. Psychiatry* 1988; **145**: 19–24.
7. Howard, K., Davidson, C., O'Mahoney, M., Orlinsky, D. and Brown, K. Patterns of psychotherapy utilization. *Am. J. Psychiatry* 1989; **146**: 775–778.
8. Lavik, N. Utilization of mental health services over a given period. *Acta Psychiatrica Scand* 1983; **67**: 404–413.
9. Mustard, C., Derksen, S. and Tararyn, D. Intensive use of mental health care. *Can. J. Psychiatry-Rev. Can de Psychiatrie* 1996; **41**: 93–101.
10. Ford, D., Anthony, J., Nestadt, G., Romanoski, A. The General Health Questionnaire by interview: performance in relation to recent use of health services. *Med. Care* 1989; **27**: 367–375.
11. Perry, J., Lavori, P. and Hoke, L. A Markov model for predicting levels of psychiatric service use in borderline and antisocial personality disorders and bipolar type II affective disorder. *J. Psychiatric Res.* 1987; **21**: 215–232.
12. Smith, M. and Loftus-Rueckheim, P. Service utilization patterns as determinants of capitation rates. *Hospital Community Psychiatry* 1993; **44**: 49–53.
13. Duan, N., Manning, W., Morris, C. and Newhouse, J. A comparison of alternative models for the demand for medical care. *J. Business Econ. Stat.* 1983; **1**: 115–126.
14. Pohlmeier, J. and Ulrich, V. An econometric model of the two-part decisionmaking process in the demand for health care. *J. Human Resources* 1995; **30**: 129–160.
15. Watts, C.A., Scheffler, R.M. and Jewell, N.P. Demand for outpatient mental health services in a heavily insured population: the case of the Blue Cross and Blue Shield Association's Federal Employees Health Benefits Program. *Health Services Res.* 1986; **21**: 267–289.
16. Horgan, C.M. The demand for ambulatory mental health

services from speciality providers. *Health Services Res.* 1986; **21**: 291–319.

17. Scheffler, R. and Miller, A. Demand analysis of mental health service use among ethnic subpopulations. *Inquiry* 1989; **26**: 202–215.

18. Haas-Wilson, D., Cheadle, A. and Scheffler, R. The demand for mental health services: an episode of treatment approach. *Southern Econ. J.* 1989; **56**: 219–232.

19. Wells, K.B., Keeler, E. and Manning, W.G. Patterns of outpatient mental health care over time: some implications for estimates of demand and for benefit design. *Health Services Res.* 1990; **24**: 773–789.

20. Holmes, A. and Seb, P. Provider choice and use of mental health care: implications for gatekeeper models. *Health Services Res.* 1998; **33**: 1262–1284.

21. Kronick, R., Dreyfus, T., Lee, L. and Zhou, Z. Diagnostic risk adjustment for Medicaid: the Disability Payment System. *Health Care Financing Rev.* 1996; **17**: 7–33.

22. Weiner, J., Dobson, A., Maxwell, S., Coleman, K., Starfield, B. and Anderson, G. Risk-adjusted Medicare capitation rates using ambulatory and inpatient diagnoses. *Health Care Financing Rev.* 1996; **17**: 77–99.

23. Laird, N. Nonparametric maximum likelihood estimation of a mixing distribution. *J. Am. Stat. Assoc.* 1978; **73**: 805–811.

24. Heckman, J.J. and Singer, B. A method of minimizing the distributional impact in econometric models for duration data. *Econometrica* 1984; **52**: 271–320.

25. Heckman, J.J., Robb, R. and Walker, M. Testing the mixtures of exponentials hypothesis and estimating the mixing distribution by the method of moments. *J. Am. Stat. Assoc.* 1990; **85**: 582–589.

26. Gritz, M. The impact of training on the frequency and duration of employment. *J. Economet.* 1993; **57**: 21–51.

27. Wedel, M., Desarbo, W., Bult, J. and Ramaswamy, V. A latent class poisson regression model for heterogeneous count data. *J. Appl. Economet.* 1993; **8**: 397–411.

28. Geweke, J. and Keane, M. Mixture of normals probit models, 1997; 237. Federal Reserve Bank of Minneapolis Staff Report.

29. Morduch, J. and Stern, H. Using mixture models to detect sex bias in health outcomes in Bangladesh. *J. Economet.* 1997; **77**: 259–276.

30. Wang, P., Cockburn, I. and Puterman, M. Analysis of patent data – a mixed Poisson regression model approach. *J. Business Econ. Stat.* 1998; **16**: 27–36.

31. Deb, P. and Trivedi, P. Demand for medical care by the elderly: a finite mixture approach. *J. Appl. Economet* 1997; **12**: 313–336.

32. Manning, W. The logged dependent variable, heteroscedasticity, and the retransformation problem. *J. Health Econ.* 1998; **17**: 283–295.

33. SAS Institute. *SAS Language and Procedures – Introduction* (1st edn). SAS Institute: Cary, NC, 1990.

34. Sin, C.-Y. and White, H. Information criteria for selecting possibly misspecified parametric models. *J. Economet.* 1996; **71**: 207–225.

35. Andrews, D. Chi-square diagnostic tests for econometric models. *J. Economet.* 1988; **37**: 135–156.

36. Sakata, S. and White, H. High breakdown point conditional dispersion estimation with application to S&P 500 daily returns volatility. *Econometrica* 1998; **66**: 529–568.

37. National Center for Health Services Research and Health Care Technology Assessment. *National Medical Expenditure Survey, 1987.* Westat Inc., Rockville, MD, 1989.

38. Olfson, M. and Pincus, H. Measuring outpatient mental health care in the United States. *Health Affairs* 1994; **13**: 172–180.

39. Ettner, S., Frank, R., McGuire, T., Newhouse, J. and Notman, E. Risk adjustment of mental health and substance abuse payments. *Inquiry* 1998; **35**: 223–239.

40. Health Care Financing Administration. Data Fact Sheet, 1999. http://www.hcfa.gov/medicare/datafact.htm [17 November 1999].

41. Newhouse, J. Patients at risk: health reform and risk adjustment. *Health Affairs* 1994; **13**: 132–146.

42. Cameron, A.C. and Johansson, P. Count data regression using series expansions: with applications. *J. Appl. Economet.* 1997; **12**: 203–223.

43. Blough, D.K., Madden, C.W. and Hornbrook, M.C. Modeling risk using generalized linear models. *J. Health Econ.* 1999; **18**: 153–171.

7

Latent Class versus Two-part Models in the Demand for Physician Services Across the European Union

SERGI JIMÉNEZ-MARTÍN[1], JOSÉ M. LEBEAGA[2] AND MAITE MARTÍNEZ-GRANADO[1]

[1]*Universidad Carlos III de Madrid, Getafe, Spain and* [2]*UNED, Madrid, Spain*

INTRODUCTION

During the last two decades, many European countries have been reviewing their health systems. Table 7.1 shows that the health systems differ across EU countries in many respects: as the type of payment and functional role of the physicians, the governments contribution to health expenditure and the amount of co-payments of the patients of the health expenditure. Similarities in the reforms undertaken are in the changing role of the state in health care, the decentralization of the systems, the changing role of public health provision and the increase in patients' choice (selection of doctors and hospitals). The implementation of any of these reforms requires a clear knowledge of the characteristics that determine the demand for health across the EU countries. However, estimates of health demand are known to depend on the empirical specification used in the analysis. If such specifications do not correspond to the underlying behavioural structures that drive the demand of health, policy recommendations based on their estimation may not have the desired effects.

This paper addresses this issue and estimates demand for health equations for the twelve EU countries listed in Table 7.1 (France, Finland and Sweden are excluded from the analysis because of the lack of adequate and/or sufficient data). The goal is to provide evidence on the suitability of different econometric specifications for count equations collecting both number of visits to general practitioners (GP) and specialists (SP).

Theoretical analyses of medical care utilization suggest two main empirical approaches for modelling the demand of health. The first approach takes the traditional consumer theory and views this demand as patient determined. One-step econometric models for count data (Poisson or negative binomial) have been estimated as a counterpart of these theoretical models although the empirical results contradicted the theory in many cases (see Grossman [1] or Wagstaff [2]). The second approach uses a principal–agent set-up in which the physician (agent) determines the frequency of a treatment once the patient (principal) has made an initial contact. Empirical counterparts of this second generation of theoretical models are the so called two-part econometric models (TPM): the first part of the econometric specification treats the decision to seek care as a binary choice outcome and the second part treats the number of visits of the individuals to physicians as a truncated count model (see Cromwell and Michell [3] or Pohlmeier and Ulrich [4]). However, the more recent empirical evidence suggests that TPM can not separately identify the parameters driving the two decision processes described above (Santos-Silva and Windmeijer [5]). A widespread alternative to TPM are latent class models (LCM). LCM are based on the standard count data specification described above (Poisson or negative binomial) but they allow for the presence of unobservable heterogeneity among individuals, dividing the population among frequent and infrequent health care users. The distribution function of the unobservable characteristics is approximated by a finite mixture distribution function (Heckman and Singer [6]). The results of Deb and Trivedi [7,8], Deb

Econometric Analysis of Health Data. Edited by Andrew M. Jones and Owen O'Donnell

Table 7.1 Some characteristics of National Health Systems of EU countries

Country	Doctors type of payment[a,c]	GP gatekeepers[a]	Physicians/1000[b]		Total health expenditure (as % GDP)[b]		Public participation in total health expenditure[b]	
			1995	1996	1995	1996	1995	1996
Germany	F	No	3.4	3.4	10.2	10.6	78.1	78.3
Denmark	F	Yes	2.9	2.9	8.2	8.3	82.6	82.4
Netherlands	C	Yes	2.6	2.6	8.9	8.8	72.5	67.7
Belgium	F	No	3.4	3.4	8.2	8.6	88.7	88.8
Luxembourg	F	No	2.8	2.9	6.3	6.4	92.4	92.8
UK	C	Yes	1.6	1.6	7.0	7.0	84.9	83.7
Ireland	C	Yes	2.1	2.1	7.4	7.2	72.7	72.5
Italy	C	Yes	5.4	5.5	8.0	8.1	67.7	67.8
Greece	S	No	3.9	4	8.3	8.3	58.7	58.7
Spain	S	Yes	4.1	4.2	7.0	7.1	78.3	78.5
Portugal	S	Yes	3	3	7.7	7.7	65.3	66.7
Austria	F	No	2.7	2.8	8.9	8.9	71.9	70.5

[a]*Source*: WHO (1997).
[b]*Source*: Health Data OECD (2000).
[c]F, fee for service: C, capitation; S, salary.

and Holmes [9] and Deb [10] suggest that these LCM perform better than the TPM both in count equations and also in equations for health care expenditures. Note that other modelling alternatives to the TPM could be used instead of the LCM, e.g. the joint Generalized Method of Moments estimation of the parameters of the two processes using the conditional mean of the total demand, as in Santos-Silva and Windmeijer [11].

Using maximum likelihood we estimate two alternative econometric models: TPM and LCM. We estimate equations for GP and for SP services, separately for males and females and for the 12 European countries in Table 7.1. The results from the econometric specifications are then compared and the performance of the models tested. We use a sample of males and females drawn from the three available waves of the European Community Household Panel (ECHP). Although the ECHP focuses on household income and living conditions across EU15 countries it also collects the necessary information to estimate demand for health equations. In particular it collects information about the general health situation of the individuals (self-perceived health status, chronic conditions, whether the individual was admitted as in-patient in a hospital or whether the individual is hampered by their health condition in its daily activities) and more importantly, it records the individuals' number of visits to a GP and to a SP during the previous year.

The novelty of this paper is that it uses a homogeneous and comparable data set to estimate a common model of health services for a group of European countries. It makes two contributions to the literature on demand for health. First, this paper provides economic and statistical

evidence on the more appropriate econometric specification for GPs and SPs health decision and count equations. The distinction between the demand of services from these two types of physicians allows us to distinguish cases in which TPM perform better than LCM which is different from previous findings in the literature (Deb and Trivedi [7,8], Deb and Holmes [9], and Deb [10]). In particular, the TPM are more appropriate to model the visits to a SP and in countries where the access to them is not direct but requires first visiting a GP. A possible explanation of this finding is as follows. The econometrician has access to data on the number of visits to a physician during a given period of time (say 1 week or, as in our case, 1 year) but not to the number of visits to the physician during an illness spell, as the TPM models require. Our result suggests that TPM tend to perform better when the data used in the estimation is less likely to violate the single illness spell assumption, as it happens with the number of visits to a SP. Second, it sheds some light on the empirical determinants of demand for physician services in Europe. There is little empirical evidence on the demand for health across Europe. Exceptions are Pohlmeier and Ulrich [4], who estimate demand for health equations for Germany, Santos-Silva and Windmeijer [11] for the UK and Vera-Hernández [12] for Catalonia. These papers use different data sets and different model specifications, which makes the results difficult to compare.

The rest of the paper contains four sections. In section 2 we set up the model in a theoretical framework, specify it and explain the econometric techniques. Section 3 describes the data source. The model specification tests, a cross-validation exercise and some empirical results are reported in section 4. Section 5 contains the conclusions. Finally the data Appendix describes the variables used.

THEORETICAL FRAMEWORK, SPECIFICATION AND ESTIMATION PROCESSES

Throughout the analysis we assume that medical care (measured as the number of visits to a physician) is purchased and used as an input in the household production function of health. The demand of medical services is in this context a derived demand, because services are not consumed *per se* but required to maintain or improve upon a certain health status. The patient perceives the marginal product of the different medical services in order to take his or her decisions about contacting different physicians. In general, the consumer (the patient) decides whether to visit a physician by comparing the marginal benefits and marginal costs of improving their health. The duration of the treatment would be decided on a second stage by both the patient, and more importantly the physician. This second stage can be accommodated in the context of a principal–agent framework in which the agent (physician) could induce or not demand for his or her services. Since the agent does not only offer their services but can act as the principal's advisor, inducement could take place because of asymmetric information between the patient and the physician (see for instance, Kenkel [13] and Grytten and Sørensen [14]).

Although probably this simple decision process can adequately describe visits to a GP, this is not the case for visits to the specialist. The reason is that a visit to the GP is also a compulsory step for visiting a specialist, both being normally covered by the National Insurance systems (see Table 7.1). At a second stage, the GP decides upon a possible visit to a specialist and the specialist decides at a third stage the number of visits. No attempt to model this type of complex and interrelated process has been made in this paper given the data we use. Moreover, throughout the paper we assume that the individual only suffers an illness spell during the period covered by the survey, which seems to be an important assumption concerning the econometric models (see Santos-Silva and Windmeijer [5]). This hypothesis is a necessary one for TPM and our main aim for estimating LCM is not to impose it on the data. In addition to these considerations, the lack of sufficient data in the ECHP does not allow to estimate a full structural model. On the contrary, we assume a reduced form as follows:

$$I_{iljk} = f_{1iljk}(Z_{iljk}, \varepsilon_{1iljk}) \tag{7.1}$$

$$Y_{iljk} = f_{2iljk}(X_{iljk}, \varepsilon_{2iljk}) \tag{7.2}$$

where $I_{iljk} = \mathbf{1}(Y_{iljk} > 0)$ is the binary index used for the first decision (latent variable) with $\mathbf{1}(A)$ indicating the occurrence of event A. Y_{iljk} is the number of visits of individual i, belonging to country k and group j to physician l (l = GP and SP) and we omit the time sub-index, t, for simplicity. Note that Y_{iljk} only takes non-negative integers as values. Finally, X and Z are conditions of both dependent variables that can have common elements and $\varepsilon_1, \varepsilon_2$ are error terms.

Suppose that we have a sample of N_{ljk} observations on (Y_{ljk}, w_{ljk}), where the vector of covariates w_{ljk} includes variables both in X and Z that, following Winkelman [15], may be disjoint or overlapping. We also assume that $Y_{iljk} = 0$ for N_{ljk0} observations and $Y_{iljk} > 0$ for N_{ljk+} and $N_{ljk} = N_{ljk0} + N_{ljk+}$. We are interested in explaining the conditional expectation of the number of visits to physician l by individual i, belonging to group j and country k, Y_{iljk}, given the covariates. In the TPM this expectation can be decomposed in two terms: the probability of observing a positive outcome (part one or first hurdle) times the conditional expectation of Y_{iljk} given that it is positive (part two or second hurdle). This decomposition is made in two parametric models. The first component is usually estimated assuming a discrete choice model (probit or logit). The second component can be seen as a count data model (Poisson or negative binomial).

The most common specification for the count model is the Poisson regression. However, there are some undesired features of the model (because of data characteristics or failures from Poisson distribution, see Cameron and Trivedi [16,17]) and one of them is the equality of mean and variance conditional on the explanatory variables. This equi-dispersion property generally appears as restrictive in empirical applications. A negative binomial (NB) model could be assumed for the data generating process to overcome the previous assumption (see Hausmann *et al.* [18] or Cameron and Trivedi [19]). Under these circumstances, if Y_{iljk} follows a Poisson distribution with mean λ_{ljk}, we can write the probability of y_{iljk} visits of patient i (belonging to group j in country k) to physician l as:

$$P(Y_{iljk} = y_{iljk}/\lambda_{iljk}) = \frac{e^{-\lambda_{iljk}}\lambda_{iljk}^{y_{ijkt}}}{y_{iljk}!} \quad y_{iljk} = 0, 1, 2, \ldots \tag{7.3}$$

where $\lambda_{iljk} = E(y_{iljk}/X_{iljk}, \varepsilon_{2iljk}) = \exp(X_{iljk}'\beta + \varepsilon_{2iljk})$, and ε_{2iljk} represents unobserved heterogeneity which is uncorrelated with the X's by assumption. On the other hand, the NB can be written as a mixture of a Poisson and Gamma distributions. If we specify λ_{iljk} as a Gamma distribution and make the integration over λ_{iljk}, we obtain a NB for Y_{iljk} (see Cameron and Trivedi [16,17], for details).

$$P(Y_{iljk} = y_{iljk}) = \int_0^\infty P(Y_{iljk} = y_{iljk}/\lambda_{iljk}) f(\lambda_{iljk}) d\lambda_{iljk}$$

$$= \frac{\Gamma(y_{iljk} + v_{iljk})}{\Gamma(y_{iljk} + 1)\Gamma(v_{iljk})} \left(\frac{v_{iljk}}{v_{ljk} + \theta_{ijkl}}\right)^{v_{\kappa v\lambda\mu}} \left(\frac{\theta_{iljk}}{v_{iljk} + \theta_{iljk}}\right)^{y_{iljk}}$$

(7.4)

Γ being a Gamma distribution with parameters y_{iljk} and v_{iljk}. The moments of the resulting NB are $E(Y_{iljk}) = \theta_{iljk}, \theta_{iljk} > 0$ and $\text{Var}(Y_{iljk}) = \theta_{iljk} + \frac{1}{v_{iljk}}\theta_{iljk}^2$ where we must understand $E(.)$ and $\text{Var}(.)$ as conditional on covariates. Since $\theta_{iljk} > 0$, the distribution derived in this way allows for over-dispersion. Moreover, v_{iljk} permits to introduce a stochastic error term that captures unobserved heterogeneity and possible measurement errors. Finally, we could include conditioning variables through θ_{ljk}, v_{ljk} or both. In fact modelling in different ways the variance yields different NB models. In this work we consider the NB2, in the terminology of Cameron and Trivedi [17].

However, the behaviour of individuals concerning decisions and counts of visits to physicians, at least in the light of the data or previous work with the ECHP by Jiménez-Martín et al. [20], seems to follow a double decision process: a process where the individual decides to go to the practitioner and a process where the practitioner has the decision to determine the length of the treatment. The patient is also competent in this second stage for many reasons: (i) a visit to a GP, for instance, could have the sole purpose of obtaining information in order to know to which specialist she needs to go (the agent acts as the patient's advisor); (ii) although the GP has the facility to send patients to the specialist in most of the countries, an individual can decide not to go; (iii) the patient can also decide the number of visits independently of the opinion of the physician.

From an econometric viewpoint it is very important to note that the results provided by the previous models are correct only when the process governing the discrete part of the model (the zero observations) and the process describing the positive counts are the same. Even when the same determinants appear as important in the two parts of the decision process, their effects and interpretations could be different. In this work we use, as in Pohlmeier and Ulrich [4], the hurdle models for count data proposed by Mullahy [21]. Unlike Mullahy, we assume that the underlying distribution for the first stage is normal and we model that decision by a probit. For the

second stage, as suggested by a previous exploration of the same data set, we opt for an NB process. If we further assume absence of zeros in the second stage using a truncated distribution for this second process, we can write the log-likelihood function for the sample as:

$$L_{TPMl} = \sum_{k=1}^K \left(\sum_{i\in N_{k0}} \ln P(I_{iljk} = 0 | Z_{iljk}; \beta_{1ljk}, \sigma_{1ljk}^2) \right.$$

$$+ \sum_{i\in N_{k1}} \ln (1 - P(I_{iljk} = 0 | Z_{iljk}; \beta_{1ljk}, \sigma_{1ljk}^2))$$

$$+ \sum_{i\in N_{k1}} \ln P(Y_{iljk} | X_{iljk}; \beta_{2ljk}, \sigma_{2ljk}^2)$$

$$\left. - \sum_{i\in N_{k1}} \ln P(Y_{iljk} \geq 1 | X_{iljk}; \beta_{2ljk}, \sigma_{2ljk}^2) \right)$$

$$l = GP, SP$$

(7.5)

where the first two terms in Equation 7.5 govern the binary outcome and the last two terms the number of visits once the first decision has been taken. The second hurdle is governed by a truncated NB distribution. Note that although we maintain sub-index j, it does not vary in this model. Given the nature of the data that we have, the Zero Inflated Model (see Cameron and Trivedi [16,17] or Mullahy [21]) is not reasonable since we know that a patient decides to contact a physician just when she makes a visit. Therefore, the count for those that decide to visit a physician in the first stage is always at least 1. The likelihood implicit in Equation 7.5 has been expressed as the product of two parametrically independent likelihood functions for each country. The errors of the two parts of the model can be assumed to be correlated, although this would imply the use of a different method of estimation (for instance, a Simulated Method of Moments, as in Winkelman [15]). This specification of the log-likelihood function for all the sample allows us to test among different models by imposing simple restrictions on the parameters (for instance, pooled estimates are easily obtained by imposing appropriate restrictions in the parameters of Equation 7.5).

A second problem we would like to deal with concerns the impossibility of distinguishing different illness spells in the data during the period information is collected. This is known as the excess zeros problem (Cameron and Trevedi [16,17] or Mullahy [21]). Although TPM allow to deal with this problem by means of zero inflated NB, i.e. without truncation at the second stage as above, they only permit mixing with respect to zeros and not with respect to positives, whereas the problem of unique spell affects both positives and zeros. One could account for this deficiency by using recent proposals in the health economics literature of Deb and Trivedi [7,8]. LCM are expressed as mixing distributions and in particular finite mixtures distributions. The log-likelihood function for these models, when considering data from several countries, is given by,

$$L_{LCMl} = \sum_{k=1}^{K} \sum_{i=1}^{N_k} \ln \left[\sum_{j=1}^{J} p_{ljk} f_{iljk}(Y_{lijk} \mid X_{iljk}; \delta_{lijk}) \right]$$
$$l = GP, SP \qquad\qquad (7.6)$$

where p_{ljk} and $f_{iljk}(.)$ are respectively the mixing probability and the density corresponding to group j, country k and physician l and δ_{ljk} is the set of parameters to estimate. Note that the specification is restricted to the case in which the number of groups is homogeneous across countries. The mxing probabilities are unknown parameters to be estimated jointly with the rest of parameters of the model. In order to identify all the parameters we estimate subject to the restriction $1 = \Sigma_{j=1}^{J} p_j$. If we specify $f(.)$ as in Equation 7.4, the LCM allows for overdispersion. As in the case of Equation 7.5, this general specification of the log-likelihood function for all the sample allows us to specify a variety of testing procedures as simple restrictions on the parameters of the model (for instance, equality of the coefficients across countries and equality of the coefficients across groups).

This approach has a number of advantages with respect to TPM. First, the possibility of modelling unobserved heterogeneity, which is accommodated in the model through the density and permits unobservables to affect the different types of groups in different ways. Second, the approach is semiparametric because it does not require distributional assumptions for the mixing variable and as noted by Heckman and Singer [6], finite mixture models may provide good numerical approximations even if the underlying mixing distribution is continuous. They are also useful if the data shows multimodality.

It is also worthwhile to mention that the LCM analysis suffers from a few disadvantages. While TPM are natural extensions of economic models (in the principal–agent framework, for instance), LCM are forced by statistical reasoning. This model has a long history in statistics (Everitt and Hand [22]) but it is a very new proposal in health economics. Second, it is sometimes difficult to estimate (by maximum likelihood) due to over-parameterization since the mixing distribution has to be estimated jointly with the rest of parameters of the model. There are, however, several recent approaches to deal with the estimation using the EM procedure (Böhning [23]). Third, misspecification of the density is as possible in LCM as it is in TPM. Moreover, they are not nested and we cannot answer whether the better adjustment of

LCM to the data is only a question of over-parameterization, i.e. the subsets of observations belonging to the different groups defined are statistically different. In our view, unobserved heterogeneity is much more related to economic issues (differences in tests, preferences, etc.) than to statistical ones.

DATA AND VARIABLES

The data that we use is a sample of males and females drawn from waves 1 to 3 of the ECHP. This panel survey (see Peracchi [24] for a description of the features of the ECHP), which has been carried out since 1994, contains valid information, for the purposes of this paper, on 12 European countries. Given the reduced time span of the panel we pool the three waves and use the longitudinal nature of the data only to construct some explanatory variables as explained below.

Despite that the ECHP focuses on household income and living conditions across EU15 countries it still provides interesting information on individual health and related issues. Apart from the traditionally asked questions on health status, such as self-statement on global health or whether the person is hampered in daily activities, the survey includes some additional ones. More specifically, it records whether the individual has any chronic physical or mental health problem, illness or disability. Individuals are also asked if they have been admitted to a hospital as in-patients (the number of nights spent in a hospital as in-patient are confidential information for Germany and therefore will not be used in this study). Finally, the survey collects information on how many times an individual has consulted a doctor, a dentist or an optician during the past 12 months (visits to a doctor, optician or dentist are aggregated for the first wave) which allows us to construct some measures of demand as the quantity of health services purchased.

Let us concentrate on the latter peices of information namely the counts of visits to GPs and SPs. Table 7.2 shows crude descriptive information on the zeros and positive counts in the 12 countries that are analyzed herein. Several remarks are in order as regards contacting a physician. First, women more often visit doctors than men. Although we do not report these figures in the paper, this is so at practically all ages, as shown in Jiménez-Martín et al. [20]. In all countries individuals more often visit a GP than an SP. There is more overdispersion of GP counts than of SP counts. Notable differences are detected by country, sex and kind of physician. Several reasons can be behind these figures. First, there seems to be a strong relationship between visits to a GP and per capita income, since individuals do visit a GP

Table 7.2 Descriptive statistics of visits counts by sex and country

Country		General practitioner		Specialist	
		Female	Male	Female	Male
Germany	0 visits (%)	21.63	26.31	29.39	54.00
	1 visit (%)	13.85	17.87	18.31	15.23
	Mean	4.457	3.644	3.618	2.269
	st-dev	7.586	7.190	6.972	5.827
Denmark	0 visits (%)	20.74	36.80	69.22	76.41
	1 visit (%)	19.80	25.93	12.64	11.29
	Mean	3.287	1.936	1.040	0.679
	st-dev	5.139	3.772	2.978	2.299
Netherlands	0 visits (%)	24.46	37.32	61.39	70.02
	1 visit (%)	19.76	24.54	11.52	10.93
	Mean	3.149	1.897	1.903	1.170
	st-dev	4.657	3.633	5.054	3.460
Belgium	0 visits (%)	15.98	21.31	39.59	62.96
	1 visit (%)	14.08	19.87	20.54	14.67
	Mean	4.368	3.314	2.282	1.301
	st-dev	6.311	5.483	4.295	3.446
Luxembourg	0 visits (%)	19.34	24.25	23.19	56.50
	1 visit (%)	15.87	20.75	26.72	16.50
	Mean	3.155	2.539	2.712	1.496
	st-dev	3.610	3.752	4.137	3.370
UK	0 visits (%)	16.88	30.25	64.22	70.04
	1 visit (%)	14.83	23.26	12.77	11.73
	Mean	4.217	2.554	1.146	0.934
	st-dev	5.534	4.326	3.169	2.756
Ireland	0 visits (%)	26.37	42.49	77.03	83.04
	1 visit (%)	16.16	19.64	8.31	7.99
	Mean	3.617	2.259	0.771	0.460
	st-dev	5.985	4.898	2.331	1.897
Italy	0 visits (%)	24.30	36.02	58.61	74.29
	1 visit (%)	12.52	15.88	16.05	11.22
	Mean	3.851	2.648	1.296	0.777
	st-dev	5.915	4.940	3.084	2.672
Greece	0 visits (%)	53.01	61.74	62.03	75.92
	1 visit (%)	10.75	11.07	9.49	6.71
	Mean	1.676	1.195	1.501	1.023
	st-dev	3.311	2.554	3.342	3.499
Spain	0 visits (%)	33.96	44.84	53.79	69.56
	1 visit (%)	13.69	16.47	16.65	11.35
	Mean	3.681	2.354	1.792	1.141
	st-dev	6.804	5.306	4.081	3.635
Portugal	0 visits (%)	33.35	48.32	60.56	77.72
	1 visit (%)	10.39	13.30	11.81	7.81
	Mean	3.172	1.888	1.349	0.714
	st-dev	4.784	3.201	3.117	2.234
Austria	0 visits (%)	11.24	15.39	16.47	41.62
	1 visit (%)	17.75	22.24	30.08	26.01
	Mean	4.611	3.707	2.911	2.060
	st-dev	7.299	5.965	5.532	4.919

substantially less frequently in southern countries and Ireland. Second, the pattern for visits to the specialist is less clear and differences may respond to accessibility criteria, which varies from country to country. And third, the differences by sex are more evident in the case of visits to SP than in GP visits, probably because of the type of physicians that the specialists include.

The explanatory variables used in the estimation can be divided in three groups (see the Data Appendix for a detailed description). The first group is formed by variables that affect the individual's health perception. It includes age and its square, and income and its square. It also includes variables which try to pick the individuals' health endowments or stocks (see Anderson and Burkhauser [25] for details on measures and problems of health variables): a dummy for self-perceived good health, a dummy for suffering a chronic condition, a dummy for individuals that were accepted as in-patients at a hospital, and a dummy for individuals hampered in their daily activities. Finally, this group of variables also include measures of the time opportunity cost, that is, variables relating job status (dummies for employment, self-employment, unemployment, and retirement; dummies for part-time jobs) and variables relating the family structure of the individual (marital status, household size, and dummy for heads of the household). We consider a second group of variables that is composed by those that affect the probability of having a health shock and the knowledge of this likelihood (dummy for high education), occupation (dummies for professional workers, for clerical workers, and for services workers; dummy for doing any type of supervisory job; dummy for working in the public sector), and risk of the job (dummy that equals one if the individual perceives their job as risky).

In our empirical application, all the job, income, and health-related variables are lagged, since they may be endogenous to the processes of utilization of health services. However, there is a notorious exception, since it is not possible to have a lagged indicator of the chronic health condition because it was not asked for in the first wave of the survey. This does not cause major problems (except through persistent individual heterogeneity) since the chronic conditions today and yesterday are practically collinear.

RESULTS AND DISCUSSION

This section discusses the model selection and main results of the estimation. We organize it into three subsections. The first one presents a set of tests that are used to select the econometric specification that fits better the modelling of the visits to GPs and to SPs. The next one reports a cross-validation analysis of the results in the previous section. The last one briefly summarizes the results of the independent estimation by country of the preferred models.

MODEL SELECTION

We first discuss the performance of two econometric specifications, a TPM and a LCM characterized by a finite mixture distribution with two points of support (that is, a LCM with two components or latent classes). The models are estimated by maximum likelihood by country and separately for males and females. The reason to estimate the models by country is that several tests show that homogeneous models are not supported by the data. For instance, in Table 7.3 the comparison of the sum

Table 7.3 Model selection and specification testing

GP	Log-L: Male		Log-L: Female		AIC: Males		AIC: Females	
	TPM	LCM2	TPM	LCM2	TPM	LCM2	TPM	LCM2
Germany	15 509.32	15 365.05	17 408.72	17 212.45	31 120.65	30 836.1	34 919.43	34 530.9
Denmark	6776.382	6737.44	8882.01	8816.929	13 654.76	13 580.88	17 866.02	17 739.86
Netherlands	11 616.83	11 517.37	15 884.59	15 781.16	23 335.65	23 140.74	31 871.18	31 668.32
Belgium	9690.668	9641.132	11 828.39	11 722.26	19 483.34	19 388.26	23 758.78	23 550.52
Luxembourg	3105.134	3068.428	3530.205	3504.675	6312.269	6242.856	7162.41	7115.351
UK	9129.753	9091.48	13 111.01	13 193.45	18 361.51	18 288.96	26 324.01	26 492.9
Ireland	11 104.38	11 040.6	13 842.94	13 776.57	22 310.76	22 187.2	27 787.89	27 659.14
Italy	26 910.96	26 733.21	32 188.7	32 023.89	53 923.92	53 572.42	64 479.4	64 153.79
Greece	10 591.94	10 623.10	13 814.71	13 844.21	21 285.87	21 352.21	27 731.43	27 794.42
Spain	20 531.2	20 386.96	25 943.59	25 816.3	41 164.4	40 879.93	51 989.17	51 738.61
Portugal	13 380.59	13 458.38	18 078.64	18 087.9	26 863.19	27 022.76	36 259.28	36 281.8
Austria	5200.213	5149.338	5909.753	5836.512	10 502.43	10 386.68	11 921.51	11 779.87
Sum of statistics								
GP not gatekeeper	*55 714.1*	*55 380.63*	*38 683.96*	*38 644.42*	*88 704.6*	*88 206.1*	*105 493.6*	*104 771.1*
GP gatekeeper	*87 833.27*	*87 448.07*	*46 424.86*	*46 455.93*	*199 614.2*	*198 690.9*	*256 576.9*	*255 733.5*
Sum het. models	*143 547.4*	*142 812.5*	*180 423.3*	*179 616.3*	*288 318.8*	*286 897*	*362 070.5*	*360 504.6*
Pooled estimates								
All countries	*144 750.7*	*144 511.4*	*182 546.7*	*181 669.3*	*289 603.4*	*289 172.8*	*365 195.4*	*363 488.7*
Specialist	TPM	LCM2	TPM	LCM2	TPM	LCM2	TPM	LCM2
Germany	11 654.88	11 616.76	15 867.92	15 793.36	23 411.77	23 339.51	31 837.84	31 692.71
Denmark	3568.955	3569.196	4769.909	4775.523	7239.909	7244.392	9641.818	9657.047
Netherlands	7742.829	7758.996	10 999.51	10 999.74	15 587.66	15 623.99	22 101.02	22 105.48
Belgium	5805.509	5766.917	8985.694	8966.915	11 713.02	11 639.83	18 073.39	18 039.83
Luxembourg	2291.633	2268.542	3287.04	3277.868	4685.265	4643.085	6676.08	6661.737
UK	5116.85	5108.83	6952.288	6932.71	10 335.7	10 323.66	14 006.58	13 971.42
Ireland	4237.657	4259.97	5736.805	5774.681	8577.314	8625.94	11 575.61	11 655.36
Italy	13 249.31	13 216.62	19 328.78	19 302.30	26 600.14	26 539.23	38 759.56	38 710.59
Greece	7926.225	7990.46	12 433.84	12 468.06	15 954.45	16 086.92	24 969.67	25 042.12
Spain	13 160.99	13 167.09	18 781.98	18 746.06	26 423.97	26 440.19	37 665.96	37 598.11
Portugal	7091.107	7134.228	11 906.61	11 985.52	14 284.21	14 374.46	23 915.22	24 077.04
Austria	3262.886	3242.745	4718.412	4729.305	6627.772	6591.49	9538.824	9564.61
Sum of statistics								
GP not gatekeeper	*68 376.38*	*67 901.27*	*56 292.41*	*56 235.25*	*62 392.3*	*62 300.8*	*91 095.8*	*91 001.0*
GP gatekeeper	*112 046.9*	*111 715*	*67 476.38*	*67 526.79*	*109 048.9*	*109 171.9*	*157 665.8*	*157 775.1*
Sum het. models	*85 108.83*	*85 100.35*	*123 778.8*	*123 752.2*	*171 441.2*	*171 472.7*	*248 761.6*	*248 776.1*
Pooled estimates								
All countries	*85 985.31*	*86 208.52*	*124 831.4*	*125 557.8*	*172 072.6*	*172 567*	*249 764.8*	*251 265.7*

Countries without gatekeeper: Germany, Netherlands, Belgium, Luxembourg, Greece and Austria. With gatekeeper: the rest of the countries.

of the likelihood from a fully heterogeneous model against an homogeneous model strongly rejects the latter (see Jiménez-Martín et al. [20] for further details). The reason to estimate the models by sex is that differences in behaviour regarding the demand of health can be expected, in particular differences on the visits to the specialist which for females may be related to fertility. In addition, we have conducted tests on the equality of the coefficients among the male and female specifications and the results confirm significant differences in 10 out of 12 countries in the GP equation and in all 12 countries in the SP equations. The utilization behaviour differ for reasons different to fertility or gender specific diseases as some tests confirm. The results of such tests are available upon request.

The specification of the TPM consists of a probit for the first part (which represents the contact decision) and a truncated NB for the second part (which represeents the frequency of the visits). The specification of the LCM allows for a different constant term, a different over-dispersion parameter, and different slope coefficients in the two components (LCM2). This last specification of the LCM was preferred to more restrictive ones in which only the constant or the constant and the over-dispersion parameter were allowed to vary across classes. However, it should be noted that although enriching the specifications using additional heterogeneous parameters help explain better the demand for health services, there is a quantitatively small gain (in terms of likelihood) for using the LCM2 instead of a specification where only the constant and the over-dispersion parameter vary (see Jiménez et al. [20]). This finding suggests that could be a problem of over-parameterization that makes the unrestricted model more likely to be preferred.

To compare the performance of both the TPM and the LCM models we use the Akaike Information Criterion (AIC) and the Bayesian Information Criterion (BIC). The former is defined as $AIC = -2 \ln L + 2K$ and the latter as $BIC = -2 \ln L + K \ln(N)$, where $\ln L$ is the value of the log-likelihood function for either the TPM or the LCM, K the number of parameters estimated and N the sample size. We prefer those models with bigger values of log-likelihood and smaller values of AIC and BIC. The absolute values of $\ln L$ and AIC for each specification are reported in Table 7.3. The values of BIC, which always give the same results than AIC, are available upon request.

In the GP equation, both the AIC and the BIC criteria clearly favour LCM when comparing the aggregated values of the tests. They also support LCM when making comparisons for individual countries, just with the exceptions of Greece and Portugal in the equations for males and UK, Greece and Portugal in equations for females.

The result is not as clear in the SP equations as it is in the GP ones. We do not reject the TPM model both in the case of males and females in at least six out of 12 countries (Denmark, the Netherlands, Greece and Portugal are always in the list of countries where the TPM adequately reflect the individuals' decisions as regards utilization of health services). More importantly the AIC (and BIC) tests favour TPM for both men and women in the aggregate measures we present, that is when adding up the country specific AIC (BIC).

The results are highly coherent with the existent econometric theory on the topic. Santos-Silva and Windmeijer [5] point out that the poor performance of the TPM is due to the violation of the single illness spell hypothesis on which those models are based. For Germany they show evidence about the violation of this single-spell assumption. In our data set the visits to GPs are more likely to suffer from a multi-spell problem (see Table 7.2) and in line with Santos-Silva and Windmeijer [5] the TPM performs poorly relatively to the LCM. Visits to SPs are however less frequent than visits to a GP and consequently less likely to suffer from the same problem. This is especially true in our data for countries in which the GP act as a *gatekeeper*, as a first stage before accessing SPs (see Table 7.1). We see from the results that for males four out of the six countries for which the LCM are preferred to the TPM (Germany, Belgium, Luxembourg and Austria) do not have GPs acting as gatekeepers. This is not surprising since visits to SPs and GPs have a similar structure in those countries (see Table 7.2). For females the same results than for males hold in Germany, Belgium and Luxembourg. Greece does not use the figure of the gatekeeper, although for this country the TPM are preferred to the LCM for both the visits to GP and to SP. However there is a lower frequency of visits to GPs and SPs in Greece than in the rest of countries without a gatekeeping mechanism: 63.8% of the women and 72.8% of men visited their GP at most once during the year previous to the interview and 71.5% of the women and 82.7% visited a SP at most once during the year previous to the interview. That could explain the direction of the test for this country. As it can be seen from the last two rows of Table 7.3, if we estimate the model on an aggregate of countries using the gatekeeping criteria, the results are even clearer: TPM are preferred to LCM for modelling SP services in countries in which GPs act as gatekeepers of the health care system.

CROSS-VALIDATION

In the case of complicated models, in-sample model selection methods may induce over-fitting and consequently

Table 7.4 Cross-validation analysis

	TPM preferred (AIC) (%)				$\ln L_{TPM} - \ln L_{LCM}$			
	GP		SP		GP		SP	
	Training Sample	Holdout Sample	Training Sample	Holdout Sample	Training Sample	Holdout Sample	Training Sample	Holdout Sample
Males								
Germany	0	1	0	8	−114.91	−28.62	−30.97	−6.12
Denmark	1	24	2	74	−29.59	−4.84	−6.74	5.61
Netherlands	0	1	98	51	−75.34	−22.14	13.41	0.03
Belgium	1	17	9	34	−40.35	−5.24	−24.28	0.02
Luxembourg	0	39	0	55	−26.77	0.80	−14.72	5.07
UK	1	28	26	53	−28.63	−2.59	−2.20	3.89
Ireland	0	14	98	87	−49.76	−12.06	16.94	9.14
Italy	0	1	2	25	−141.36	−36.85	−25.79	−5.77
Greece	100	82	99	98	24.45	8.24	15.90	8.63
Spain	1	2	66	50	−113.31	−28.70	5.63	2.33
Portugal	100	97	100	91	56.29	17.10	36.25	11.17
Austria	5	48	11	44	−69.71	1.32	−12.11	5.59
All	0	0	50	85	−608.99	−113.58	−28.67	39.59
GP not Gatekeeper	0	5	29	73	−227.28	−23.49	−66.18	13.19
GP Gatekeeper	0	0	86	69	−381.71	−90.08	37.51	26.40
Females								
Germany	0	0	0	0	−155.06	−39.17	−58.02	−15.70
Denmark	0	2	63	71	−54.22	−16.15	2.95	9.71
Netherlands	1	0	28	55	−80.99	−24.01	−0.45	2.64
Belgium	1	1	1	33	−89.94	−20.71	−16.41	−0.35
Luxembourg	0	36	29	64	−21.15	−0.42	−12.26	3.55
UK	0	0	9	42	−93.12	−23.07	−12.40	0.68
Ireland	0	2	100	93	−51.26	−12.44	34.94	14.22
Italy	1	2	2	33	−132.34	−30.82	−22.80	−1.50
Greece	96	93	100	97	39.09	13.50	64.25	18.01
Spain	0	0	2	20	−101.38	−25.16	−26.39	−5.33
Portugal	67	53	100	97	9.21	2.09	43.67	16.04
Austria	0	9	80	53	−57.74	−12.51	−36.15	−6.68
All	0	0	47	74	−788.89	−188.87	−39.06	35.29
GP not Gatekeeper	0	0	41	51	−284.79	−59.31	−58.59	−1.18
GP Gatekeeper	0	0	63	81	−504.10	−129.57	19.53	36.46

The cross-validation exercise has been replicated 100 times. TPM preferred % denotes the percentage of replications for which TPM are preferred to LCM according to the AIC.

not choosing the best model. This bias can be avoided by splitting the initial sample into two sub-samples and using the first sub-sample (the training sample) to estimate the model and the second sub-sample (the hold-out sample) to forecast comparisons.

In order to make a cross-validation study, we carried out the following exercise. We divided the whole sample in a training sample consisting in 80% randomly chosen observations from the initial sample while the remaining 20% constituted the hold-out sample. The TPM and LCM parameters were estimated on the training sample and the measures of performance, log-likelihood and AIC, calculated using the parameter estimates both for the training and hold-out samples. The summary of the results of repeating this experiment 100 times are presented in Table 7.4, in which we show the number of times in which TPM was preferred to LCM according to each criteria.

In general, the results are completely coherent with the results in the previous section for both males and females. In the training sample, LCM are preferred to TPM in visits to GPs for most countries (exceptions are again

Table 7.5a Visits to the GP: LCM (males)

	Germany	Denmark	Netherlands	Belgium	Luxembourg	UK	Ireland	Italy	Greece	Spain	Portugal	Austria
Age	−0.043	−0.050	−0.067*	0.006	−0.082	0.020	0.080*	−0.016	0.029	−0.072+	0.024	−0.045
Age squared/100	0.060*	0.063	0.074*	−0.013	0.107	−0.015	−0.090+	0.041*	−0.027	0.100+	−0.014	0.051
Head of household	0.071	−0.082	0.262	0.098	−0.124	−0.119	−0.166	0.038	0.224+	0.033	−0.046	−0.043
Married	−0.020	−0.398	0.202	−0.008	0.715+	−0.289*	0.098	−0.048	−0.099	−0.104	0.327+	0.089
Divorced	−0.192	0.003	0.416	0.208	0.481	0.097	1.144*	−0.390	−0.003	0.088	0.051	0.116
Household size	−0.002	0.020	−0.015	−0.073+	0.084	0.078	−0.054	0.017	0.002	0.000	−0.042+	0.038
High education	0.131	−0.273	−0.335+	−0.235+	−0.440	0.182	0.058	−0.151	0.006	0.012	−0.088	0.482
Employed	0.228	−0.091	−0.268	0.047	−0.848+	−0.245	0.398	−0.026	−0.067	0.006	0.146	0.084
Self-employed	0.159	−0.418	0.300	0.062	−0.687*	−0.246	−0.121	−0.027	0.081	0.024	0.075	−0.365
Unemployed	0.552*	0.675*	0.106	0.718+	−0.951+	−0.091	0.132	0.143	0.165	−0.058	−0.244*	0.846*
Retired	0.445*	0.088	0.706+	0.502+	−1.370+	−0.392	−0.369	0.287*	0.428+	0.206*	0.171*	0.552+
Part time job	−0.284	−0.484	−0.394	0.239	1.836	−6.134	−0.445	0.015	−0.374	0.107	0.136	−0.193
Professional	−0.040	0.119	−0.061	−0.264+	−0.068	−0.505+	−0.127	−0.096	0.169+	−0.169+	−0.184+	−0.295*
Clerical	−0.399+	−1.362	0.192	0.112	0.272	−0.248	−0.108	0.047	0.015	0.105	0.128	−0.512*
Services	−0.275	0.272	−0.269	0.334*	−0.169	−0.466	−0.273	0.096	0.034	0.047	0.002	0.259*
No supervisory job	0.201+	0.284	0.093	0.021	0.050	0.228	−0.019	0.202+	0.156	0.055	−0.206+	−0.178
Household income	0.171+	0.797	0.057	−0.012	−0.158*	−0.058	−0.004	−0.068	−0.051	0.016	0.015	0.229+
H. Income squared/100	−1.739+	−15.70	−0.264	0.407	0.565	0.442	−0.021	0.143	0.450	−0.395	0.526*	−2.711+
Public Sector	−0.108	−0.323	−0.025	0.219+	0.451	−0.048	−0.386*	0.069	0.051	0.202+	0.044	0.268*
Good health	−0.465	−0.493+	−0.445+	−0.765+	−0.561+	−0.254*	−0.252	−0.218+	−0.260+	−0.426+	−0.360+	0.318+
Chronic illness	0.630+	0.608+	0.818+	0.675+	0.693+	0.657+	1.339+	0.789+	0.824+	0.644+	0.769+	0.798+
Hampered	0.287+	0.395	0.222	0.055	0.239	0.626	0.391	0.397+	0.208+	0.320+	0.243+	0.500+
In hospital	0.286+	0.350	0.477+	0.400+	0.326	0.144	0.326	0.480+	0.063	0.413+	0.432+	0.253*
Risk at job	0.240*	−0.268	−0.069	0.159	0.374	0.120	−0.284	−0.087	0.117*	0.007	−0.075+	0.158
Constant 1	0.961+	0.715+	0.969+	1.832+	0.180	1.288*	−0.488	0.791+	−1.748+	−0.934+	−1.502+	−2.371+
Ln alpha 1	1.539+	1.543	2.026+	0.298+	2.950+	−0.328	1.178+	1.198+	−0.146	1.811+	−0.198	2.361+
Age	−0.038+	−0.068+	−0.012	−0.019	−0.039	−0.039+	−0.011	0.024+	0.278+	−0.011	0.007	−0.033+
Age squared/100	0.057+	0.071+	0.022	0.040*	0.064+	0.049+	0.021	−0.006	−0.212+	0.030	0.012	0.047+
Head of Household	−0.015	0.087	−0.136	−0.083	0.122	0.050	0.252+	−0.065	−0.285*	0.075	0.147	−0.019
Married	0.130*	0.110	0.283+	0.040	−0.093	0.020	0.086	0.036	0.939+	0.036	−0.034	0.167+
Divorced	0.123	0.320*	0.189	−0.011	−0.224	0.116	0.143	0.149	0.417	0.169	−0.100	0.014
Household size	0.023	0.031	0.012	0.013	−0.048	0.024	−0.016	−0.027+	−0.083+	0.025	−0.066	−0.042+
High education	0.018	−0.068	−0.031	0.103	0.156	−0.105*	0.090	−0.132*	−0.674+	−0.196*	−0.235+	−0.185+
Employed	−0.184+	0.187	−0.016	−0.131	−0.080	−0.160*	−0.270+	−0.136*	−0.247	−0.007	−0.077	0.118
Self-employed	−0.507+	−0.240	−0.473+	−0.725+	−0.737+	−0.389+	−0.341+	−0.264+	−0.240	−0.137	−0.221	−0.070
Unemployed	−0.194	0.497+	−0.046	−0.397+	−0.338	−0.127	0.096	−0.093	−0.547+	0.114	0.350	0.369
Retired	−0.172	0.408+	0.086	−0.146	0.080	0.008	−0.014	−0.069	−0.196	0.250	−0.154	0.172
Part time job	−0.305	0.259	−0.088	0.160	−0.684+	0.260+	0.080	−0.136	0.802+	−0.385	−0.052	−0.005
Professional	−0.143+	0.062	0.073	−0.163+	−0.120	0.134+	0.009	−0.022	−0.343+	0.064	0.340+	0.050
Clerical	0.092	0.167	−0.008	−0.055	−0.066	0.141	0.094	−0.036	−0.192	−0.101	0.159	0.007
Services	0.014	−0.081	0.251+	0.033	0.144	0.144	0.076	−0.146+	−0.159	−0.329+	0.041	−0.192+
No supervisory job	0.053	−0.090	−0.003	−0.032	−0.095	−0.104*	0.002	0.029	0.089	0.028	0.157	0.014
Household income	−0.083+	0.010	−0.082+	−0.045	0.081	−0.006	0.021	0.016	0.154	−0.066	0.326+	0.088+
H. income squared/100	0.376+	0.040	0.118	0.170	−0.645	−0.054	−0.046	−0.397	−1.930	0.118	−7.939+	−0.998+
Public sector	0.088*	0.059	0.010	0.042	0.043	0.075	−0.015	0.041	0.527+	0.157	−0.068	0.126+
Good health	−0.522+	−0.523+	−0.201+	−0.531+	−0.338+	−0.491+	−0.451+	−0.327+	−0.352+	−0.335+	−0.360+	−0.333+
Chronic illness	0.489+	0.509+	0.656+	0.355+	0.206*	0.926+	1.245+	0.944+	0.965+	0.872+	1.053+	0.551+
Hampered	0.175+	0.338+	0.217+	0.231+	0.125	0.102	0.231+	0.171+	−0.121	0.509+	0.180	0.285+
In hospital	0.293+	0.259+	0.226+	0.332+	0.070	0.259+	0.445+	0.170+	0.215	0.387+	0.566+	0.231+
Risk at job	−0.057	0.209+	0.093	−0.098	0.080	−0.076	0.125	0.117+	−0.342+	−0.025	0.084	−0.009
Ln alpha 2	1.856+	1.592+	0.472*	−1.629+	1.467+	−0.740+	−0.381+	−1.128+	−8.633+	0.571	−0.355	1.237+
Constant 2	−1.253+	−0.781+	−1.109+	1.526+	−2.370+	1.314+	0.562+	0.201	1.186+	1.375+	1.370+	−1.120+
Prob group 1	0.388+	0.209+	0.299+	0.382+	0.368+	0.132+	0.210+	0.401+	0.285+	0.498	0.473	0.052+
Log-L	15365.05	6737.44	11517.37	9641.132	3068.428	9091.48	11040.6	26733.21	10623.10	20386.96	13458.38	5149.338
LR test (β1 = β2; d.f. = 24)	36.39	33.62	45.95	66.42	61.14	41.46	20.87	27.91	122.69	32.28	38.89	32.23

Level of significance: + and * denote significance at the 5% and 10% levels.

Table 7.5b Visits to the GP: LCM (Females)

	Germany	Denmark	Netherlands	Belgium	Luxembourg	UK	Ireland	Italy	Greece	Spain	Portugal	Austria
Age	0.010	-0.044	0.002	-0.053+	-0.038	-0.075+	-0.058+	0.009	0.040+	-0.049+	0.048+	-0.004
Age squared/100	-0.011	0.032	-0.018	0.061+	0.056	0.063+	0.047+	0.003	-0.018	0.070+	-0.042+	0.006
Head of household	-0.141	0.239+	-0.081	0.013	0.010	0.101	0.035	-0.009	0.017	0.154*	0.008	0.081
Married	-0.062	-0.207	0.328+	0.496+	0.136	0.298+	0.569+	0.248+	0.374+	0.196+	0.203+	0.123
Divorced	-0.051	-0.217	0.543+	0.689+	0.356	0.282+	1.025+	0.221+	0.395+	-0.057	0.170+	0.236
Household size	-0.084+	0.013	0.015	0.030	0.014	0.018	-0.045+	-0.030+	-0.031*	0.007	-0.033+	-0.082+
High education	-0.383+	-0.106	-0.112	-0.153*	-0.407	-0.230+	-0.074	-0.096	-0.175*	-0.099	-0.254+	-0.364
Employed	-0.406+	-0.165	-0.106	-0.333*	0.013	-0.032	0.091	-0.096	-0.014	-0.227	0.045	-0.274
Self-employed	-0.409	-0.175	-0.311	-2.011+	-0.325	-0.044	-0.263	0.017	-0.096	-0.094	-0.033	-0.200
Unemployed	-0.095	0.142	-0.049	0.094	-0.671	0.088	0.040	0.078	0.196+	-0.078	0.016	0.165
Retired	-0.007	0.042	-0.645	-0.010	-0.284	0.143	0.168	0.145+	0.141*	0.745+	0.039	0.202
Part time job	0.064	-0.227	-0.206+	-0.153	0.012	-0.173+	-0.158	0.024	-0.111	0.064	-0.060	-0.078
Professional	-0.007	0.111	0.053	0.052	-0.320	0.084	-0.030	-0.139+	0.088	-0.346+	-0.256+	0.328*
Clerical	0.112	0.008	0.089	0.201	0.154	-0.017	-0.169	-0.048	0.024	-0.311+	-0.164+	0.270
Services	0.005	0.030	0.025	0.254	0.423	0.188	0.238	0.063	0.099	-0.158	-0.108*	-0.095
No supervisory job	0.148	-0.002	0.095	0.249+	-0.462+	-0.068	0.005	0.137+	0.034	0.137	0.010	0.334
Household income	-0.020	0.057	-0.016	0.023	0.026	-0.048	-0.144+	-0.026	0.019	-0.021	0.012	0.115
H. income squared/100	0.403	-0.259	-0.032	-0.299	-0.365	0.179	1.010+	-0.066	-0.108	-0.342	0.058	-1.124
Public sector	0.085	0.041	-0.114	-0.075	0.636+	0.074	0.154	0.156+	0.232*	0.291+	-0.164+	-0.223
Good health	-0.658+	-0.756+	-0.449+	-0.482+	0.009	-0.409+	-0.276+	-0.287+	-0.243+	-0.368+	-0.433+	-0.721+
Chronic illness	0.478+	0.226+	0.736+	0.584+	0.551+	0.542+	1.022+	0.776+	0.779+	0.674+	0.601+	0.355+
Hampered	0.199*	0.454+	0.123	0.218+	-0.045	0.067	0.274+	0.040	-0.079	0.272+	0.145+	0.180
In hospital	0.263+	0.279+	0.147	0.173	-0.207	0.481+	0.436+	0.172+	0.123	0.185+	0.234+	0.130
Risk at job	-0.046	0.276	0.194	-0.206	-0.244	-0.061	-0.067	0.028	0.173*	-0.032	0.000	0.180
Constant group 1	2.139+	3.015+	0.457+	2.361+	0.153	3.480+	0.319+	-1.977+	-0.939	1.733+	-0.062	-0.093
Ln alpha 1	0.869+	0.208*	1.415+	0.284*	1.528*		2.888+	0.714+	-2.012+	-1.134+	-1.488+	2.324+
Age	-0.042+	-0.053+	-0.029+	-0.039*	-0.035*	-0.052+	-0.025	-0.011	0.028	-0.035+	-0.068+	-0.010
Age squared/100	0.059+	0.045+	0.032*	0.050*	0.043*	0.051+	0.022	0.024*	0.004	0.051+	0.082+	0.021
Head of household	0.060	-0.111*	-0.099	0.008	-0.042	-0.011	0.086	0.059	0.270*	-0.170*	0.001	0.064
Married	0.076	0.185+	-0.005	-0.059	-0.147	0.198+	0.496+	0.235+	0.140	0.242+	0.758+	0.153*
Divorced	0.083	0.159	0.001	-0.074	-0.259*	0.220+	0.633+	0.140	0.074	0.388+	0.707+	0.256+
Household size	0.056+	-0.133+	-0.066+	-0.056+	0.008	-0.066+	-0.031*	-0.011	0.025	-0.001	-0.062+	0.010
High education	-0.140+	0.047	-0.093	0.001	0.115	-0.055	0.104	-0.120	0.158	-0.330+	-0.136	-0.076
Employed	0.177+	0.285+	-0.207+	0.240+	-0.039	0.069	-0.187	-0.007	0.080	0.109	0.168	0.086
Self-employed	-0.004	-0.074	-0.251	0.380+	0.139	-0.174	0.007	-0.128	0.248	0.032	0.040	-0.142
Unemployed	0.174+	0.084	0.059	-0.022	-0.052	-0.004	0.022	0.016	-0.054	0.144*	0.006	0.337+
Retired	0.232+	0.007	0.182	0.115	-0.169	-0.212+	0.326	0.036	-0.074	-1.411+	0.317*	0.102
Part time job	-0.060	0.058	0.156+	-0.034	-0.041	-0.013	-0.102	-0.167+	0.107	0.039	0.163	-0.082
Professional	-0.208+	-0.258+	-0.067	-0.251+	-0.161	0.006	-0.013	-0.039	-0.882+	-0.172	0.206	-0.255+
Clerical	-0.228+	-0.259+	-0.068	-0.352+	-0.028	-0.122	0.087	0.066	-0.312	-0.073	0.150	-0.021
Services	-0.134	-0.199*	0.038	-0.085	-0.308	0.015	-0.030	-0.001	-0.526*	-0.278+	0.160	-0.115
No supervisory job	0.100*	-0.047	0.033	-0.032	0.197	0.104*	0.259+	0.032	0.005	0.082	-0.128	0.109
Household income	-0.029	0.051	-0.012	-0.005	-0.004	0.018	0.004	-0.168+	0.054	-0.113+	0.010	0.070*
H. income squared/100	0.103	-0.061	0.009	0.009	-0.169	-0.260	0.003	1.323+	-2.101	0.062	-1.711	-0.884+
Public sector	0.044	-0.037	0.178+	0.019	-0.041	-0.064	-0.123	0.025	-0.025	0.057	-0.204	0.025
Good health	-0.399+	-0.424+	-0.513+	-0.577+	-0.555+	-0.484+	-0.549+	-0.375+	-0.622+	-0.607+	-0.229+	-0.295+
Chronic illness	0.580+	0.639+	0.574+	0.414+	0.482+	0.740+	1.037+	0.809+	0.822+	0.654+	0.878+	0.614+
Hampered	0.125+	0.068	0.061	0.205+	0.269+	0.194+	0.107	0.317+	0.170	0.349+	0.148	0.193+
In hospital	0.199+	0.249+	0.317+	0.424+	0.414+	0.302+	0.342+	0.259+	0.364+	0.282+	0.408+	0.344+
Risk at job	0.111	-0.141	0.117	0.075	0.230	-0.108	0.071	0.194+	-0.251	0.089	0.403+	0.003
Constant group 2	-1.500+	-1.366+	1.921+	-1.728+	2.020+	2.234+	1.402+	1.566+	1.605+	0.969+	1.318+	0.765+
Ln alpha 2	1.677+	2.390+	-1.457+	2.414+	-2.195+	-1.494+	-1.068+	0.522+	-1.042+	1.912+	1.584+	-1.795+
Prob group 1	0.430+	0.340+	0.430+	0.406+	0.398	0.392+	0.424+	0.443+	0.410+	0.427*	0.403+	0.286+
Log-L	172121.245	8816.929	15781.16	11722.26	3504.675	13193.45	13776.57	32023.89	13844.21	25816.3	18087.9	5836.512
LR test (β1 = β2; d.f. = 24)	44.447	48.05	42.06	24.20	31.46	54.06	37.39	45.66	48.17	37.21	44.19	22.84

Level of significance: + and * denote significance at the 5% and 10% levels.

Table 7.6a Visits to the specialist: TPM (males)

	Germany	Denmark	Netherlands	Belgium	Luxembourg	UK	Ireland	Italy	Greece	Spain	Portugal	Austria
First stage												
Age	−0.027+	−0.020	−0.044+	0.006	−0.014	−0.034+	−0.001	−0.001	0.013	−0.032+	−0.017	−0.010
Age squared/100	0.033+	0.024	0.056+	0.027	0.038	0.038+	0.001	0.002	0.001	0.041+	0.019	0.023
Head of household	0.067	0.082	0.042	−0.177+	0.033	0.048	0.022	0.064	0.065	0.036	0.037	−0.022
Married	0.159+	0.119*	0.143+	0.014	0.028	0.111*	0.200+	0.117+	0.068	0.099+	0.259+	0.114
Divorced	0.084	0.043	0.181*	−0.101	0.008	0.016	−0.118	0.184*	0.212*	0.075	0.027	−0.243
Household size	−0.046+	−0.033	−0.037+	−0.036+	−0.037	−0.032*	−0.034+	−0.052+	−0.011	−0.017*	−0.042+	−0.073+
High education	0.127+	−0.021	−0.039	0.127+	0.034	0.077	0.108	−0.033	−0.056	0.079+	−0.019	0.496+
Employed	−0.207+	−0.116	0.035	−0.170*	−0.087	−0.161*	−0.039	−0.041	0.007	−0.025	−0.074	−0.255+
Self-employed	−0.364+	−0.278+	−0.111	−0.167	−0.289	−0.213+	−0.225+	−0.141+	−0.081	−0.123+	−0.083	−0.484+
Unemployed	−0.145	−0.025	−0.091	−0.341+	−0.091	−0.082	−0.254+	−0.087	−0.063	−0.074	−0.075	−0.109
Retired	−0.147	−0.365+	0.105	−0.057	−0.183	0.044	0.020	0.010	0.233+	−0.093	0.019	−0.438+
Part time job	0.056	0.076	−0.036	0.070	−0.553	−0.164	0.041	−0.188+	−0.178*	0.032	0.135	0.071
Professional	0.161+	−0.059	0.115+	0.231+	0.088	0.094	0.059	0.123+	0.056	0.086+	0.170+	0.216+
Clerical	0.111	−0.205+	0.308+	0.012	0.031	−0.110	0.089	0.137+	−0.025	0.093	0.252+	0.309+
Services	0.182+	−0.057	0.035	−0.071	−0.260	0.122	−0.035	0.008	0.035	−0.057	0.170+	0.142
No supervisory job	0.052	0.075+	0.012	0.026	−0.100	−0.117+	−0.049	−0.084+	0.013+	−0.021	−0.093	−0.029
Household income	0.057+	−0.064+	−0.017	−0.363	0.075+	0.068+	0.095+	0.117+	0.103+	0.046+	0.230+	0.007
H. income squared	−0.290+	0.023	0.064	0.104*	−0.372*	−0.372+	−0.292+	−0.612+	−1.560+	−0.003	−1.421+	0.108
Public sector	0.122+	−0.367+	0.008	−0.422+	0.070	0.024	−0.030	−0.014	0.165+	0.175+	0.185+	0.059
Good health	−0.270+	0.392+	−0.308+	0.470+	−0.245+	−0.187+	−0.273+	−0.205+	−0.312+	−0.238+	−0.233+	−0.081
Chronic illness	0.478+	0.152*	0.752+	0.188+	0.495+	0.792+	0.847+	0.924+	1.215+	0.714+	0.943+	0.457+
Hampered	0.120+	0.298+	0.081	0.631+	0.281+	0.217+	0.057	0.150+	0.050	0.205+	0.077	0.236+
In hospital	0.316+	−0.009	0.741+	−0.015	0.298+	0.497+	0.481+	0.436+	0.318+	0.584+	0.347+	0.278+
Risk at job	0.015	−0.275	0.024	−0.142	0.167	0.004	0.021	−0.008	0.021	−0.083+	0.086	−0.221*
Constant	0.317		0.187		−0.134	−0.091	−1.061+	−0.784+	−1.439+	−0.103	−0.874+	0.432
Second Stage												
Age			0.015	−0.073*		0.055*	0.051	0.012		0.010	−0.010	0.025
Age squared/100	−0.004	−0.096+	−0.024	0.082	−0.035	−0.077+	−0.077*	−0.010	−0.028	−0.020	0.010	−0.031
Head of household	0.023	0.114+	−0.095	−0.105	0.064	−0.105	0.425+	0.066	0.026	0.055	−0.088	−0.027
Married	0.083	0.070	0.062	0.044	−0.199	0.088	−0.254	−0.235	−0.248+	0.093	0.123	−0.235
Divorced	−0.064	−0.094	0.104	0.106	0.057	0.284	−0.829+	−0.234	0.102	0.512	0.210	−0.034
Household size	−0.124	0.475	0.032	0.004	0.220	−0.074+	−0.137+	0.043	0.160	−0.049+	−0.009	−0.150+
High education	0.060*	0.115	−0.058	−0.284+	0.145	0.111	−0.069	0.024	0.118	−0.032	0.271	0.143
Employed	−0.130	−0.365+	−0.085	0.216	−0.075	0.353*	−0.716+	−0.359*	−0.575+	−0.007	0.389+	0.156
Self-employed	0.186	0.807+	−0.295	0.259	−0.432	0.180	−0.473+	−0.398+	−0.228	−0.084	0.002	−0.330
Unemployed	0.267	0.543	0.053	−0.035	0.176	0.237	−0.247	−0.074	−0.315	0.113	0.033	0.011
Retired	−0.142	0.841+	0.514*	−0.018	−0.324	0.229	−0.706+	−0.090	0.013	−0.129	0.090	−0.325
Part time job	0.144	0.432	0.008	−0.152	1.527*	0.222	−0.197	0.340	−0.040	−0.379	0.225	−0.666
Professional	−0.340	−0.529	0.087	−0.234	−0.137	−0.213	−0.265	−0.085	0.087	−0.118	−0.085	0.047
Clerical	−0.117	−0.088	−0.026	0.342	0.025	−0.106	0.262	−0.242	−0.118	−0.284	0.121	0.536*
Services	−0.011	−0.724+	−0.271	−0.054	0.109	−0.238	−0.377	−0.048	0.111	−0.111	0.062	−0.008
No supervisory job	0.320*	−0.355	0.151	−0.168	0.317+	−0.272*	0.255	0.266+	0.507+	−0.053	−0.439+	−0.567+
Household income	0.042	0.144	0.036	−0.130	0.034	−0.045	0.098	−0.114*	0.080	−0.012	0.034	0.147
H. income squared	0.003	0.044	−0.455	1.390	−0.017	0.776*	−0.315	0.966	−0.561	−0.302	−0.292	−1.556
Public sector	0.029	−0.775	0.028	0.280*	−0.403+	0.110	0.037	0.024	−0.127	−0.030	−0.154	−0.045
Good health	−0.290+	−0.129	−0.191*	−0.545+	−0.536+	−0.254+	−0.247	−0.200*	−0.288+	−0.281+	−0.320+	−0.611+
Chronic illness	0.693+	−0.321	0.828+	0.682+	0.621+	0.954+	1.065+	0.604	+1.072+	0.703+	0.804+	1.089+
Hampered	0.308+	0.621+	0.214+	−0.001	−0.056	0.096	−0.139	0.220*	0.033	0.314+	0.161*	0.223
In hospital	0.564+	0.376+	0.056	0.568+	0.597+	0.321+	0.361+	0.449+	0.546+	0.571+	0.307+	0.324*
Risk at job	−0.037	0.246	0.330+	−0.052	0.531*	−0.277*	0.153	−0.079	0.028	0.305+	0.284*	−0.322
Constant	−0.585	−1.426	−0.425	1.663+	0.861	−1.054*	−0.557	−8.753	+1.363+	−0.327	0.370	−2.968
Ln(alpha)	1.875+	3.723	1.541+	1.650+	0.624+	1.124+	1.341+	10.338+	0.427+	2.011+	0.402+	4.877
Log-L	11654.88	3568.955	7742.829	5805.509	2291.633	5116.85	4237.657	13249.31	7926.225	13160.99	7091.107	3262.886
LR test (β1 = β2; d.f. = 25)	198.35	72.92	339.16	165.59	49.64	193.13	188.79	692.33	801.17	486.52	325.47	150.69

Level of significance: + and * denote significance at the 5% and 10% levels.

Table 7.6b Visits to the specialist: TPM (females)

	Germany	Denmark	Netherlands	Belgium	Luxembourg	UK	Ireland	Italy	Greece	Spain	Portugal	Austria
First stage												
Age	-0.017	0.005	-0.038 +	0.019	-0.022	-0.001	-0.017	0.001	-0.008	0.005	0.020 +	0.037*
Age squared	0.002	-0.007	0.041 +	-0.031	0.013	-0.034	0.009	-0.010	-0.004	-0.010	-0.031 +	-0.062 +
Head of household	0.068	0.050	0.035	-0.054	0.059	-0.081	0.063	0.053	0.068	0.030	0.013	0.086
Married	0.411 +	-0.059	0.317 +	0.266 +	0.474 +	0.084	0.529 +	0.411 +	0.627 +	0.327 +	0.321 +	0.386 +
Divorced	0.203 +	0.022	0.196 +	0.388 +	0.222	0.128	0.436 +	0.361 +	0.540 +	0.156 +	0.176 +	0.133
Household size	-0.089 +	-0.087 +	-0.048 +	-0.100 +	-0.077 +	-0.059 +	-0.067 +	-0.106 +	-0.079 +	-0.074 +	-0.075 +	-0.099 +
High education	0.245 +	0.058	0.053	0.134 +	0.374 +	0.057	0.064	0.072	0.036	0.075*	0.284*	0.198
Employed	-0.034	-0.009	-0.031	-0.308 +	0.119	-0.032	0.078	-0.118 +	-0.071	0.005	-0.112	0.026
Self-employed	-0.178	-0.366 +	-0.287 +	-0.295 +	0.119	-0.229 +	0.172	0.097*	-0.024	-0.113*	-0.172 +	-0.156
Unemployed	0.093	-0.122	0.054	-0.099	0.071	-0.123	0.055	-0.038	0.023	-0.027	-0.009	0.092
Retired	0.211 +	-0.171	0.346	-0.010	0.036	0.035	-0.196	0.021	0.105	-0.001	0.156 +	0.050
Part time job	-0.017	0.015	0.080	-0.029	-0.028	-0.032	-0.006	0.028	-0.050	0.008	0.057	0.079
Professional	0.183 +	0.082	0.042	0.429 +	-0.036	0.192 +	0.085	0.185 +	0.023	0.086	0.235 +	-0.024
Clerical	0.068	0.030	0.001	0.325 +	0.089	0.176 +	0.075	0.180 +	0.117	0.008	0.350 +	0.378 +
Services	0.075	-0.047	-0.036	-0.095	0.174	0.136*	0.068	0.103*	-0.042	-0.050	0.201 +	-0.014
No supervisory job	0.042	-0.188 +	-0.043	0.137 +	-0.200	-0.007	-0.058	0.039	0.161 +	-0.017	-0.013	-0.041
Household income	0.064 +	0.115 +	0.051*	0.116 +	0.075 +	0.048 +	0.126 +	0.141 +	0.121 +	0.123 +	0.255 +	0.097 +
H. income squared	-0.278 +	-0.227 +	-0.363	-0.547 +	-0.315	-0.139	-0.642 +	-0.632 +	-1.290 +	-0.462 +	-1.819 +	-0.215 +
Public sector	0.067	0.046	0.097*	-0.068	0.027	0.012	-0.004	-0.003	0.113*	0.023	0.135 +	0.142
Good health	-0.064	-0.180 +	-0.289 +	-0.280 +	-0.153	-0.254 +	-0.232 +	-0.166 +	-0.259 +	-0.220 +	-0.085 +	-0.063
Chronic illness	0.403 +	0.434 +	0.684 +	0.389 +	0.233 +	0.686 +	0.851 +	0.787 +	1.066 +	0.669 +	0.623 +	0.300 +
Hampered	0.178 +	0.123*	0.168 +	0.133*	-0.057	0.199 +	0.063	0.107 +	0.125 +	0.173 +	0.047	0.009
In hospital	0.075	0.170 +	0.513 +	0.417 +	0.332 +	0.478 +	0.518 +	0.373 +	0.158 +	0.368 +	0.398 +	0.225 +
Risk at job	-0.005	-0.120	0.052	-0.019	0.038	-0.052	0.160*	0.009	-0.065	0.064	0.171 +	0.188
Constant	0.841 +	-0.516 +	0.237	-0.064	1.027 +	-0.413	-0.717 +	-0.260*	-0.412 +	-0.299 +	-0.984 +	0.303
Second stage												
Age	-0.059 +	0.025	0.006	-0.026	-0.012	0.035	-0.013	-0.087 +	-0.058 +	-0.069 +	-0.007	-0.034
Age squared	0.041 +	-0.032	-0.026	0.001	-0.013	-0.066 +	-0.013	0.076 +	0.049 +	0.058 +	-0.005	0.021
Head of household	0.051	0.248 +	-0.150	0.036	0.632 +	0.012	-0.135	0.265 +	0.132	0.118	0.054	0.028
Married	0.550 +	-0.156	0.177	0.366 +	0.405 +	0.185	0.265	0.688 +	0.543 +	0.537 +	0.234 +	0.496 +
Divorced	0.293 +	-0.597 +	0.146	0.159	0.485*	0.148	0.237	0.491 +	0.596 +	0.390 +	-0.048	0.616 +
Household size	-0.181 +	0.046	-0.082 +	-0.106 +	-0.099 +	-0.138 +	-0.092 +	-0.078 +	-0.107 +	-0.095 +	-0.031*	-0.105 +
High education	-0.054	-0.204	0.063	0.207 +	0.392 +	0.166	0.035	-0.014	0.191 +	-0.171	0.082	0.126
Employed	-0.076	0.013	-0.375 +	0.100	0.135	-0.089	0.157	0.143	-0.125	-0.122	0.077	-0.002
Self-employed	-0.485 +	0.513	0.150	0.326*	-0.358	-0.409	-0.172	0.403 +	-0.106	-0.127	-0.093	-0.352 +
Unemployed	-0.018	0.288	-0.218 +	-0.114	-0.022	-0.012	-0.012	0.175*	-0.052	-0.065	0.195	0.395
Retired	-0.120	0.221	0.174	0.135	-0.429*	0.124	0.483	-0.036	0.259 +	0.655	0.232 +	0.175
Part time job	0.047	-0.187	-0.241 +	-0.139	-0.263	0.108	-0.067	0.012	-0.044	0.356 +	0.123	-0.291 +
Professional	-0.026	0.069	0.145	-0.193	-0.345*	0.236	0.284	-0.022	-0.032	0.086	0.320 +	0.408 +
Clerical	-0.013	-0.376*	0.234	-0.264*	-0.645 +	-0.110	0.150	-0.258 +	-0.037	0.216	0.250 +	0.479 +
Services	0.021	0.218	0.074	-0.415 +	-0.182	0.223	0.090	-0.194	0.134	-0.030	0.294 +	0.022
No supervisory job	-0.037	0.275*	0.355 +	0.174	-0.015	0.175	-0.074	0.000	0.109	0.052	-0.214 +	-0.097
Household income	0.105 +	-0.183 +	0.003	0.010	0.099 +	0.037	0.107*	-0.007	0.207 +	0.102 +	0.069	0.037
H. income squared	-0.583 +	0.429 +	-0.264	-0.156	-0.676 +	-0.005	-0.552	-0.078	-1.920 +	-1.070 +	-0.508	-0.348
Public sector	0.062	0.205	-0.070	0.047	0.034	-0.137	0.229	0.085	-0.034	0.247*	-0.078	0.113
Good health	-0.363 +	-0.437 +	-0.331 +	-0.411 +	-0.509 +	-0.337 +	-0.424 +	-0.309 +	-0.415 +	-0.458 +	-0.259 +	-0.474 +
Chronic illness	0.753 +	0.445 +	0.755 +	0.490 +	0.474 +	0.674 +	0.491 +	0.863 +	0.813 +	0.579 +	1.011 +	0.934 +
Hampered	0.444 +	0.145	0.158	0.389 +	0.124	0.147	-0.047	0.240 +	-0.004	0.288 +	-0.017	0.337 +
In hospital	0.308 +	0.353 +	0.404 +	0.586 +	0.635 +	0.363 +	0.489 +	0.356 +	0.266 +	0.415 +	0.336 +	0.423 +
Risk at job	-0.038	-0.225	-0.187	-0.240*	0.153	-0.002	-0.332*	0.067	-0.119	-0.231*	0.177*	0.091
Constant	2.392 +	-0.689	0.942 +	1.497 +	0.854 +	-0.089	1.219 +	1.843 +	2.074 +	1.685 +	0.626 +	1.092 +
Ln(alpha)	1.008 +	2.206 +	1.242 +	1.012 +	0.957	0.918 +	0.811 +	1.224 +	0.135	1.676 +	0.304 +	1.045 +
Log-L	15 867.92	4769.909	10 999.51	8985.694	3287.04	6952.288	5736.805	19 328.78	12 433.84	18 781.98	11 906.61	4718.41
LR test (β1 = β2; d.f. = 25)	213.01	118.14	325.04	161.22	130.16	179.86	273.21	392.80	476.29	433.12	290.36	416.54

Level of significance: + and * denote significance at the 5% and 10% levels.

Table 7.A1 Mean of the variables by sex and country

	Male														Female													
---	All	st-d	G	DK	NL	B	L	UK	IRL	I	GK	SP	P	A	All	st-d	G	DK	NL	B	L	UK	IRL	I	GK	SP	P	A
Observations	79959	—	7109	3877	6599	4562	1577	5599	6265	13564	8384	11492	8083	2648	82974	—	7192	4032	7281	4924	1624	5969	6182	13776	8882	11844	8569	2699
Visits to GP: observ.	77648	—	6906	3872	6597	4458	1571	4737	6251	13554	8110	11242	8029	2320	81705	—	7056	4026	7277	4836	1613	5514	6169	13764	8812	11684	8826	2428
Visits to GP: frequency	0.610	0.488	0.737	0.632	0.626	0.787	0.757	0.697	0.575	0.640	0.383	0.552	0.517	0.846	0.719	0.449	0.784	0.793	0.755	0.840	0.807	0.831	0.736	0.757	0.470	0.660	0.667	0.888
visits to GP: uncond. mean	2.394	4.805	3.645	1.936	1.898	3.314	2.540	2.556	2.258	2.644	1.199	2.358	1.869	3.711	3.526	5.807	4.456	3.285	3.139	4.372	3.156	4.214	3.613	3.848	1.676	3.683	3.151	4.603
Visits to SP: observ.	77114	—	6883	3871	6595	4376	1570	4740	6244	13552	8109	11240	8031	1903	81558	—	7049	4028	7277	4781	1613	5514	6164	13759	8812	11684	8533	2344
Visits to SP: frequency	0.293	0.455	0.460	0.236	0.300	0.370	0.435	0.300	0.170	0.257	0.241	0.304	0.223	0.584	0.445	0.497	0.706	0.308	0.386	0.604	0.768	0.358	0.230	0.414	0.380	0.462	0.394	0.835
Visits to SP: uncond. mean	1.072	3.433	2.263	0.676	1.170	1.300	1.483	0.935	0.459	0.781	1.027	1.143	0.714	2.061	1.720	4.113	3.592	1.040	1.908	2.286	2.709	1.147	0.770	1.302	1.502	1.797	1.357	2.902
Age	40.23	13.23	41.6	40.5	40.8	40.19	40.90	41.20	38.80	39.70	41.39	39.19	39.77	40.22	40.449	13.12	41.77	40.51	40.14	40.14	39.88	40.89	39.9	39.9	40.93	39.82	41.38	40.75
Age-squared	1793	1095	1906	1795	1807	1766	1825	1858	1696	1756	1897	1722	1774	1803	1808	1092	1905	1800	1758	1767	1741	1829	1730	1769	1858	1773	1900	1835
Head of the house	0.675	0.468	0.719	0.702	0.869	0.568	0.778	0.776	0.629	0.630	0.715	0.648	0.596	0.506	0.191	0.393	0.285	0.427	0.197	0.146	0.195	0.255	0.140	0.123	0.142	0.143	0.176	0.384
Married	0.682	0.466	0.741	0.719	0.783	0.737	0.744	0.697	0.598	0.628	0.708	0.631	0.673	0.697	0.705	0.456	0.764	0.739	0.777	0.722	0.749	0.714	0.655	0.668	0.730	0.656	0.690	0.712
Sep.-divorced-widowed	0.030	0.171	0.041	0.061	0.034	0.051	0.046	0.065	0.015	0.016	0.018	0.021	0.023	0.030	0.081	0.273	0.088	0.110	0.077	0.113	0.080	0.123	0.065	0.053	0.075	0.071	0.091	0.099
Size of the household	3.645	1.507	3.073	2.790	3.153	3.320	3.380	3.094	4.485	3.806	3.716	4.054	3.983	3.698	3.561	1.493	2.986	2.809	3.052	3.266	3.344	3.058	4.476	3.739	3.616	3.965	3.818	3.588
Educated (college)	0.171	0.377	0.283	0.320	0.210	0.284	0.201	0.261	0.137	0.075	0.183	0.179	0.036	0.062	0.141	0.348	0.123	0.323	0.155	0.298	0.110	0.211	0.118	0.060	0.172	0.156	0.041	0.065
Employed	0.580	0.494	0.717	0.729	0.718	0.627	0.682	0.633	0.514	0.508	0.433	0.508	0.589	0.662	0.392	0.488	0.503	0.643	0.424	0.474	0.442	0.524	0.345	0.319	0.308	0.254	0.413	0.443
Self-employed	0.157	0.364	0.064	0.075	0.055	0.113	0.087	0.147	0.201	0.180	0.324	0.149	0.189	0.108	0.054	0.227	0.026	0.030	0.021	0.030	0.030	0.050	0.026	0.061	0.081	0.053	0.104	0.076
Retired	0.081	0.272	0.049	0.068	0.049	0.059	0.028	0.084	0.119	0.101	0.069	0.131	0.053	0.033	0.084	0.277	0.062	0.107	0.145	0.054	0.017	0.027	0.041	0.089	0.104	0.110	0.064	0.030
Unemployed	0.064	0.245	0.082	0.056	0.023	0.070	0.134	0.047	0.033	0.096	0.083	0.032	0.061	0.118	0.046	0.209	0.067	0.084	0.003	0.068	0.046	0.058	0.006	0.070	0.045	0.004	0.063	0.083
Part-time	0.021	0.145	0.010	0.023	0.028	0.014	0.013	0.028	0.031	0.022	0.033	0.020	0.013	0.010	0.094	0.292	0.144	0.124	0.185	0.121	0.122	0.177	0.083	0.060	0.051	0.047	0.054	0.099
Professional	0.231	0.421	0.320	0.334	0.413	0.266	0.284	0.313	0.220	0.141	0.209	0.164	0.136	0.220	0.153	0.360	0.244	0.269	0.215	0.145	0.237	0.214	0.131	0.098	0.108	0.098	0.113	0.123
Clerk	0.064	0.245	0.053	0.045	0.057	0.125	0.075	0.070	0.039	0.103	0.049	0.042	0.048	0.056	0.092	0.289	0.111	0.146	0.098	0.140	0.130	0.158	0.085	0.096	0.056	0.045	0.060	0.117
Services employee	0.056	0.230	0.030	0.046	0.042	0.036	0.056	0.051	0.052	0.060	0.060	0.070	0.078	0.066	0.079	0.270	0.084	0.145	0.079	0.057	0.068	0.103	0.078	0.056	0.060	0.067	0.106	0.113
Not supervisory job	0.361	0.480	0.387	0.448	0.430	0.357	0.390	0.243	0.337	0.171	0.313	0.331	0.137	0.355	0.283	0.451	0.378	0.480	0.328	0.361	0.321	0.238	0.248	0.243	0.191	0.197	0.351	0.310
Household income	2.410	1.641	2.698	2.666	2.486	3.090	4.532	2.771	2.865	2.190	1.870	2.093	1.640	3.350	2.299	1.607	2.541	2.529	2.400	2.949	4.447	2.585	2.751	2.117	1.773	2.017	1.552	3.155
Household income sq.	8.498	24.139	9.958	11.04	7.983	12.74	27.00	10.78	11.96	6.512	5.116	6.226	4.154	14.79	7.867	20.885	9.022	9.049	7.685	11.96	26.80	9.701	11.00	6.197	4.648	5.944	3.952	13.37
Pub.	0.169	0.374	0.215	0.212	0.183	0.211	0.199	0.161	0.173	0.171	0.159	0.119	0.137	0.186	0.145	0.352	0.198	0.360	0.155	0.206	0.150	0.198	0.120	0.124	0.083	0.078	0.130	0.140
Good health	0.764	0.425	0.747	0.859	0.821	0.819	0.763	0.742	0.872	0.697	0.836	0.739	0.655	0.783	0.719	0.449	0.729	0.828	0.769	0.760	0.711	0.743	0.850	0.639	0.812	0.689	0.544	0.775
Chronic illness	0.164	0.376	0.224	0.241	0.200	0.133	0.190	0.249	0.142	0.096	0.103	0.173	0.170	0.191	0.172	0.378	0.217	0.281	0.222	0.126	0.179	0.276	0.150	0.090	0.109	0.178	0.203	0.165
Hampered	0.137	0.344	0.185	0.135	0.173	0.124	0.181	0.162	0.115	0.114	0.104	0.108	0.164	0.173	0.153	0.360	0.176	0.179	0.202	0.148	0.181	0.184	0.125	0.124	0.115	0.130	0.146	0.140
At hospital	0.069	0.254	0.105	0.054	0.054	0.091	0.115	0.074	0.069	0.067	0.056	0.061	0.041	0.105	0.086	0.280	0.123	0.109	0.089	0.107	0.139	0.112	0.101	0.075	0.056	0.067	0.045	0.140
Risk at job	0.106	0.307	0.088	0.087	0.071	0.085	0.056	0.147	0.088	0.119	0.162	0.122	0.073	0.061	0.064	0.245	0.068	0.072	0.053	0.061	0.020	0.088	0.048	0.067	0.092	0.058	0.054	0.039

Greece and Portugal) while the TPM are preferred to LCM in visits to the SP for a set of countries (the Netherlands, Ireland, Greece, Italy, Spain and Portugal for males, and Denmark, Ireland, Greece, Spain and Portugal for females) and for the aggregation of the countries in which there are not direct access to SPs. Furthermore, the forecasting power of the TPM turns out to be better than expected as the LCM are more often rejected in the hold-out sample. Together the in-sample and cross-validation results cast some doubts about the general superiority of the LCM over the TPM and provide strong evidence on the fact that the traditional failure of the TPM may be due to the violation of the single illness spell requirement.

A FEW COMMENTS TO RESULTS FROM COUNTRY-SPECIFIC ESTIMATES

Our country specific results are presented in Tables 7.5a, 7.5b, 7.6a and 7.6b. They suggest both important regularities and differences across countries. Among the latter we find statistically significant differences in the behaviour of men and women specially in the decision to visit and the number of visits to SPs. As regards the effect of the quadratic age controls, we find important differences by gender, country and type of doctor.

Among the regularities we stress, first, that the health stock variables are major determinants of the utilization of health services, both for males and females, for GPs and SPs and for the contact and frequency stages of the decision process. Their effect is similar in the GP and SP count equations: good self-perceived health has a negative effect on the frequency of the visits (also on the probability of contacting the SP), and the rest of dummy variables, which act as indicators of a low health endowment, have a positive effect on the frequency of the visits to them (and also on the probability of contacting a SP). Among all health-related variables, the dummy for individuals hampered in their activities is the one less significant across countries. The results for females are slightly less precise but go in the same direction.

Second, we do not find any effect of income on the number of visits to the GP, although income has a concave effect on the decision to contact a SP. The positive effect of income on the frequency of visits to the SP for females could be explained as a form of induced demand. Finally, as regards demographics, we find that household size negatively affects the use of health services, thus indicating economies of scale in the production of health within the household. Education and some occupation variables show a mixed effect of income (positive) and efficiency (negative) in the production of health.

CONCLUDING REMARKS

In this work we analyze both the decision to visit a GP and an SP for a sample of EU countries using data from the ECHP. The major novelty of this chapter is that it uses a homogeneous and comparable data set to estimate a common model of demand for physician services for a group of European countries. It contributes to the literature on utilization of health services, because it provides economic and statistical evidence on the more appropriate econometric specification for GPs and SPs health demand equations, based on intuition, and tested using a battery of diagnostics and a cross-validation exercise.

We have obtained indirect evidence that the multi-spell problem, which is present in the ECHP, may crucially influence the validity of TPM and LCM. In particular, our results suggest that LCM are more appropriate than TPM in the GP equations, more likely to suffer from the multi-spell problem in our data set, while evidence of the opposite is found as regards SP equations, since visits to SPs are less likely to suffer from the multi-spell problem.

ACKNOWLEDGEMENTS

We are very grateful for many helpful comments from the participants in the 9th Health and Econometrics Workshop and specially to Raquel Carrasco, Eddy van Doorslaer, Daniele Fabbri, Berthold Herrendorf, Andrew Jones, Owen O'Donnell, and two anonymous referees. This study was supported by an unrestricted educational grant from The Merck Foundation, the philanthropic arm of Merck & Co. Inc., Whitehouse Station, New Jersey, USA, and by DGES PB98-1058-C03-02/03.

DATA APPENDIX

The variables included in the analysis are grouped in the following five categories:

1. *Personal and household characteristics*:
- Marital status: two dummies, one taking value 1 if the individual is married, and the other equalling 1 if the individual is separated/divorced/widowed.
- A dummy for the individual being head of the household, dated in wave −1.
- Age and its square.
- Education: a dummy for the individual having a third level of education recognized.
- Household size.

2. *Labour force status characteristics*:

- Dummies controlling for self-employment, unemployment, retired part-time job and, working in the public sector, dated in wave -1.
- Occupational dummies: professionals, clerks, services workers, dated in wave -1.
- Risk at job, dated in wave -1.

3. *Health-related variables*:

- A dummy if the individual reports himself as having good health, dated in wave -1.
- A dummy for individuals having a chronic physical or mental health problem, current (since it was not asked for in the first wave of the survey).
- A dummy if the individual is hampered in daily activities by any physical or mental health problem, illness or disability, dated in wave -1.
- A dummy for individual was admitted as in-patient in a hospital during the previous year, dated in wave -1.

4. *Income variables*:

- Household income and its squared (in 10^5 PPP units), dated in wave -1.

In Table 7.A1 we present summary statistics by sex and by sex and country.

REFERENCES

1. Grossman, M. *The Demand for Health – A Theoretical and Empirical Investigation*. New York: Columbia University Press, 1972.
2. Wagstaff, A. The demand for health. Some new empirical evidence. *J. Health Econ.* 1986; **5**: 195–233.
3. Cromwell, J. and Michell, J. Physician-induced demand for surgery. *J. Health Econ.* 1986; **1**: 293–313.
4. Pohlmeier, W. and Ulrich, V. An econometric model of the two-part decision making in the demand for health care. *J. Human Res.* 1995; **30**: 339–361.
5. Santos-Silva, J.M.C. and Windmeijer, F. Two-part multiple spell models for health care demand. IFS WP Series No. W99/2,1999.
6. Heckman, J.J. and Singer, B. A method of minimizing the distributional impact in econometric models for duration data. *Econometrica* 1984; **52**: 271–320.
7. Seb, P. and Trivedi, P.K. Demand for medical care by the elderly in the United States: a finite mixture approach. *J. Appl. Econometrics* 1999; **12**: 313–336.
8. Deb, P. and Trivedi, P.K. The structure of demand for health care: latent class versus two-part models. Mimeo, 1999.
9. Deb, P. and Holmes, A.M. Estimates of use and costs of behavioural health care: a comparison of standard and finite mixture models, *Health Econ.* 2000; **9**: 475–489.
10. Deb, P. Building a better mousetrap: a finite mixture model for health care expenditures. Mimeo, 2000.
11. Santos-Silva, J.M.C. and Windmeijer, F. Endogeneity in count data models: an application to demand for health care. *J. Appl. Econometrics* 1997; **12**: 281–294.
12. Vera-Hernández, A.M. Duplicate coverage and demand for health care. The case of Catalonia, *Health Econ.* 1999; **8**: 579–598.
13. Kenkel, D.S. Consumer health information and the demand for medical care. *Rev. Econ. Stat.* 1990; **22**: 587–595.
14. Grytten, J. and Sørensen, R. Type of contract and supplier-induced demand for primary physicians in Norway. *J. Health Econ.* 2001; **20**: 379–393.
15. Winkelmann, R. Count data models with selectivity. *Econometrics Rev.* 1998; **17**: 339–359.
16. Cameron, A.C. and Trivedi, P.K. Econometric models based on count data: comparisons and applications of some estimators and tests. *J. Appl. Econometrics* 1986; **1**: 29–53.
17. Cameron, A.C. and Trivedi, P.K. *Regression Analysis of Count Data*. Cambridge: Cambridge University Press, 1998.
18. Hausman, J., Hall, B.H. and Griliches, Z. Econometric models for count data with an application to the patents-R&D relationship. *Econometrica* 1984; **52**: 909–938.
19. Cameron, A.C. and Trivedi, P.K. Regression-based tests for over-dispersion in the Poisson model. *J. Econometrics* 1990; **46**: 347–364.
20. Jiménez-Martínez, S., Labeaga, J.M. and Martínez-Granado, M. An empirical analysis of the demand for physician services across the European Union. WP 01/07, Instituto de Estudios Fiscales, 2001.
21. Mullahy, J. Specification and testing of some modified count data models. *J. Econometrics* 1986; **33**: 341–365.
22. Everitt, B.S. and Hand, D.J. *Finite Mixture Distributions*. London: Chapman and Hall, 1981.
23. Böhning, D. A review of reliable maximum likelihood algorithms for semiparametric mixture models. *J. Stat. Planning Inference* 1995; **47**: 5–28.
24. Peracchi, F. The European Community Household Panel: a review. *Empirical Econ.* 2000, in press.
25. Anderson, K. and Burkhauser, R. The retirement-health nexus: a new measure of an old puzzle. *J. Human Res.* 1985; **20**: 315–330.

8

Proportional Treatment Effects for Count Response Panel Data: Effects of Binary Exercise on Health Care Demand

MYOUNG-JAE LEE[1] AND SATORU KOBAYASHI[2]

[1]*Sunkyunkwan University, Seoul, South Korea and* [2]*University of Tsukuba, Ibaraki, Japan*

INTRODUCTION

Rapidly increasing health care cost is a serious financial problem for most developed countries. There are at least three ways to reduce the health care cost. The first is revamping the whole health care system, which, however, takes time and often faces strong resistance from the parties concerned. The second is making minor changes in copayment rates or in health insurance coverage; most health care studies estimate the health care demand elasticity with respect to the copayment rates, and (quasi-) experimental evidence suggests about 20% (Phelps [1]) although many other numbers have also appeared in the literature. The third is health promotion programmes, which encourage people to adopt a healthy lifestyle and thus aim to reduce health care demand. There are many aspects in a healthy lifestyle: no drinking, no smoking, wearing a seat belt, exercise and so on. In this paper, we focus on exercise: our goal is finding effects of exercise on health care demand, which is a count response (the number of doctor office visits or hospitalization days). Note that it is not always the unhealthy that demand health care: healthy people may demand more health care, e.g. if they are more concerned about health.

The literature on *exercise effects on health care demand* is thin although there are countless papers on *exercise effect on health*, because health has so many dimensions. Leigh and Fries [2] observed 1558 Bank of America retirees for 12 months and analysed relationships between healthy habits and subsequent medical costs. Their results suggest that healthy habits such as absence of smoking, excessive drinking and excess body mass and

increased exercise and seat belt use were associated with roughly $372–598 of direct cost saving and $4298 of total cost saving per person per year in the nominal term in the year of their survey. Hofer and Kats [3] showed that there is a positive association between the number of healthy behaviours and use of preventive services such as Pap smears, dental care and physical exams; this shows that health concern matters. Both studies, however, pay no attention to 'endogeneity problems', one of which is that health habits including exercise may be chosen with health care usage taken into account. Huijsman *et al.* [4] mention the difficulties in analysing the effect of exercise on health care demand in their English summary (the paper is written in Dutch).

For our analysis, we use a 'two-wave' panel data drawn from the Health Retirement Study. A single wave consists of over 10 000 relatively old individuals. This is observational non-experimental data, and is thus subject to biases due to non-random selection of treatment (i.e. exercise). However, using non-experimental data seems unavoidable: even if one can do a randomized experiment, it will be virtually impossible to force the subjects to do exercise (a partial compliance problem) exactly as prescribed. Worse yet, since exercise should be done over some period of time, it will be impossible to control for other factors; the most problematic would be the risk-taking behaviour of the subjects: since they do exercise, they may feel that they can afford to smoke or drink, just as seat belt use can lead to faster driving. Despite being observational, our data has some advantages. First, the size of the data is quite big, and even after removing observations with missing or imputed values, still a size-

Econometric Analysis of Health Data. Edited by Andrew M. Jones and Owen O'Donnell

able number of observations remain. Second, the data are in panel form and this has the following well-known advantage over cross-section data.

Suppose we are interested in the effect of marriage on health care demand. If we use cross-section data, we can compare two people, one married and the other not. The two people may differ in observed variables, which can be controlled for by regression analysis or conditioning (or grouping) approach; if not controlled for, the observed difference can cause an 'overt bias'. The two people may differ also in unobserved variables, which can cause a 'covert bias'. In panel data, we can compare a single individual before and after the marriage, and thus there is less room for changes in observed or unobserved variables, meaning less overt or covert bias. Putting it differently, one's past is the better control for one's future than somebody else's future is.

For old people, most of them have been married for a long time. There may very well be an unobserved trait characterizing people (un-)married long-term. The trait may be (i) a cause (say, genes) for long-term (un)married life, or (ii) an outcome of long-term (un)married life. If (ii) is the case, we will be measuring a long-term effect of marriage on health care demand by comparing married and unmarried groups in cross-section data; the long-term effect consists of the short-term 'just-married' effect and the effect of staying in the marriage for a long time. If (i) is the case, the cross-section data will give a biased estimate (due to genes) for the short-run effect. In a panel data spanning over a couple of years, we can control for (or eliminate) the unobserved trait so long as it is time-invariant over the span. That is, the panel data estimate will render the short-term effect regardless of (i) or (ii). If, however, two panel waves are far apart so that the unobserved trait becomes time-variant, this advantage of the panel data may not hold.

The rest of the paper is organized as follows. In the next section, we introduce conditional and marginal treatment effects for count data, which will be the basis for drawing conclusions later. In the third section, data is described in detail. In the fourth section, regression estimators used in this paper are presented. In the fifth section, we present our first data analysis using conditioning (or grouping) approaches after selecting a few important variables to control for. In the sixth section, we present the second analysis using regression models. In the final section, conclusions are drawn. The advantage of the conditioning approaches relative to the regression approaches is allowing for unknown (non-parametric) ways the conditioned variables can influence health care demand, whereas the disadvantage is that we cannot condition on too many variables (a dimension problem in practice); these are why we apply both.

CONDITIONAL AND MARGINAL TREATMENT EFFECTS FOR COUNT RESPONSE

Consider an observed response variable y_i for an individual i and two treatments 0 and 1, with 0 being the base (or no) treatment and 1 being the new treatment of interest. Let $y_{ji}, j = 0, 1$, denote the 'potential' outcome when individual i receives treatment j exogenously (i.e. when treatment j is forced upon i rather than self-selected by i). Typically only one outcome is observed while the other (called 'counter-factual') is not; e.g. for the effects of a PhD education on lifetime earnings, only one treatment (PhD education or not) is available per person. The individual treatment effect is $y_{1i} - y_{0i}$, which is however not identified. In the rest of this paper, often we will omit i indexing individuals.

Ideally, one would like to know the joint distribution for (y_0, y_1), which is a tall order however. A little less ambitious goal would be knowing the distribution of $y_1 - y_0$ as in Heckman et al. [5]; but even this is hard. Then one can look for some aspects of $y_1 - y_0$, and the most popular choice is the mean effect $E(y_1 - y_0)$, because $E(y_1 - y_0) = E(y_1) - E(y_0)$: the mean of $y_1 - y_0$ can be found from the two marginal means. This is thanks to the linearity of $E(\cdot)$, which does not hold in general for other functions such as quantiles. Although a headway for median effect has been made by Lee [6], quantile effects are not identified in general unless strong assumptions are imposed on (y_0, y_1). Nonetheless, considering quantile effects brings up the obvious point: there are many different interesting treatment effects other than $E(y_1 - y_0)$. One extreme example is an income policy that takes away incomes from all but one person and gives them all to the single person; here the mean effect is zero while median effect will be substantial. In the literature (e.g. Heckman et al. [7]), indeed, the fact that there are many interesting treatment effects has been emphasized, but the focus has been on various conditional mean effects such as the mean effect on the treated, on the participants and so on. In the following, we introduce two mean-based 'proportional' treatment effects; they are applicable for any y, but particularly well suited for count responses with an exponential regression function. We start with a cross-section model, and then move on to panel data.

Let d_i and x_i denote an exercise variable and a covariate vector, respectively for individual i. What is observed is

$$x_i, d_i, y_i (= (1 - d_i)y_{0i} + d_i y_{1i}), \quad i = 1, \ldots, N$$

Suppose that the potential response variables satisfy

$$E(y_{ji} | x_i) = \exp(z_i'\eta + j \cdot m_i'\alpha), \quad j = 0, 1 \qquad (8.1)$$

where m_i is a $k_m \times 1$ vector of components of x_i interacting with exercise while z_i is a $k_2 \times 1$ vector of components of x_i, and η and α are conformable parameter vectors; both z_i and m_i always include 1. As an example of m_i, a dummy variable for heart-related illnesses may interact with exercise, for people with heart problems tend to consult their doctors for exercise.

Define a 'conditional (on x_i) treatment effect' of exercise on y_i as

$$E(y_{1i} - y_{0i} | x_i)/E(y_{0i} | x_i)$$
$$= E(y_{1i} | x_i)/E(y_{0i} | x_i) - 1 = \exp(m_i'\alpha) - 1 \qquad (8.2)$$

This effect differs from the usual conditional effect $E(y_{1i} - y_{0i} | x_i)$ by the denominator $E(y_{0i} | x_i)$, which removes the multiplicative term $\exp(z_i'\eta)$ common to both $E(y_{1i} | x_i)$ and $E(y_{0i} | x_i)$. In the usual linear regression, say $E(y_{ji} | x_i) = z_i'\eta + j \cdot m_i'\alpha$, such common terms do not appear in the difference $E(y_{1i} - y_{0i} | x_i)$; the advantage of Equation 8.2 is, regardless of whether y_{ji} is a count response or not, removing multiplicative as well as additive terms common for $E(y_{0i} | x_i)$ and $E(y_{1i} | x_i)$. Equation 8.2 shows the proportional change relative to the base level $E(y_{0i} | x_i)$, and it varies across i: we can get as many as N individual effects. Equation 8.2 is bounded from below by -1; this is natural, for one cannot decrease health care demand by more than the current level of the demand. In the usual regression analysis, one would say that the exercise has no effect if $\alpha = 0$: this implies $\exp(m_i'\alpha) - 1 = 0$. In representing the effect of the treatment, $\exp(m_i'\alpha) - 1$ is better than α, for it is a proportional change free of z_i and it takes the values of the interaction terms into account as well.

For an 'unconditional (or marginal) effect', m_i should be removed; one choice is integrating m_i out:

$$E\{\exp(m_i'\alpha) - 1\} \qquad (8.3)$$

the sample version of which is the arithmetic average $(1/N)\Sigma_i\{\exp(m_i'\alpha) - 1\}$. For the exponential model, however, a better way to remove m_i than the arithmetic average is the geometric average: with $\bar{m} \equiv (1/N)\Sigma_i m_i$,

$$\left\{\prod_{i=1}^{N} \exp(m_i'\alpha)\right\}^{1/N} - 1 = \exp(\bar{m}'\alpha) - 1 \qquad (8.4)$$

which is the same as the conditional effect with m_i evaluated at $\bar{m}$. An estimate for this marginal, or (geometric) average, effect is

$$\exp(\bar{m}'a_N) - 1$$

where a_N is a consistent estimator for α. We will use this as *the* treatment effect of interest in the remainder of this paper.

Once we get the marginal effect, we will want to construct a confidence interval (CI) for $\exp(\bar{m}'\alpha) - 1$. Taking $\bar{m}$ as an evaluation point, we will ignore the error $\bar{m} - E(m)$ and focus only on the error $a_N - \alpha$; it goes without saying that $\exp(\bar{m}'a_N) - 1$ is consistent for $\exp(E(m)'\alpha) - 1$. Let $\beta \equiv (\eta', \alpha')'$, and suppose, for some estimator b_N for β, we have

$$\sqrt{N}(b_N - \beta) \rightarrow N(0, C)$$

for an asymptotic variance matrix C consistently estimated by C_N. There are a number of valid asymptotic CIs for the marginal effect, but we will use the following *asymmetric* 95% CI: with $\hat{m} \equiv (0_{k_z}', \bar{m}')'$ where 0_{k_z} is the $k_z \times 1$ zero vector,

$$[\exp\{\hat{m}'b_N - 1.96(\hat{m}'C_N\hat{m}/N)^{1/2}\} - 1,$$
$$\exp(\hat{m}'b_N) - 1 + 1.96\exp(\hat{m}'b_N)(\hat{m}'C_N\hat{m}/N)^{1/2}]$$

note that $\hat{m}'b_N = \bar{m}'a_N$ and $\hat{m}'\beta = \bar{m}'\alpha$. The upper bound was based upon the usual Taylor's expansion of $\exp(\hat{m}'\beta) - 1$ around $\hat{m}'\beta = \hat{m}'b_N$ and the lower bound was obtained by applying the transformation $\exp(\cdot) - 1$ to $\hat{m}'b_N - 1.96(\hat{m}'C_N\hat{m}/N)^{1/2}(\leq \hat{m}'b_N)$. Observe that the lower bound was bounded below by -1 as $\exp(\hat{m}'\beta) - 1$ is, while the upper bound with 1.96 replaced by -1.96 does not respect this bound -1, which explains why we used the asymmetric CI.

So far, we took consistent estimator b_N as given, which we deal with now. Assume

$$E(y | x, d) = \exp(z'\eta + d \cdot m'\alpha) \qquad (8.5)$$

Under Equation 8.1, it will be shown shortly that Equation 8.5 is equivalent to

$$E(y_j | x, d = j) = E(y_j | x), \quad j = 0, 1 \qquad (8.6)$$

which is the usual no 'selection bias' (or the mean-independence of y_j from d given x) condition: d is allowed to be related to y_j but only through x. With (5), it is easy to find b_N; e.g. a non-linear least squares estimator for β using Equation 8.5 will do. Turning to the equivalence between Equation 8.5 and Equation 8.6, first Equation 8.5 implies Equation 8.6 because

$$E(y_j | x, d = j) = E(y | x, d = j)$$
$$= \exp(z'\eta + j \cdot m'\alpha) = E(y_j | x) \qquad (8.7)$$

second, Equation 8.6 implies Equation 8.5 because

$$E(y \mid x, d) = (1 - d) \cdot E(y \mid x, d = 0)$$
$$+ d \cdot E(y \mid x, d = 1)$$
$$= (1 - d) \cdot E(y_0 \mid x, d = 0)$$
$$+ d \cdot E(y_1 \mid x, d = 1)$$
$$= (1 - d) \cdot E(y_0 \mid x) + d \cdot E(y_1 \mid x)$$
$$= \exp(z'\eta + d \cdot m'\alpha) \tag{8.8}$$

Although it is easy to find a consistent estimator under no selection bias (i.e. no endogeneity of d), zero selection bias may not be plausible. In panel data, there is a simple way to relax this assumption. Consider panel data, and assume, analogously to Equation 8.5,

$$E(y_{it} \mid x_{it}, d_{it}, \delta_i) = \exp(z'_{it}\eta + d_{it} \cdot m'_{it}\alpha + \delta_i) \tag{8.9}$$

where the additional subscript t is attached to all observed variables, and δ_i is a time-invariant unobserved term possibly related to components of x_{it}. Analogously to Equation 8.1, suppose

$$E(y_{jit} \mid x_{it}) = \exp(z'_{it} + j \cdot m'_{it}\alpha), \quad j = 0, 1 \tag{8.10}$$

Under Equation 8.10, analogously to Equation 8.5 and Equation 8.6, Equation 8.9 is equivalent to (omitting i)

$$E(y_{jt} \mid x_t, d_t = j, \delta) = E(y_{jt} \mid x_t, \delta) \tag{8.11}$$

d_t is allowed to be related to y_{jt} through δ as well as x_t, which is weaker than Equation 8.6. Since

$$E(y_t \mid x_t, d_t)$$
$$= \exp(z'_t\eta + d_t \cdot m'_t\alpha) \cdot E(\exp(\delta) \mid x_t, d_t) \tag{8.12}$$

so long as $E(\exp(\delta) \mid x_t, d_t)$ is not a constant, the simple cross-section non-linear least squares estimator of y_t on x_t and d_t will be inconsistent. But in the panel data literature, '(first-)difference'-type estimators for β allow δ to be related to x_t and d_t in an arbitrary fashion.

Regardless of consistent estimation, the conditional treatment effect Equation 8.2 applies also to panel data: the conditional treatment effect at time t is, invoking Equation 8.10,

$$E(y_{1t} - y_{0t} \mid x_t)/E(y_{0t} \mid x_t)$$
$$= E(y_{1t} \mid x_t)/E(y_{0t} \mid x_t) - 1 = \exp(m'_{it}\alpha) - 1 \tag{8.13}$$

Since the cross-section sample mean $\bar{m}_t$ varies over time,

evaluating Equation 8.13 at $\bar{m}_t$ shows the varying marginal effect of the treatment.

As well known, in (first-)difference panel data estimators, the coefficients of time-invariant regressors are not identified. This means that $E(t_{1t} - y_{0t} \mid x_t)$ is not identified so long as there is a single time-invariant regressor. Our conditional effects Equation 8.2 and Equation 8.13 were in fact designed anticipating this problem: since exercise is time-variant, the interaction terms are all time-variant, and consequently α is identified even for (first-)difference panel estimators.

DATA DESCRIPTION: HEALTH RETIREMENT STUDY

The Heath and Retirement Study (HRS) from the Health and Retirement Study Research Center in University of Michigan is a nationwide longitudinal study focusing on health, retirement and economic status of people born mainly between 1931 and 1941. This survey has been held every 2 years since 1992. Wave 1 (1992) and wave 2 (1994) complete releases are available as of 1 October 1999. The sample size of wave 1 and 2 is 12 652 and 11 596, respectively, and there are 11 522 subjects who participated in both surveys. The final data used for our analysis consists of 8484 subjects in each wave, after removing subjects with either missing or imputed values in the variables selected for our analysis. Table 8.1 lists the variables used, with their summary statistics provided in Table 8.2.

In HRS, two health care use variables are available: the number of doctor visits (VIS) and hospital days (HOS); here doctors include specialists (psychiatrists included too) as well as general practitioners. But HOS has too many zeros (88.6%), and as such it does not seem to be appropriate for our regression approaches. We will use only VIS for our regression approaches later, while both VIS and HOS will be used for the conditioning (grouping) approaches. In wave 1, VIS and HOS were asked for the last 12 months, but they were asked in wave 2 for the interval since the wave 1 interview. The interval varies across individuals. To deal with this problem, we redefined wave 2 response y_{i2} as y_{i2}/τ_i where τ_i is the interval for individual i with $\tau_i = 1$ for 1 year interval so that wave 1 response y_{i1} can be taken as $y_{i1}/1$. Since the frequency in 2 years may not be twice the frequency in 1 year, which is a 'duration dependence', we will use τ_i and τ_i^2 as a regressor for our empirical analysis to account for the duration dependence. The mean and standard deviation (SD) of τ_i in wave 2 are 1.89 and 0.19, respectively.

In HRS, there are two variables on exercise: light exercise (LEX) and vigorous exercise (VEX). LEX includes walking, dancing, gardening, golfing, bowling, etc., and

Table 8.1 Variables (other than responses and exercises)

τ: Interval between interviews (years)
Age (year)
Married $(1, 0)$
Job dummy $(1, 0)$
Work hour (per week)
Income ($1000)
Schooling (year)
Male $(1, 0)$
Race $(1, 0)$: Rc1: white
    Rc2: black
    Rc3: Asian
    Rc4: Hispanic
    R54: Native American
Hypertension $(1, 0)$
Diabetes $(1, 0)$
Lung diseases $(1, 0)$
Heart diseases $(1, 0)$
Emotion/Nerve problem $(1, 0)$
Arthritis/Rheumatism $(1, 0)$
Pain $(1, 0)$
Residence $(1, 0)$: Rs1: New England
    Rs2: Middle Atlantic
    Rs3: East North Central
    Rs4: West North Central
    Rs5: South Atlantic
    Rs6: East South Central
    Rs7: West South Central
    Rs8: Mountain
    Rs9: Pacific

J1: Managerial specialty operation
J2: Professional specialty operation and technical support
J3: Sales
J4: Clerical, administrative support
J5: Service: private household, cleaning, building
J6: Service: protection
J7: Service, food preparation
J8: Health services
J9: Personal services
J10: Farming, forestry
J11: Mechanics and repair
J12: Construction trade and extractors
J13: Precision production
J14: Operators: machine
J15: Operators: transport, etc.
J16: Operators: handlers, etc.
J17: Member of armed forces
Health insurance $(1, 0)$: H1: Medicare
H2: Medicaid
H3: CHAMPS/VA
H4: Other government plan
H5: Group insurance

VEX includes aerobics, running, swimming, bicycling, etc. The question on exercise in wave 1 asks the frequency for the last 12 months in five categories:

Never, less than once a month,

1–3 times a month,

1–2 times a week, 3 or more a week

The question in wave 2 asks the frequency for the interval since the wave 1 interview: 'How often do you participate in physical activity?' and 'What interval was that?' We converted the frequency here into one appropriate for the five categories. But then we found that some categories are not well defined with too few observations, and that people change their exercise habits too much across two waves, which may be a recollection error. Given below are the transition probabilities for exercise: in a given row, the transition probabilities from a given exercise category at wave 1 to the categories at wave 2 are presented (thus, the sum in a given row in one):

LEX transition matrix

$t = 1 \backslash t = 2$	0	1	2	3	4
0	0.433	0.019	0.081	0.136	0.331
1	0.212	0.059	0.184	0.171	0.373
2	0.130	0.041	0.165	0.234	0.429
3	0.084	0.012	0.126	0.265	0.513
4	0.061	0.005	0.045	0.165	0.723

VEX transition matrix

$t = 1 \backslash t = 2$	0	1	2	3	4
0	0.626	0.044	0.151	0.079	0.099
1	0.423	0.083	0.248	0.137	0.109
2	0.282	0.055	0.323	0.213	0.127
3	0.232	0.036	0.258	0.287	0.187
4	0.195	0.027	0.123	0.273	0.381

Table 8.2 Summary statistics for variables

	Wave 1					Wave 2				
	Mean	SD	Min.	Med.	Max.	Mean	SD	Min.	Med.	Max.
HOS	0.60	3.40	0	0	91	0.65	2.88	0	0	76
VIS	3.64	6.01	0	2	80	3.34	4.91	0	2	78
τ (interview interval)	1	0	1	1	1	1.89	0.19	1.31	1.88	2.60
LEX	0.75	0.44	0	1	1	0.78	0.41	0	1	1
VEX	0.24	0.43	0	0	1	0.30	0.46	0	0	1
Age	55.31	5.49	23	55	82	57.31	5.49	25	57	84
Married	0.83	0.38	0	1	1	0.81	0.39	0	1	1
Job dummy	0.69	0.46	0	1	1	0.64	0.48	0	1	1
Work hour	27.88	21.38	0	40	95	25.52	21.79	0	35	95
Income	55.72	48.78	−1.08	46	625.2	60.03	87.20	−4.9	42.28	1570
Schooling	12.19	3.18	0	12	17	12.19	3.18	0	12	17
Male	0.46	0.50	0	0	1	0.46	0.50	0	0	1
Hypertension	0.36	0.48	0	0	1	0.41	0.49	0	0	1
Diabetes	0.10	0.30	0	0	1	0.12	0.32	0	0	1
Lung diseases	0.07	0.26	0	0	1	0.09	0.28	0	0	1
Heart diseases	0.11	0.31	0	0	1	0.14	0.35	0	0	1
Emotion/Nerve	0.10	0.29	0	0	1	0.13	0.33	0	0	1
Arthritis/Rheumatism	0.36	0.48	0	0	1	0.44	0.50	0	0	1
Pain	0.23	0.42	0	0	1	0.25	0.43	0	0	1
H1	0.06	0.23	0	0	1	0.09	0.29	0	0	1
H2	0.03	0.17	0	0	1	0.04	0.19	0	0	1
H3	0.05	0.22	0	0	1	0.05	0.22	0	0	1
H4	0.00	0.07	0	0	1	0.01	0.10	0	0	1
H5	0.72	0.45	0	1	1	0.72	0.45	0	1	1

LEX = 1 and VEX = 1 columns have too small probabilities compared with the other columns. Also, the tables show too much variation in exercise habits over 2 years.

Facing these problems, we converted the five categories into two: (0, 1, 2) becomes 0 while (3, 4) becomes 1; it may take at least once a week frequency for the exercises to be effective. With the conversion, 75% (24%) of the people do LEX (VEX) in wave 1, and the new transition matrices are:

LEX: (0, 1, 2) to 0, (3, 4) to 1

$t = 1 \backslash t = 2$	0	1
0	0.438	0.562
1	0.144	0.856

VEX: (0, 1, 2) to 0, (3, 4) to 1

$t = 1 \backslash t = 2$	0	1
0	0.786	0.214
1	0.423	0.577

One should not be too wary of this construction of the dummy variables: we are merely redefining LEX and VEX as 'doing exercise at least once a week'. Had we constructed the dummy variables differently, we would be defining LEX and VEX (i.e. the treatments) differently, and consequently measuring the effects of different treatments. For instance, if we define exercise as at least once a month, we should transform the five categories into two by (0, 1) to 0 and (2, 3, 4) to 1, in which case the transition matrix becomes

LEX: (0, 1,) to 0, (2, 3, 4) to 1

$t = 1 \backslash t = 2$	0	1
0	0.369	0.631
1	0.086	0.914

VEX: (0, 1,) to 0, (2, 3, 4) to 1

$t = 1 \backslash t = 2$	0	1
0	0.620	0.380
1	0.267	0.733

Here, the right-most columns have more probability masses than those in the preceding two matrices, because exercise = 1 becomes easier with the 'easier' transformation. In most of our empirical analysis later, we will use the dummy variables (0, 1, 2) to 0 and (3, 4) to 1; when we present regression results, we will show the estimates for the other dummy variables ((0, 1) to 0 and (2, 3, 4) to 1) as well.

Turning to the other variables, the average age of wave 1 is 55.31 indicating an old population; we added two to the first wave age to get the second wave age, because the actual second wave age that depends on the interview date was not available. The age in wave 1 ranges from 23–82 because the respondents include spouses and partners. The majority of the respondents are married: 83 and 81% in wave 1 and wave 2, respectively.

We use job dummy, work hour, income and job title (17 categories) as job-related variables. Simply having a job or not may matter, say for mental health and for staying active. A high work-hour means less chance to visit doctors; the average work-hour per week among the workers in wave 1 is 27.88 while the national average is 34.8 (Bureau of Labor Statistics). Income includes all kinds of household income, not only wage and pension but also capital gain (or loss); the average household income and the median is $57 877 and $44 220, respectively. Job categories matter for health care demand; e.g. blue-collar workers are subject to higher risk for job-related injuries. For confidentiality, however, job categories in HRS have been aggregated and available only in 17 categories; their summary statistics are omitted to save space.

Schooling, top-coded at 17, shows the highest grade competed; it is time-invariant in our data. There are 3906 males and 4578 females. The race variable consists of five categories: 'White', 'Black', 'Asian or Pacific Islander', 'Hispanic' and 'American Indian or Alaskan Native'. The majority in the samples is White (74%), followed by Black (15%), Hispanic (9%), Asian (1%) and American Indian (1%). The proportions are not too far from the census proportions: according to 1997 US Bureau of Census, they are 72.6%, 12.1%, 11.0%, 3.6% and 0.7%, respectively.

There are a large number of diseases and it is impossible to know exactly what kind of disease each respondent has. Hypertension, diabetes, lung diseases, heart diseases, emotion/nerve problems, arthritis/rheumatism and pain are used as disease variables. Lung disease dummy includes chronic bronchitis and emphysema. Heart disease dummy includes heart attack, coronary heart disease, angina and congestive heart failure. Emotion/nerve dummy includes emotional, nervous and psychiatric problems. Those who have a cancer or experienced a stroke are removed from the data, because they may be too different in terms of health care demand from the rest of the population (admittedly, this decision is somewhat arbitrary). All disease variables show whether one has *ever* gotten the disease or not; using *ever* variables instead of the *current* status alleviates the endogeneity problem of the disease variables. All disease variables increase over time. Smoking variables are available, but unreliable: the past smokers show the maximum number of cigarettes per day and how long ago they quit, whereas the current smokers show only the average number of cigarettes per day but not when they started smoking. Thus, those who tried smoking only once in a high school day and quit on the same day has the maximum smoking equal to one, which is also the case for a regular smoker smoking one cigarette per day. Smoking will not be used in our empirical analysis.

Health care demand may be affected by residence because each state has its own health care policy. For confidentiality, however, the residence variables in HRS have been aggregated to 11 regions, two of which have no respondents: 'US NA state' and 'Not in a Census Division'. The remaining nine regions are shown in Table 8.1. The residence is available only in wave 1; in wave 2, there is a question whether the respondent has moved since wave 1 interview; less than 10% answered yes. But it is unlikely that many of them moved out of their regions. For these reasons, we treat residence as time-invariant. To save space, summary statistics for residence are omitted.

Health insurance matters for health care. About 16% of the subjects are covered by public health insurance: Medicare (for the old and the handicapped), Medicaid (for the poor) and CHAMPS/VA (for military retirees). About 72% are covered by insurance bought through their or their partner's companies or unions.

REGRESSION ESTIMATORS

In this section, we describe the regression estimators used in this paper; more discussion can be found, e.g. in Cameron and Trivedi [8] and Lee [9]. First, cross-section regression estimators are presented, pooling two waves into one big cross-section, which entails that independence assumption across observations may fail. This is often called a 'group structure' problem: each individual is a group with two observations possibly related to each other. Second, panel regression estimators are described. In the literature, two strains of panel estimators are available: 'random-effect' and 'fixed-effect'; we will use only the latter in this paper, for it allows relationships between a time-invariant error δ_i and regressors while the former does not unless strong parametric assumptions are invoked. Allowing the relationships is our only route through which regressor endogeneity issue is addressed. Although all methods described in this section were applied to our data, only about half the results will be reported later for different reasons.

Let y_{it} be the observed count response variable for individual i at time t. Poisson regression specifies that y_{it} given x_{it} is drawn from Poisson(λ_{it}), where

$$\lambda_{it} \equiv \exp(x'_{it}\beta) \qquad (8.14)$$

x_{it} is a $k_x \times 1$ vector of regressors, and Poisson(λ_{it}) denotes Poisson distribution with parameter λ_{it}; the probability of y_{it} given x_{it} is given by

$$f(y_{it}|x_{it}) = \frac{\exp(-\lambda_{it})\lambda_{it}^{y_{it}}}{y_{it}!}, \quad y_{it} = 0, 1, 2, \ldots$$

Further assuming that $(y_{it}, x'_{it})'$, $t = 1, 2, i = 1, \ldots, N$ are *iid* (independent and identically distributed), the Poisson maximum likelihood estimator (MLE) maximizes the log-likelihood function:

$$\sum_{i=1}^{N} \sum_{t=1}^{T} [-\ln(y_{it}!) - \exp(x'_{it}\beta) + y_{it}x'_{it}\beta] \qquad (8.15)$$

the first derivative is

$$\sum_{i=1}^{N} \sum_{t=1}^{T} \{y_{it} - \exp(x'_{it}\beta))\}x_{it} \qquad (8.16)$$

The Poisson MLE includes the restriction

$$E(y_{it}|x_{it}) = V(y_{it}|x_{it}) = \lambda_{it}$$

In reality, the conditional variance often tends to be bigger than the conditional mean; this is called an 'over-dispersion' problem. Ignoring this problem renders too small standard errors. Since Equation $8.16 = 0$ is a sample moment condition, the estimator using Equation $8.16 = 0$ only under $E(y_{it}|x_{it}) = \lambda_{it}$ without specifying the likelihood is a method of moment estimator (MME); we will use this MME, not the Poisson MLE. The MME does not require the *iid* assumption across t, while the Poisson MLE requires *iid* across t as well as i. In the MME, the asymptotic variance is to be estimated by

$$\left(\sum_i \partial s_i(\beta)/\partial b\right)^{-1} \cdot \sum_i s_i(\beta)s'_i(\beta) \cdot \left(\sum_i \partial s_i(\beta)/\partial b'\right)^{-1},$$

$$\text{not by } \left(\sum_i s_i(\beta)s'_i(\beta)\right)^{-1} \qquad (8.17)$$

where $s_i(b) \equiv \Sigma_{t=1}^{T}\{y_{it} - \exp(x'_{it}b)\}x_{it}$.

One way to allow for over-dispersion while staying within MLE framework is introducing unobserved heterogeneity, say ε_{it}. Suppose $y_{it}|(x_{it}, \varepsilon_i)$ follows Poisson($\tilde{\lambda}_{it}$),

$$\tilde{\lambda}_{it} \equiv \exp(x'_{it}\beta + \varepsilon_{it})$$

$\exp(\varepsilon_{it})|x_{it}$ follows $\gamma(\psi_{it}, \psi_{it})$, $\psi_{it} = (1/\alpha)\lambda_{it}k$, $\alpha > 0$, where $\gamma(a, b)$ denotes γ distribution with parameters a and b, and α and β are parameters to estimate, while k is typically set at 0 or 1. With ε_{it} integrated out, $y_{it}|x_{it}$ follows a negative binomial distribution with parameters $\psi_{it}/(\lambda_{it} + \psi_{it})$ and ψ_{it} (denoted as NB($\psi_{it}/(\lambda_{it} + \psi_{it})$, ψ_{it})): for $\Gamma(s) \equiv \int_0^\infty z^{s-1}e^{-z} dz$ with $s > 0$,

$$f(y_{it}|x_{it}) = [\Gamma(y_{it} + \psi_{it})/\{\Gamma(\psi_{it})\Gamma(y_{it} + 1)\}]$$
$$\cdot \{\psi_{it}/(\lambda_{it} + \psi_{it})\}^{\psi_{it}} \cdot \{\lambda_{it}/(\lambda_{it} + \psi_{it})\}^{y_{it}}$$

NB with $k = 1$ ($k = 0$) is called NB1 (NB2). This distribution allows over-dispersion:

$$E(y_{it}|x_{it}) = \lambda_{it} \text{ and } V(y_{it}|x_{it}) = \lambda_{it} + \alpha\lambda_{it}^{2-k}$$

The variance is linear in λ_{it} if $k = 1$, and quadratic if $k = 0$, which explains the names NB1 and NB2; either way, the variance is greater than the mean. For NB1, $\psi_{it}/(\lambda_{it} + \psi_{it}) = 1/(1 + \alpha)$ is a constant between 0 and 1; for NB2, $\psi_{it}/(\lambda_{it} + \psi_{it})$ is not a constant but $\psi_{it} = 1/\alpha$ is. The Poisson MLE is included as a limiting case when $\alpha \to 0^+$ since $E\{\exp(\varepsilon_{it})|x_{it}\} = 1$ and $V\{\exp(\varepsilon_{it})|x_{it}\} = \alpha\lambda_{it}^{-k}$.

Assuming that $(y_{it}, x'_{it})'$, $t = 1, 2, i = 1, \ldots, N$ are *iid*, the NB log-likelihood function to maximize for α and β is

$$\sum_{i=1}^{N} \sum_{t=1}^{T} [\ln(\Gamma(y_{it} + \psi_{it})) - \ln(\Gamma(\psi_{it})) - \ln(\Gamma(y_{it} + 1))$$
$$+ \psi_{it}(\ln(\psi_{it}) - \ln(\lambda_{it} + \psi_{it}))$$
$$+ y_{it}(\ln(\lambda_{it}) - \ln(\lambda_{it} + \psi_{it}))]$$

There are different ways to parametrize NB (e.g. Winkelmann and Zimmermann [10]), and we followed Deb and Trivedi [11]. For our empirical analysis later, we will report the NB2 result, but not the NB1, for the maximized log-likelihood value was bigger for NB2. Since NB2 is based upon stronger assumptions than the MME, we will focus on the MME when we interpret our empirical findings.

One problem with cross-section analysis is that there may be an unobserved variable related to regressors and the response variable at the same time, which renders cross-section estimates inconsistent in general unless the unobservable variable is integrated out as in NB1 in a fully parametric framework. For example, some people tend to be (genetically) weak or always worrying that they use health care more often than others; such genetic factor or tendency can be related to regressors. Those unobserved components, if time-invariant as genes, can be controlled for (i.e. eliminated) if panel data is used: the basic idea is to first-difference the model (or variables) to eliminate them. For count responses, the so-called 'conditional Poisson' (Hausman et al. [12]), being a panel version of the cross-section Poisson, does this task. The unobserved time-invariant variable δ_i, is often called 'fixed-effect', 'unit-specific effect' or 'related-effect' is the literature; following Lee [13], we will adopt the last expression 'related-effect' for δ_i from now on. There can be other sources of endogeneity, say through a time-variant error, but the methods to be used in this paper cannot deal with them; the latent-variable-based approach to allow for endogeneity in Lee [14] and a related one in Lee [15] are, in general, not applicable for count responses (see also Windmeijer and Santos-Silva [16]).

In addition to the *iid* assumption across i, imposing two assumptions that

$y_{i1}, \ldots, y_{iT}$ are independent of one another

given $x_{i1}, \ldots, x_{iT}, \delta_i$, and $y_{it} | (x_{it}, \delta_i)$

follows Poisson $(\exp(x_{it}'\beta + \delta_i))$ (8.18)

the conditional Poisson log-likelihood function to be maximized for β is

$$\sum_{i=1}^{N} \left[\ln \left\{ \left(\sum_{t=1}^{T} y_{it} \right)! \right\} - \sum_{t=1}^{T} \ln(y_{it}!) \right.$$
$$\left. + \sum_{t=1}^{T} y_{it} \left\{ \Delta x_{it1}'\beta - \ln \left(\sum_{s=1}^{T} \exp(\Delta x_{is1}'\beta) \right) \right\} \right] \quad (8.19)$$

where $\Delta x_{it1} \equiv x_{it} - x_{i1}$. The two assumptions listed ahead are the restrictive features of the conditional Poisson.

Still maintaining the *iid* assumption across i, Hausman et al. [4] assume

$y_{i1}, \ldots, y_{iT}$ are independent of one another

given $x_{i1}, \ldots, x_{iT}, \delta_i$, and $y_{it} | (x_{it}, \delta_i)$

follows NB$(p_i, \exp(x_{it}'\beta + \delta_i))$ for some p_i (8.20)

to relax the Poisson part in the conditional Poisson; since the first parameter p_i is time-invariant, the NB here is of type NB1. The resulting 'conditional negative binomial' log-likelihood function to be maximized for β is (both p_i and δ_i drop out in the conditioning)

$$\sum_{i=1}^{N} \left[\sum_{t=1}^{T} \{ \ln \Gamma(\lambda_{it} + y_{it}) - \ln \Gamma(\lambda_{it}) - \ln \Gamma(y_{it} + 1) \} \right.$$
$$+ \ln \Gamma \left(\sum_{t=1}^{T} \lambda_{it} \right) + \ln \Gamma \left(\sum_{t=1}^{T} y_{it} + 1 \right)$$
$$\left. - \ln \Gamma \left(\sum_{t=1}^{T} \lambda_{it} + \sum_{t=1}^{T} y_{it} \right) \right]$$

Wooldridge [17] shows that the conditional Poisson's restrictive assumption can be relaxed considerably. Suppose

$$E(y_{it} | x_{i1}, \ldots, x_{iT}, \delta_i) = E(y_{it} | x_{it}, \delta_i)$$
$$= \exp(x_{it}'\beta + \delta_i)$$

where the first equality is 'strict exogeneity'. So long as this holds (along with minor regularity conditions), maximizing the conditional Poisson maximand Equation 8.19 yields a $\sqrt{N}$-consistent estimator for β. This 'quasi-conditional MLE (QCL)' allows dependence among $y_{i1}, \ldots, y_{iT}$ given $x_{i1}, \ldots, x_{iT}, \delta_i$, relaxing Equation 8.18. The asymptotic variance of QCL can be estimated analogously to Equation 8.17 with s_i denoting the score function. QCL may be taken as a panel version of the MME for the Poisson MLE. Since QCL is based upon the weakest assumptions yet while allowing for a related-effect, we take QCL as our main estimator.

It is not known whether analogous relaxation of assumption is possible for the conditional negative binomial. For our empirical analysis, conditional negative binomial converged not as well as QCL, and when it did, it returned implausible values (with most absolute t-values running over 50). For these two reasons, the conditional negative binomial will not be reported later for our empirical analysis.

RESULTS OF CONDITIONING APPROACHES

In this section, we present our empirical analysis without using the exponential regression function. Here, covariates are controlled for by conditioning, and the variable of interest (exercise) is used for grouping; inferences can be then drawn from differences between the groups with different exercise habits. The advantage of this conditioning approach is that there is no need to specify the regression functional form nor distributions for the model error terms. But a disadvantage is that we cannot control for too many variables; if we do, there will be too few observations left for the groups. Not being able to control for all relevant variables means the risk of omitted variable bias. In the following section, we present regression approaches that can control for many covariates; but then, there will be the risk of misspecified models. Another disadvantage of the conditioning approach is that we will be learning only about the selected sub-population, and there is no guarantee that the findings from the sub-population can be applied to the other sub-populations. Despite this, since the effects of exercise are a concern for everybody, not just for old people, we will extract a sub-population representing relatively younger and healthier group and analyse them.

The following is for the average health care demand across exercise habits using all observations:

	LEX = 0	LEX = 1	VEX = 0	VEX = 1
HOS	0.982	0.514	0.712	0.388
VIS	4.120	3.293	3.707	2.896

People who do exercise, LEX or VEX, having lower health care demand. But since exercising people may differ from non-exercising people in other variables, this table does not show that the differences in health care demand are due to differences in exercise habits.

To better control for covariates and get a homogenous group of people, we select a healthy sub-population with age 50–57 in wave 1 and the following characteristics holding for both waves: married, all zero disease dummies, no pain, working, no public health insurance, and group insurance dummies being one. To the extent that the unobserved variables are related to these covariates, the unobserved variables and partially controlled for as well. Given that we are looking at an old population, the findings from this healthy sub-population stands a better chance to be applicable to young and healthy people, which was the main motivation to look at the particular sub-population as already mentioned. The sample size of the sub-population is 1260 ($630_{people} \times 2_{waves}$) in the pooled data.

Table 8.3 consists of four 3×2 contingency panels showing the absolute frequencies and the relative frequencies in a given column; at the bottom right of each panel is the Pearson χ^2 test statistic; for the 3×2 classification, the critical value for the test is 6.0 at size 5%. Looking at the test statistics and the relative frequencies,

Table 8.3 Results of conditioning and pooled-data

A. LEX and VIS

VIS\LEX	0: Seldom do	1: Do	Sum
0	89 (0.366)	241 (0.237)	330 (0.262)
1–5	140 (0.576)	723 (0.711)	863 (0.685)
6–	14 (0.058)	53 (0.052)	67 (0.053)
Sum	243 (1.000)	1017 (1.000)	1260 (1.000)

Test statistic: 17.831

B. VEX and VIS

VIS\VEX	0: Seldom do	1: Do	Sum
0	226 (0.271)	104 (0.244)	330 (0.262)
1–5	558 (0.670)	305 (0.714)	863 (0.685)
6–	49 (0.059)	18 (0.042)	67 (0.053)
Sum	833 (1.000)	427 (1.000)	1260 (1.000)

Test statistic: 3.118

C. LEX and HOS

HOS\LEX	0: Seldom do	1: Do	Sum
0	237 (0.975)	967 (0.951)	1204 (0.956)
1–5	5 (0.021)	45 (0.044)	50 (0.040)
6–	1 (0.004)	5 (0.005)	67 (0.005)
Sum	253 (1.000)	1017 (1.000)	1260 (1.000)

Test statistic: 2.919

D. VEX and HOS

HOS\VEX	0: Seldom do	1: Do	Sum
0	796 (0.975)	408 (0.951)	1204 (0.956)
1–5	33 (0.040)	17 (0.040)	50 (0.040)
6–	4 (0.005)	2 (0.005)	6 (0.005)
Sum	833 (1.000)	427 (1.000)	1260 (1.000)

Test statistic: 0.001

independence between VIS and LEX is rejected in the first panel while we fail to reject independence in the other panels. The relative frequencies however show that, if anything, *LEX increases both VIS and HOS*, contrary to the message of the above simple table with no covariates controlled for; the effects of VEX are not clear. We can think of some reasons for this surprising finding: enhanced health-awareness, exercise under doctors' supervision, and the reverse causal effect of more exercise following doctor visits or hospitalization.

The preceding analysis is of cross-section type. To take

Table 8.4   Exercise change and health care demand change

A. LEX and VIS changes

VIS-change\LEX change	0–0	0–1	1–0	1–1	Sum
Decreased	16 (0.308)	21 (0.276)	17 (0.270)	130 (0.296)	184 (0.292)
Same	17 (0.327)	20 (0.263)	21 (0.333)	139 (0.317)	197 (0.313)
Increased	19 (0.365)	35 (0.461)	25 (0.397)	170 (0.387)	249 (0.395)
Sum	52 (1.000)	76 (1.000)	63 (1.000)	439 (1.000)	630 (1.000)

B. VEX and VIS changes

VIS-change\VEX change	0–0	0–1	1–0	1–1	Sum
Decreased	100 (0.304)	34 (0.304)	20 (0.317)	30 (0.238)	184 (0.292)
Same	97 (0.295)	41 (0.366)	15 (0.238)	44 (0.349)	197 (0.313)
Increased	132 (0.401)	37 (0.33)	28 (0.444)	52 (0.413)	249 (0.395)
Sum	329 (1.000)	112 (1.000)	63 (1.000)	126 (1.000)	630 (1.000)

C. LEX and HOS changes

HOS-change\LEX-change	0–0	0–1	1–0	1–1	Sum
Decreased	3 (0.058)	0 (0.000)	0 (0.000)	18 (0.041)	21 (0.033)
Same	47 (0.904)	68 (0.895)	62 (0.984)	398 (0.907)	575 (0.913)
Increased	2 (0.038)	8 (0.105)	1 (0.016)	23 (0.052)	34 (0.054)
Sum	52 (1.000)	76 (1.000)	63 (1.000)	439 (1.000)	630 (1.000)

D. VEX and HOS changes

HOS-change\VEX-change	0–0	0–1	1–0	1–1	Sum
Decreased	8 (0.024)	3 (0.027)	5 (0.079)	5 (0.04)	21 (0.033)
Same	302 (0.918)	102 (0.911)	52 (0.825)	119 (0.944)	575 (0.913)
Increased	19 (0.058)	7 (0.063)	6 (0.095)	2 (0.016)	34 (0.054)
Sum	329 (1.000)	112 (1.000)	63 (1.000)	126 (1.000)	630 (1.000)

advantage of panel data, now we look at changes in exercise habits and health care demand over two waves. If a linear model were used, this would amount to first-differencing the model to get rid of all time invariants, which then would not affect analysis based on changes. Table 8.4 lists four panels, analogously to Table 8.3. There are four types of LEX or VEX across two waves: 0–0, 0–1, 1–0, and 1–1. VIS and HOS are now classified into three: decrease, the same and increase. In Table 8.5, many Pearson χ^2 test statistics are presented. For instance, the entry at row 0–1 and column 0–0 of panel A is 1.202, which is the test statistic for the 3×2 contingency panel consisting of panel A of Table 8.4 with all rows and only two columns for 0–0 and 0–1.

In Table 8.5, there are four numbers greater than the critical value 6 at 5%, but all four are for HOS. In panel C, the first significant number 6.151 is based upon too few observations as can be seen in the corresponding panel C of Table 8.4, but the second significant number 6.135 (for 0–1 and 1–1) is based upon observations not as few, and panel C of Table 8.4 indicates a *positive association between HOS increase and LEX increase*. In panel D of Table 8.5, the first significant number is 6.498 (for 0–0 and 1–0), and the corresponding panel D of Table 8.4 shows both decrease and increase in HOS, making inference difficult. The second significant number in the panel D of Table 8.5 is 8.158 for 1–0 and 1–1, but judging from the corresponding panel D of Table 8.4, the number is based upon too few observations.

In short, for the healthy sub-population with some covariates controlled for, there is a *positive association between LEX and both VIS and HOS*. For the same sub-population, looking at changes over time, we have a positive association between LEX and HOS changes.

Table 8.5 Test statistics for exercise change and health care demand change

	0–0	0–1	1–0
A. LEX and VIS changes			
0–1	1.202	—	—
1–0	0.219	0.904	—
1–1	0.094	1.561	0.191
B. VEX and VIS changes			
0–1	2.450	—	—
1–0	0.869	3.502	—
1–1	2.282	2.068	2.761
C. LEX and HOS changes			
0–1	6.151	—	—
1–0	4.386	4.545	—
1–1	0.480	6.135	4.481
D. VEX and HOS changes			
0–1	0.057	—	—
1–0	6.498	3.354	—
1–1	4.284	3.775	8.158

These findings are in sharp contrast to the message of the crude table with no covariates controlled for, and they suggest that the healthy sub-population and the remaining (unhealthy) sub-population may differ in terms of exercise effects on health care demand.

Since the above tables are based only upon 630×2 cases, now we enlarge the healthy sub-population by selecting the individuals from the pooled data with zero disease dummies (all six of them) and zero pain dummy (insurance, working, and marriage are not controlled for now). Defining $h_i = 1$ if healthy and 0 otherwise according to this definition, we get $P(h = 1) = 0.288$, and

$$E(y \mid LEX = 0, h = 0) = 4.815$$

$$> E(y \mid LEX = 1, h = 0) = 3.858$$

$$E(y \mid LEX = 0, h = 1) = 1.433$$

$$< E(y \mid LEX = 1, h = 1) = 1.643$$

considerably more information may lurk in δ for health, but δ is not observed and hence cannot be used for h. The numbers show that, for the healthy sub-population, LEX is indeed positively associated with y; for the unhealthy sub-population, LEX is negatively associated with y. Since the proportion of the healthy sub-population is low (0.288), the unhealthy sub-population effect dominates to results in the first simple table of this section.

RESULTS OF REGRESSION APPROACHES

In the preceding section, we showed our conditioning approaches for a healthy sub-population. In this section, we present three sets of regression model estimates: MME, NB2 and QCL, where MME and NB2 are for pooled cross-sections while QCL is for panel. As mentioned already, we use only VIS as health care demand in this section, since HOS has too many zeros. Thanks to the advantages of panel related-effect methods, QCL provides the most robust conclusions in the regression approaches, followed by MME, which is based upon assumptions weaker than those for NB2. NB2 results are provided (but de-emphasized) only for the sake of comparison; we will not mention NB2 any further other than noting here that they are close to the MME estimates.

Table 8.6 shows the estimates and the t-values obtained with the main exercise dummies, whereas Table 8.7 shows those with the 'easy' exercise dummies constructed from the original five categories as $(0, 1)$ to 0 and $(2, 3, 4)$ to 1; we will focus on Table 8.6. To save space, the estimates for the residence and job-dummies are omitted. As a reference, the last rows of Tables 8.6 and 8.7 show the maximized log-likelihood function values; for MME, it is the Poisson log-likelihood at MME, and for QCL, it is the conditional Poisson log-likelihood at QCL; constants irrelevant for maximization in those log-likelihoods are not included in the reported maximand values.

In Table 8.6, τ and τ^2 look insignificant for MME. But we easily reject insignificance of τ *and* τ^2, because the Wald test statistic value is 126.4 with the p-value 0.000. When only τ is included in the MME model, the coefficient (t-value) for τ is -2.73 (-11.56), meaning negative duration dependence. This shows that the small t-values for τ and τ^2 in MME are due to a high correlation between τ and τ^2. In QCL however, the duration effect is positive, contradicting the negative effect in MME.

Both LEX and VEX look insignificant in MME and QCL, but this is misleading, because some interaction terms (e.g. heart disease-LEX in MME and QCL, and emotion/nerve-VEX in QCL) are significant; so long as there is at least one significant interaction term, LEX and VEX are significant. The marginal effects for wave 1 and wave 2 are in the following table where Lower (Upper) stands for the lower (upper) bound for the 95% confidence interval, Effect is the desired marginal effect, and the numbers in (·) are the arithmetic mean effects Equation 8.3 provided here without confidence intervals only for the sake of comparison:

MME	Lower	Effect	Upper	QCL	Lower	Effect	Upper
LEX				**LEX**			
$t = 1$	−0.068	−0.027 (−0.024)	0.015	$t = 1$	−0.026	0.031 (0.034)	0.089
$t = 2$	−0.068	−0.027 (−0.023)	0.015	$t = 2$	−0.025	0.031 (0.035)	0.089
VEX				**VEX**			
$t = 1$	−0.021	−0.010 (−0.009)	0.002	$t = 1$	−0.027	−0.010 (−0.009)	0.006
$t = 2$	−0.027	−0.013 (−0.012)	0.002	$t = 2$	−0.033	−0.013 (−0.011)	0.006

None of the effects is significant. But looking at the estimates and the interval sizes on the positive and negative sides, we can say that LEX has a small negative effect of around −3% in MME and a small positive effect of around 3% in QCL, whereas VEX has a small negative effect of around −1% in both MME and QCL. The arithmetic mean effects are little different from the geometric mean effects. The effects do not change much over time; for a longer panel, the time-varying pattern of the effects would be more interesting.

How do we reconcile the difference between MME and QCL for LEX? Suppose δ_i is the unobserved trait affected by LEX; here we regard δ_i as unobserved health stock built long-term. And recall our discussion on short-term and long-term effects in the Introduction. According to the discussion, the panel estimate shows the short-term effect of LEX, while the cross-section estimate is a long-term affect consisting of the short-term effect and the effect through δ_i. The reconciliation is as follows. In the short run, with both observed health and unobserved health controlled for by the regression method and related-effect, respectively, LEX increases VIS by about 3% perhaps due to consulting doctors or enhanced health concern. But doing LEX for a long time will decrease VIS by about 6% perhaps due to improved health which can be a result of LEX itself as well as other adopted healthy life style going along with LEX. This negative effect cancels the short-term positive effect to result in the long-term effect, which is −3%. One caution is that, for the interpretation of δ_i as unobserved health stock to be coherent, we would expect a difference between short-run and long-run effects for VEX, but the table shows the identical numbers, which may be due to the statistical

insignificance; in the table presented below however, VEX is seen to have different short-run and long-run effects.

Now we turn to the estimates of MME and QCL other than those for LEX and VEX. Among the estimates significant for both MME and QCL (hypertension, lung disease, pain and heart-disease-LEX), the signs all agree, and only the magnitude of pain in MME is twice as big as that in QCL; the other magnitudes are close. As difference-type panel estimators typically have small absolute t-values, QCL's t-values are mostly smaller than those of MME; the only variable that is significant in QCL but not in MME is emotion/nerve-VEX (and diabetes-VEX). In fact, the interaction terms with VEX are all insignificant other than emotion/nerve-VEX in QCL.

Age increases y in MME while decreasing y in QCL. If we still interpret δ as unobserved health stock, then with observed and unobserved health cotrolled for, there is no reason to believe that age should increase y. Marriage has a negative effect, but insignificant and small in its magnitude. Schooling has a significant positive effect, possibly reflecting health awareness aspect. Men demand substantially lower health care than women, which is an almost universal phenomenon. All disease variables increase y other than the insignificant estimate for diabetes in QCL. Heart-disease-LEX increases y, probably because heart conditions require a doctor's supervision for exercise. Most health insurance variables increase y in MME while they are all insignificant in QCL with mixed signs.

In Table 8.7, we present the results of the same analysis but with the easy exercise dummies constructed from the five categories as (0, 1) to 0 and (2, 3, 4) to 1. Tables 8.6 and 8.7 are little different other than in some interaction terms. The marginal treatment effects are:

MME	Lower	Effect	Upper	QCL	Lower	Effect	Upper
LEX				**LEX**			
$t = 1$	−0.119	−0.063 (−0.055)	−0.006	$t = 1$	−0.037	0.044 (0.050)	0.128
$t = 2$	−0.118	−0.063 (−0.053)	−0.007	$t = 2$	−0.027	0.052 (0.060)	0.134
VEX				**VEX**			
$t = 1$	−0.037	−0.022 (−0.021)	−0.007	$t = 1$	−0.035	−0.014 (−0.014)	0.007
$t = 2$	−0.055	−0.034 (−0.033)	−0.012	$t = 2$	−0.050	−0.021 (−0.020)	0.010

Table 8.6 Estimation with the main exercise dummies

Variables	MME (*t*-value)	NB2 (*t*-value)	QCL (*t*-value)
α		0.748 (69.12)	
1	0.700 (1.08)	0.680 (1.77)	
τ	−0.075 (−0.28)	−0.040 (−0.20)	2.548 (1.76)
τ^2	−0.066 (−0.75)	−0.073 (−1.08)	−0.745 (−1.96)
LEX	−0.023 (−0.51)	0.000 (0.00)	0.068 (1.13)
VEX	−0.044 (−1.15)	−0.024 (−0.96)	−0.029 (−0.55)
Age/10	0.297 (1.40)	0.172 (1.35)	−3.141 (−1.69)
(Age/10)^2	−0.038 (−1.99)	−0.025 (−2.14)	0.042 (0.51)
Married	−0.050 (−1.58)	−0.008 (−0.39)	−0.081 (−0.74)
Job dummy	0.009 (0.09)	−0.005 (−0.08)	−0.024 (−0.14)
(Work hour)/10	−0.017 (−1.54)	−0.012 (−1.63)	0.008 (0.44)
ln(income)	0.009 (0.83)	0.009 (1.87)	0.012 (1.00)
Schooling	0.010 (2.15)	0.013 (4.87)	
Male	−0.102 (−3.50)	−0.154 (−9.62)	
White	−0.223 (−1.38)	−0.145 (−2.18)	
Black	−0.142 (−0.88)	−0.067 (−0.98)	
Hispanic	−0.163 (−1.01)	−0.114 (−1.62)	
Asian	−0.221 (−1.24)	−0.208 (−2.09)	
Hypertension	0.301 (6.04)	0.349 (12.67)	0.411 (4.17)
Diabetes	0.290 (4.83)	0.353 (8.96)	−0.186 (−1.48)
Lung disease	0.251 (3.98)	0.288 (6.31)	0.238 (1.91)
Heart disease	0.108 (1.66)	0.197 (5.32)	0.098 (0.75)
Emotion/nerve	0.211 (3.51)	0.264 (7.30)	0.152 (1.49)
Arthritis	0.242 (4.65)	0.234 (8.27)	0.046 (0.52)
Pain	0.551 (10.18)	0.604 (21.63)	0.276 (4.67)
Hypertension-LEX	−0.008 (−0.15)	−0.016 (−0.48)	−0.050 (−0.69)
Diabetes-LEX	0.051 (0.71)	0.019 (0.39)	0.057 (0.55)
Lung disease-LEX	0.060 (0.74)	0.049 (0.89)	−0.043 (−0.42)
Heart disease-LEX	0.221 (2.93)	0.195 (4.28)	0.200 (2.13)
Emotion/nerve-LEX	0.067 (0.90)	0.050 (1.13)	−0.091 (−1.01)
Arthritis-LEX	−0.077 (−1.25)	−0.044 (−1.32)	−0.013 (−0.18)
Pain-LEX	−0.106 (−1.60)	−0.124 (−3.75)	−0.104 (−1.45)
Hypertension-VEX	0.038 (0.74)	0.038 (1.08)	−0.054 (−0.79)
Diabetes-VEX	−0.005 (−0.06)	−0.016 (−0.28)	0.205 (1.88)
Lung disease-VEX	−0.065 (−0.67)	−0.013 (−0.17)	−0.091 (−0.75)
Heart disease-VEX	0.018 (0.25)	0.041 (0.77)	0.131 (1.36)
Emotion/nerve-VEX	0.083 (0.96)	0.068 (1.27)	0.309 (2.98)
Arthritis-VEX	−0.035 (−0.60)	−0.049 (−1.41)	−0.116 (−1.63)
Pain-VEX	−0.025 (−0.34)	−0.030 (−0.82)	−0.051 (−0.61)
H1	0.230 (5.03)	0.280 (9.96)	−0.076 (−1.07)
H2	0.318 (5.76)	0.346 (8.83)	0.015 (0.15)
H3	0.129 (2.50)	0.133 (3.93)	−0.120 (−1.08)
H4	0.191 (1.83)	0.174 (1.97)	0.041 (0.32)
H5	0.149 (4.94)	0.178 (9.95)	0.079 (1.17)
Maximand (no constant)	22 393.825	35 995.033	−39 257.479

The short-term effect of LEX is now about 4–5%, while the long-run effect of LEX is about −6% and significant. The VEX effects of minus 2–3% are stronger than in the preceding table; also differently from the preceding table, the long-run effect of VEX is smaller than the short-run effect. Collectively, these findings are rather surprising, because the effects are overall stronger despite the weaker definition of exercises. Nevertheless, the confidence intervals in the two tables overlap, implying that the apparent anomalies fall within the statistical margin of errors. The

Table 8.7 Estimation with the easy exercise dummies

Variables	MME (t-value)	NB2 (t-value)	QCL (t-value)
α		0.745 (69.22)	
1	0.752 (1.16)	0.749 (1.96)	
τ	−0.036 (−0.13)	−0.011 (−0.06)	2.637 (1.79)
τ^2	−0.076 (−0.85)	−0.079 (−1.18)	−0.767 (−1.99)
LEX	−0.052 (−0.90)	−0.023 (−0.72)	0.045 (0.58)
VEX	−0.075 (−2.08)	−0.060 (−2.56)	−0.057 (−1.17)
Age/10	0.276 (1.30)	0.143 (1.14)	−3.126 (−1.66)
$(\text{Age}/10)^2$	−0.036 (−1.89)	−0.022 (−1.94)	0.031 (0.38)
Married	−0.046 (−1.44)	−0.001 (−0.07)	−0.067 (−0.62)
Job dummy	0.010 (0.10)	−0.007 (−0.10)	−0.017 (−0.11)
(Work hour)/10	−0.018 (−1.60)	−0.012 (−1.62)	0.004 (0.22)
ln(income)	0.011 (0.91)	0.009 (1.89)	0.013 (1.12)
Schooling	0.011 (2.32)	0.014 (5.27)	
Male	−0.105 (−3.64)	−0.156 (−9.66)	
White	−0.230 (−1.43)	−0.143 (−2.12)	
Black	−0.153 (−0.95)	−0.070 (−1.01)	
Hispanic	−0.171 (−1.06)	−0.112 (−1.58)	
Asian	−0.247 (−1.38)	−0.216 (−2.16)	
Hypertension	0.326 (5.13)	0.392 (11.64)	0.393 (3.58)
Diabetes	0.182 (2.55)	0.246 (5.21)	−0.264 (−1.95)
Lung disease	0.181 (2.42)	0.265 (5.12)	0.277 (1.98)
Heart disease	0.109 (1.36)	0.220 (5.09)	0.071 (0.51)
Emotion/nerve	0.107 (1.53)	0.101 (2.17)	0.121 (1.03)
Arthritis	0.270 (4.10)	0.239 (7.04)	−0.028 (−0.28)
Pain	0.613 (9.01)	0.685 (20.66)	0.332 (4.52)
Hypertension-LEX	−0.044 (−0.63)	−0.077 (−1.99)	−0.029 (−0.34)
Diabetes-LEX	0.190 (2.34)	0.170 (3.08)	0.183 (1.68)
Lung disease-LEX	0.160 (1.78)	0.095 (1.59)	−0.105 (−0.90)
Heart disease-LEX	0.199 (2.24)	0.144 (2.80)	0.233 (2.28)
Emotion/nerve-LEX	0.208 (2.54)	0.262 (4.98)	−0.003 (−0.03)
Arthritis-LEX	−0.110 (−1.49)	−0.051 (−1.31)	0.059 (0.66)
Pain-LEX	−0.193 (−2.48)	−0.233 (−6.15)	−0.191 (−2.24)
Hypertension-VEX	0.038 (0.82)	0.051 (1.62)	0.005 (0.08)
Diabetes-VEX	−0.031 (−0.42)	−0.068 (−1.37)	0.044 (0.44)
Lung disease-VEX	−0.110 (−1.32)	−0.085 (−1.34)	0.007 (0.06)
Heart disease-VEX	−0.002 (−0.03)	0.037 (0.77)	0.028 (0.30)
Emotion/nerve-VEX	0.001 (0.02)	−0.005 (−0.10)	0.081 (0.83)
Arthritis-VEX	−0.006 (−0.12)	−0.020 (−0.64)	−0.026 (−0.41)
Pain-VEX	0.017 (0.26)	0.012 (0.35)	0.051 (0.72)
H1	0.221 (4.84)	0.271 (9.66)	−0.078 (−1.09)
H2	0.328 (5.93)	0.355 (9.11)	0.033 (0.34)
H3	0.134 (2.61)	0.138 (4.11)	−0.130 (−1.17)
H4	0.193 (1.85)	0.176 (2.01)	0.034 (0.27)
H5	0.153 (5.06)	0.182 (10.16)	0.081 (1.19)
Maximand (no constant)	22 504.112	36 017.682	−39 280.601

arithmetic means are more different from the geometric means than in the preceding table; also the effects are more time-variant.

Due to lack of instruments for potentially endogenous variables (e.g., job dummy, income and exercise dummies can be endogenous), the conclusions drawn in this section should be taken with the limitation of our methods in mind: the endogeneity is allowed as far as it operates through the time-invariant error δ_i. To get better answers to our questions, we need better data; e.g., if there is a randomized health intervention programme encouraging exercise, the randomization dummy can be an effective instrument for exercise.

CONCLUSIONS

In this paper, we defined and estimated various effects of exercise (binary treatments) on health care demand (count responses) using a two-wave panel: conditional and marginal effects, light-exercise and vigorous-exercise effects, and short-run and long-run effects. We found that short-run light exercise increases health care demand by 3–5%, whereas long-run light exercise decreases it by 3–6%. Also, short-run vigorous exercise decreases health care demand by 1–2%, whereas long-run vigorous exercise decreases it by 1–3%. These findings suggest that it will be hard to reduce health care cost by encouraging people to do more exercise; i.e. the health care-cost saving feature of health intervention programs or campaigns will materialize only in the long-run at best.

ACKNOWLEDGEMENTS

The authors are grateful to the editor, two anonymous referees, Barton Hamilton, Young-sook Kim, John Mullahy and Frank Windmeijer for their helpful comments.

REFERENCES

1. Phelps, C.E. *Health Economics* (2nd edn). Addison-Wesley: Reading, MA, 1997.
2. Leigh, J.P. and Fries, J.F. Health habits, health care use and costs in a sample of retirees. *Inquiry* 1992; **29**: 44–54.
3. Hofer, T.P. and Katz, S.J. Healthy behaviors among women in the United States and Ontario: The effect on use of preventive care. *Am. J. Publ. Health* 1996; **86**: 1755–1760.
4. Huijsman, R., Wielink, G. and Rigter, H. Effect van lichaamsbeweging bij ouderen: een onerzicht can recent literatuur en de mogelijkheid van economische evaluatie. *Tijdschr Gerontol Geriatr* 1994; **25**: 237–249.
5. Heckman, J.J., Smith, J.A. and Clements, N. Making the most out of program evaluations and social experiments: Accounting for heterogeneity in program impacts. *Rev. Econ. Stud.* 1997; **64**: 487–535.
6. Lee, M.J. Median treatment effect in randomized trials. *J. R. Stat. Soc. B* 2000; **62**: 595–604.
7. Heckman, J.J., Lalonde, R.J. and Smith, J.A. The economics and econometrics of active labor market programs. In *Handbook of Labor Economics*, vol. 3, Ashenfelter, A. and Card, D. (eds). Elsevier Science B.V.: Netherlands, 1999; 1865–2087.
8. Cameron, A.C. and Trivedi, P.K. *Regression Analysis of Count Data*. Cambridge University Press: Cambridge, 1998.
9. Lee, M.J. *Panel Data Econometrics: Methods-of-Moments and Limited Dependent Variables*. Academic Press: San Diego, CA (in press).
10. Winkelmann, R. and Zimmermann, K.F. Recent developments in count data modelling: Theory and application. *J. Econ. Surv.* 1995; **9**: 1–24.
11. Deb, P. and Trivedi, T.K. Demand for medical care by the elderly: A finite mixture approach. *J. Appl. Econom.* 1997; **12**: 313–336.
12. Hausman, J., Hall, B.H. and Griliches, Z. Econometric models for count data with an application to the patents – R&D relationship. *Econometrica* 1984; **52**: 909–938.
13. Lee, M.J. A root-N consistent semiparametric estimator for related-effect binary response panel data. *Econometrica* 1999; **67**: 427–434.
14. Lee, M.J. Semiparametric estimation of simultaneous equations with limited dependent variables: A case study of female labor supply. *J. Appl. Econom.* 1995; **10**: 187–200.
15. Lee, M.J. *Method of Moments and Semiparametric Econometrics for Limited Dependent Variable Models*. Springer-Verlag: New York, 1996.
16. Windmeijer, F.A.G. and Santos-Silva, J.M.C. Endogeneity in count data models: An application to demand for health care. *J. Appl. Econom.* 1997; **12**: 281–294.
17. Wooldridge, J.M. Distribution-free estimation of some nonlinear panel data models. *J. Econom.* 1999; **90**: 77–97.

9

Estimating Surgical Volume – Outcome Relationships Applying Survival Models: Accounting for Frailty and Hospital Fixed Effects

BARTON H. HAMILTON[1] AND VIVIAN H. HO[1,2]

[1]*John M. Olin School of Business, Washington University in St Louis, MO, USA and* [2]*Centre for the Analysis of Cost-Effective Care, Montreal General Hospital, Canada*

INTRODUCTION

Past studies have found that patients receiving surgery in a hospital performing a large number of surgeries have better outcomes (shorter lengths of stay; lower probabilities of in-hospital mortality) than do those undergoing surgery in a low volume hospital (see Luft *et al.* [1] for a summary of these studies). These results are particularly pertinent in the context of the current health care debate in many countries. For example, many Canadian provinces are being faced with the decision to shut down hospitals and/or reduce the number of hospital beds due to declining health care budgets. To the extent that the positive relationship between volume and outcomes is valid, these governments may actually improve outcomes by regionalizing surgery and closing low volume providers [2].

While the positive volume–outcome relationship has been strongly established, substantial debate exists in the literature as to the interpretation of this finding. Virtually all of the empirical evidence is based on comparisons of outcomes between high and low volume hospitals at a point in time. That is, if hospital A performs more surgeries than hospital B, outcomes will be better for patients admitted to A than for those admitted to B. This relationship may reflect a 'practice makes perfect' effect in which high volume providers are able to gain expertise in performing the procedure, leading to improved outcomes. On the other hand, the relationship between higher vol-

ume and better outcomes may simply represent a 'selective referral effect': high quality hospitals which have better outcomes, *ceteris paribus*, are likely to get more referrals from primary care providers. Consequently, when regressing the outcome measure on surgical volume, the estimated coefficient on surgical volume is likely to be biased, since volume is a proxy for hospital quality as well as any practice makes perfect effect. Finally, some have argued that the positive relationship reflects case-mix differences between low and high volume hospitals that are not adequately accounted for in the empirical analysis [3].

In the light of this uncertainty regarding interpretation, this paper re-examines the relationship between surgical volume and outcomes using longitudinal data on patients undergoing hip fracture surgery at acute care hospitals in Quebec between 1991 and 1993. Hip fractures are a particularly relevant case study, given that these fractures are the leading cause of hospitalization for injuries among the elderly [4], and account for a disproportionately large number of hospital bed days owing to the relatively long recovery period associated with hip surgery. In addition, examination of the volume–outcome relationship at Canadian hospitals is particularly timely, since the Canadian health care system is currently facing substantial cutbacks and reorganization and most volume–outcome studies have examined hospitals in the USA. As a result, with few exceptions little is known about the relationship in Canada [5–7].

Econometric Analysis of Health Data. Edited by Andrew M. Jones and Owen O'Donnell
© 2002 John Wiley & Sons Ltd. Previously published in *Health Economics*, Vol. 6; pp. 383–395 (1997). © John Wiley & Sons Ltd

Our empirical approach differs from that taken in previous studies, because we attempt to distinguish between the various explanations hypothesized in the literature concerning the volume–outcome relationship. First, because the same hospitals are observed over time in the sample, these longitudinal data may be exploited to account for systematic differences in quality between hospitals in a very general way using hospital-specific fixed effects [8]. The period to period fluctuation in the number of surgical procedures performed at each hospital then identifies the effect of volume on outcomes, purged of any difference in quality across hospitals that is fixed over time. Our estimates of the volume–outcome relationship thus rely on the variation in volume and outcomes *within* hospitals over time, while almost all previous studies have relied on variations in volume and outcomes *between* hospitals to estimate the relationship. The results presented in this paper thus relate more closely to one of the key questions faced by policy makers: what would happen to patient outcomes if the number of surgeries were increased (or decreased) at a given hospital?

A second feature of the empirical framework is that the outcome measures of interest, post-surgery length of stay and inpatient mortality, are allowed to be correlated by estimating a competing risk duration model in which the individual may be discharged alive or dead. Previous studies have assumed that these outcomes are independent. The primary drawback of this assumption is that if length of stay and in-hospital mortality are not independent, then one may be more likely to observe an in-hospital death for individuals with long hospital stays. To account for this possibility, the duration model allows for unobserved (to the econometrician) systematic differences in frailty among patients at the time of admission to the hospital using the non-parametric approach described in Heckman and Singer [9]. Finally, we include much more detailed controls for patient health status than have typically been used in the literature to account for case-mix differences across patients.

Using this empirical methodology, we first estimate a specification of the volume–outcome relationship which does not control for fixed differences in hospital quality. The estimation results show that higher volume is associated with an increased conditional (on time in hospital) probability of live discharge, although no significant effect is found on the conditional (on time in hospital) probability of in-hospital mortality. However, when we re-estimate the model accounting for fixed quality differences between hospitals by including hospital-specific dummy variables in the specification, the coefficient on volume shrinks in magnitude and becomes insignificantly different from zero. Consequently, better patient outcomes in larger hospitals do not appear to be based upon a volume/learning effect. Rather, the results are more consistent with the hypothesis that higher quality hospitals are able to draw more patient referrals.

The next section describes the data and presents descriptive statistics on the volume–outcome relationship, and the subsequent section outlines the statistical framework. We present our results and concluding remarks in the last two sections.

DATA AND PRELIMINARY EVIDENCE

This paper analyses data from the MED-ICHO database, which contains standardized information from hospital discharge abstracts. All acute care hospitals in Quebec report details of each discharge to the provincial Ministry of Health and Social Services. All patients admitted to acute care hospitals with a primary diagnosis of hip fracture (ICD-9 codes 820.0–820.9, fracture of neck of femur; transcervical, pertrochanteric or other unspecified) who were admitted during or after April 1990 and discharged before March 1993 are included in the sample. Because information on patients whose hospital stays were still in progress at the end of March 1993 was unavailable, we may undercount the volume of surgeries performed in February and March 1993. These patients were thus excluded from the analysis, although the results were virtually identical when they were included. Patients admitted for revision of prior hip fracture surgery were excluded from our sample (1% of original sample). In addition, 6% of patients admitted to the hospital with a hip fracture did not undergo surgery. It appears that many of these patients were admitted to hospitals that did not perform hip fracture surgery and then transfixed to another hospital. Since our goal is to examine the impact of surgical volume on post-surgical length of stay, we excluded patients not undergoing surgery from the analysis.

For each patient, data were obtained on date of surgery and date and type of discharge (live or dead) and were used to construct post-surgery length of stay. Information was also obtained on other covariates hypothesized to affect post-surgery mortality and length of stay: age, sex, marital status, type of hip fracture (transcervical, pertrochanteric, other), whether or not the patient was admitted to a teaching hospital, year of admission, median male income in postal code of residence and the number and type of comorbidities at the time of admission. Comorbidities coded as complications were not included since these may be endogenous with respect to length of stay. Information on comorbidities was used to construct a Charlson comorbidity index [10] for each patient using a coding methodology developed specifically for administrative data [11]. This index has been validated as a predictor of mortality in logitudinal studies.

MEASURING HOSPITAL SURGICAL VOLUME

Studies in the literature have typically measured surgical volume as the number of surgeries (of the particular type) performed in the hospital during the calendar year in which the patient is admitted [1]. If the number of surgeries performed in each hospital frequently fluctuates, this variable may not accurately measure the hospital's amount of cumulative experience at the time of surgery. A more appropriate volume variable designed to capture any practice makes perfect effect is a measure of the number of operations performed by hospital h in the time period *prior* to the current patient's surgery. Consequently, we construct $HVOL_{ht}$ to be equal to the total number of surgeries performed in hospital h in the 12-month period prior to the date (t) of the current patient's surgery. Because we cannot construct the number of surgeries performed at each hospital prior to April 1990, the subsequent estimates are based on the sample of hip fracture patients undergoing surgery at Quebec hospitals between April 1991 and January 1993. Finally, like almost all studies in the literature, we are unable to identify the surgeon for all the patients in the sample and hence cannot estimate the volume–outcome relationship at the surgeon level.

PRELIMINARY TABULATIONS OF BETWEEN AND WITHIN HOSPITAL DIFFERENCES

One of the primary goals of this paper is to distinguish between variations in outcomes associated with differences in volume *between* hospitals and variations in outcomes associated with fluctuations over time in volume *within* hospitals. To provide a first look at the volume–outcome relationship between hospitals, we calculated the average number of hip fracture surgeries performed per 12-month period at each hospital in the sample between April 1991 and March 1993. Mean surgical volume for the 68 hospitals was 53 surgeries per year. Using this average volume measure, we divided hospitals into three groups: low volume hospitals performing fewer than 34 surgeries on average in a 12-month period (25% of hospitals); average volume hospitals performing between 34 and 71 surgeries (50% of hospitals); and high volume hospitals performing more than 71 surgeries (25% of sample). Table 9.1 gives the average length of stay, fraction of patients dying in-hospital, the average number of comorbidities and Charlson index value by volume category. The first row indicates that patients at low volume hospitals had an average length of stay of 31 days, with 9.4% dying in-hospital. Moving down the rows of the table, increasing surgical volume is associated with lower average lengths of stay and mortality rates. For example, length of stay is almost 10 days shorter at a high volume hospital than at a low volume hospital. Column 3 suggests that at least part of this decline could reflect differences in case mix between hospitals: high volume hospitals appear to have patients with significantly fewer comorbidities. However, column 4 indicates no significant difference in the average Charlson index score across volume quartiles. Finally, the last column of Table 9.1 investigates the relationship between a commonly cited measure of hospital quality, whether the hospital is university affiliated and volume. Using this measure, high volume hospitals appear to be of higher quality. Consequently, some of the positive relationship found between volume and average hospital outcomes is likely to reflect differences between hospitals in quality and case-mix.

Given the large variations between hospitals in surgical volume and outcomes shown in Table 9.1, our next task is

Table 9.1 Differences in outcomes and case-mix between hospitals, by volume

| Average number of surgeries performed | Averages | | | | Fraction of hospitals university affiliated |
	Length of stay (days) (1)	Fraction died in hospital (2)	Number of comorbidities (3)	Charlson index (4)	
(Low) <34	31.0	0.094	2.77	0.56	0.29
(Average) 34–71	25.9	0.083	2.37	0.55	0.47
(High) >71	21.8	0.065	1.90	0.54	0.67
Significance test: p-value[a]	0.000	0.001	0.000	0.683	0.000

[a] p-value is from a test of the null hypothesis of equality of means across volume categories.

to describe the relationship between changes over time in volume and outcomes within hospitals. To do so, we construct the percentage difference between the number of surgeries performed at the hospital in the 12 months prior to date t and the average number performed per 12-month period at the hospital over the entire sample. Thus, for each hospital at each date, we are able to determine whether volume is above, equal to or below its long-term average. We then divide this variable into three categories: hospitals whose volume at date t was 10% or more below its sample average (20% of sample); hospitals whose volume at date t was within $\pm 10\%$ of its sample average (60% of sample); and hospitals whose volume was more than 10% above its sample average at date t (20% of sample). Once hospitals are classified into periods of high, average and low volume, we calculate the differences between mean outcomes (and case-mix) for patients admitted to a particular hospital at date t and the average outcome at that hospital over the same period. Table 9.2 examines whether hospitals performing an above or below average (for the particular hospital) number of surgeries as of date t also have above or below average outcomes and case mix for that particular period.

The first row of Table 9.2 shows that in hospitals with surgical volumes at date t more than 10% below their sample mean, average length of stay and in-hospital mortality are both above the hospitals' sample average, but the difference is small and insignificant. The remainder of columns 1 and 2 indicate surprisingly that patients admitted during high volume periods have increased hospital durations, although mortality is lower. Nevertheless, these differences are statistically insignificant. Columns 3 and 4 show very small differences in hospital case mix when hospitals perform above or below the average number of surgeries as of date t. The final column shows that hospitals experiencing relatively large fluctuations in volume are less likely to be university affiliated, but again the variation is small. Consequently, comparison of Tables 9.1 and 9.2 suggests that the relationship between

outcomes and volume primarily reflects differences between hospitals, although it is not clear to what extent this results from case mix and quality differences. From these simple tabulations, it does not appear to be the case that a hospital performing more surgeries in the 12 months prior to period t than its sample average experiences significantly improved outcomes.

METHODOLOGY

While the summary statistics presented in Tables 9.1 and 9.2 are suggestive, they do not simultaneously control for the multiple factors which may affect outcomes. This section presents the empirical framework for examining the impact of hospital surgical volume on the duration of hospital stay after hip fracture and the probability of inpatient mortality. This framework is constructed to address two potential pitfalls in the estimation of the relationship between surgical volume and outcomes: (1) the possible correlation between length of stay and inpatient mortality; and (2) fixed differences between hospitals, such as quality, which may also be correlated with volume.

Turning to the first issue, length of stay and discharge destination are estimated jointly using a duration model with multiple destinations. Studies in the literature have estimated separate length of stay and inpatient mortality regressions, hence assuming that these events are independent. If this assumption is false, these regressions potentially yield incorrect inferences regarding the effect of surgical volume on outcomes. For example, suppose that higher volume leads to shorter lengths of stay, but has no effect on in-hospital mortality conditional upon length of stay. A separate regression of mortality on volume may still yield a significant effect, since high volume leads to shorter lengths of stay and in-hospital deaths are less likely to be observed for patients with shorter lengths of stay when the outcomes are positively correlated. Conse-

Table 9.2 Differences in outcomes and case-mix across periods within hospitals, by differences in volume

Percentage difference in period t volume from hospital sample average	Period t difference from hospital sample average				Fraction of hospitals university affiliated
	Length of stay (days) (1)	Fraction died in hospital (2)	Number of comorbidities (3)	Charlson index (4)	
(Below) < -10	0.50	0.006	0.05	0.02	0.51
(Average) -10 to 10	-0.39	-0.002	-0.03	0.002	0.56
(Above) > 10	0.63	-0.002	0.03	0.01	0.48

Tests of the null hypothesis that the elements in columns 1–4 equal zero cannot be rejected in any case.

quently, the empirical framework must allow for the potential non-independence between the unobservables affecting length of stay and mortality.

Denote the duration of a hospital stay by m and suppose that there exist two mutually exclusive and exhaustive destinations indexed by $r = a$ (discharged alive from hospital), d (died in hospital). Let $\delta_r = 1$ if the patient is discharged to destination r and zero otherwise. The building block of the analysis is the transition intensity, $\lambda_r(m)$, defined as:

$$\lambda_r(m) = \lim_{\Delta m \to 0^+}$$

$$\frac{Pr[m < M \leq m + \Delta m, \delta_r = 1 | M \geq m]}{\Delta m} \quad (9.1)$$

which is the probability that the patient is discharged to destination r after m days in hospital, conditional upon surviving in the hospital for at least m days. Suppose the transition intensities depend upon a vector of individual and hospital characteristics recorded at the date t when patient i is admitted to hospital h, X_{iht}. Note that X_{iht} includes a measure of surgical volume, HVOL_{ht}. The probability of observing an exit to r after a hospital stay of length m is then

$$f_r(m_{iht} | X_{iht}) = \lambda_r(m_{iht} | X_{iht})$$

$$\prod_{j \in a, d} \exp\left[- \int_0^{m_{iht}} \lambda_j(u | X_{iht}) du \right], r = a, d \quad (9.2)$$

The first term on the right-hand side of Equation 9.2 is the transition intensity representing the probability that the patient is discharged after m days in hospital to destination r given that his or her length of stay is $\geq m$. The second term, the survivor function, is the probability that the individual survives at least to time m in the hospital and hence did not exit either alive or dead prior to m. The product of the quantities defined in Equation 9.2 across individuals provides the basis for the likelihood function.

ACCOUNTING FOR UNOBSERVED PATIENTS FRAILTY

Unobserved patient characteristics are likely to impact both the live discharge and in-hospital mortality transition intensities. For example, frailer patients are less likely to be discharged alive and also more likely to die in hospital. The typical approach used in the duration literature to account for unmeasured individual heterogeneity is to suppose that the transition intensities depend on a

scalar random variable v in addition to observed characteristics [12,13]. In our case, the unmeasured characteristics v could reflect the unobserved health status of the patient at the time of admission to the hospital, which affects outcomes. The estimation approach conditions on v and integrates it out of the likelihood function.

We are now able to construct the likelihood of observing a post-surgery length of stay of m and a discharge to destination r, conditional upon both measured and unmeasured characteristics. Let $G(v)$ be the distribution function of v. Using Equation 9.2, if the length of stay transition intensities are allowed to depend upon v, the likelihood function for the model is given by:

$$L = \prod_i \int f_a(m_{iht} | X_{iht}, v)^{\delta_{ia}} f_d(m_{iht} | X_{iht}, v)^{\delta_{id}} dG(v) \quad (9.3)$$

The first term of Equation 9.3 is the probability of observing a stay of m_{iht} days that results in a live discharge from hospital h for individual i admitted at date t, while the second term is the probability of observing a stay of m_{iht} days ending in an in-hospital death. The integral in Equation 9.3 reflects the fact that v is not observed and must be integrated out.

ACCOUNTING FOR FIXED DIFFERENCES BETWEEN HOSPITALS

As noted in the Introduction, much controversy exists in the literature as to whether the positive volume–outcome relationship reflects a practice effect or differences in hospital quality. Some studies have attempted to account for quality differences by including proxies for quality, such as whether the hospital is university affiliated or offers certain facilities, in cross-sectional regressions [1]. However, hospitals may differ in a wide variety of quality dimensions and it is unlikely that a set of three or four variables will fully capture variations in quality between hospitals.

The estimation strategy employed in the chapter to address this issue is similar to that of Farley and Ozminkowski [8] and relies on longitudinal hospital data. If hospitals differ in quality and these hospital-specific differences persist over the T periods in the sample, quality differences across hospitals may be accounted for by including a dummy variable for each hospital in the specification. It does not seem unreasonable to assume that hospital quality is relatively constant over a few years. Variables typically used in the literature to measure hospital quality, such as university affiliation and whether the hospital offers particular services, generally remain unchanged during a time period of this length. The coefficients on the hospital dummy variables indicate which hospitals have above or below average outcomes after controlling for observed patient characteristics and the number of surgeries performed at the hospital in the past 12 months. Hence, the hospital fixed effects reflect variations in outcomes *between* hospitals during the entire sample period. The volume coefficient is then identified by the relationship between outcomes and surgical volumes *within* hospitals over time. For example, a positive coefficient estimate on volume in the live discharge transition intensity when hospital specific dummies are included in the model implies that a hospital performing more surgeries in period $t + 1$ than in period t would also have improved outcomes (shorter lengths of stay) in period $t + 1$, on average. When the hospital indicators are excluded from the model, the coefficient on volume will reflect both differences between high and low volume hospitals and differences within hospitals over time.

SPECIFICATION OF FUNCTIONAL FORMS

The final step in the construction of the empirical model involves the specification of the functional form of the transition intensities in Equation 9.3. We follow a common approach and adopt a proportional hazards specification. In addition, the unmeasured component is allowed to have different factor loadings in each transition intensity function, so that

$$\lambda_r(m_{iht} \mid X_{iht}, v) = \exp(X_{iht}\beta_r + \theta_{hr} + \pi_r v)\lambda_{0r}(m_{iht})$$
$$r = a, d \qquad (9.4)$$

where θ_{hr} denotes the hospital-specific fixed effect and $\lambda_{0r}(m)$ represents the baseline transition intensity function. Measured and unmeasured characteristics thus shift the transition intensity above or below its baseline. Not all of the factor loading in Equation 9.4 are identified, so π_a is normalized to 1. We also considered an alternative specification which allowed for separate heterogeneity components, v_a and v_d, for the live and dead discharge transition intensities, respectively (all the π_r are set to 1 in this case). However, the results were virtually identical with those presented below using this alternative specification, so we adopted the simpler one factor specification of the frailty distribution.

A variety of parametric and non-parametric methods are available to estimate the baseline transition intensity [12]. Some guidance as to the appropriate functional form may be gained by examining the empirical transition intensities, shown in Figure 9.1. A parsimonious specification of the baseline transition intensity which allows for the non-monotonic behaviour shown in the

figure and which yields a reasonable fit of the data is the log–logistic distribution:

$$\lambda_{0r}(m) = \frac{\rho_r \alpha_r m^{\alpha_r - 1}}{1 + \rho_r m^{\alpha_r}} \alpha_r > 0, \rho_r > 0. \qquad (9.5)$$

When $\alpha_r > 1, \lambda_{0r}(m)$ has an inverted U shape reaching a maximum at $m = [(\alpha_r - 1)/\rho_r]^{1/\alpha_r}$. Equation 9.5 allows the parameters of the baseline transition intensities to differ for each destination.

Estimation of the model requires that a functional form be chosen for $G(v)$. Pickles and Crouchley [13] describe a variety of specifications for $G(v)$. We adopt the non-parametric approach suggested by Heckman and Singer [9] and assume that $G(v)$ may be approximated by a discrete distribution with a finite number of points of support. The location of the points of support and their associated probability mass are estimated jointly with the other parameters of the model. With this specification of $G(v)$, the likelihood function may be written as

$$L = \prod_i \sum_{k=1}^{K} \omega_k f_a(m_{iht} \mid X_{iht}, \theta_h, v_k)^{\delta_{ia}}$$
$$f_d(m_{iht} \mid X_{iht}, \theta_h, v_k)^{\delta_{id}} \qquad (9.6)$$

where $v_k, K = 1, ..., K$ are the points of support with associated probabilities ω_k which sum to one. Empirical applications have shown that the value of K required to non-parametrically represent $G(v)$ is usually small, generally $K = 3$ or 4.

EMPIRICAL RESULTS

This section presents the estimation results from the empirical model described above. Primary interest focuses on the impact of $HVOL_{ht}$ on outcomes. To make our estimates comparable to those in the literature, we use the natural logarithm of $HVOL_{ht}$ in the specifications, although the results are similar when $HVOL_{ht}$ is used as a regressor. To account for differences across patients, indicators for gender and marital status are included in X_{iht}, as are patient age and income as measured by median male income in 1988 in the postal code of residence. Given the concern in the literature regarding the possible correlation between patient case-mix and surgical volume, we include substantially more variables describing the patient's health status at the time of hospital admission than is typically found in the literature: X_{iht} includes indicator variables for whether the patient has 0, 1, 2, 3 or 4–5 comorbidities (the omitted category is 6+ comorbidities), in addition to 10 dummy variables correspond-

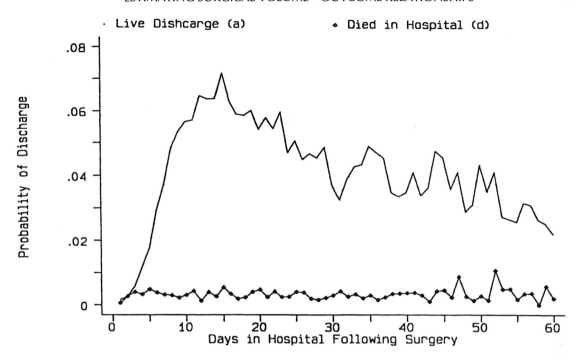

Figure 9.1. Empirical transition intensities, by destination

ing to the comorbid conditions which make up the Charlson index. Finally, we include indicators for the type of fracture and the year in which the surgery was performed. The year dummies capture any common trend across hospitals in outcomes over time.

Tables 9.3 and 9.4 present the parameter estimates of the length of stay transition intensities from the competing risk model. Positive coefficients indicate that an increase in the variable implies an increase in the transition intensity. Regarding the frailty distribution, the data indicated clustering around three points, so that $G(v)$ was approximated by a finite distribution with three points of support ($K = 3$).

Table 9.3 presents the parameter estimates of the determinants of length of stay resulting in a live discharge (columns 1 and 2) and an in-hospital death (columns 3 and 4). The odd-numbered columns correspond to a specification which excludes the hospital dummies, while the even-numbered columns allow for fixed differences across hospitals. Both specifications allow for unmeasured (by the econometrician) differences across patients. Turning first to the live discharge transition intensities, the positive and precisely estimated coefficient on $\log(\text{HVOL}_{ht})$ in column 1 implies that after controlling for other potential confounders, such as demographic characteristics and observed comorbidities, patients undergoing surgery at a

high volume hospital have a significantly higher probability of leaving the hospital on day m, conditional upon having survived in hospital at least m days. This is consistent with studies in the literature (e.g. Hughes *et al.* [14]) showing that hospitals performing a large number of hip fracture surgeries have shorter lengths of stay in the USA. The remainder of the coefficient estimates indicate that older patients and those in poorer health at the time of admission have lower conditional probabilities of leaving the hospital on any particular day. Finally, the estimates of the baseline hazard parameters ρ and α imply that the live discharge transition intensity initially increases with length of stay, peaks at approximately 20 days and then declines thereafter.

The estimates in column 2 of Table 9.3 indicate that the surgical volume-live discharge relationship found in the first column primarily reflects fixed differences between hospitals rather than a within-hospital effect. When hospital fixed effects are included in the specification, the coefficient on volume in the live discharge transitions declines substantially and is insignificant. Consequently, if the average hospital performs 10 more surgeries in the previous 12 months than its sample 12 month average, the conditional probability of live discharge will not change significantly. On the other hand, the hospital indicator variables, which capture permanent differences

Table 9.3 Proportional hazard estimates (baseline hazard specification: log–logistic)

| Variable | Exit destination | | | |
| | Live discharge (a) | | Died in hospital (d) | |
	(1)	(2)	(3)	(4)
Log(HVOL$_{ht}$)	0.245	−0.085	−0.013	−0.329
	(8.306)	(−0.806)	(−0.124)	(−0.941)
Age	−0.017	−0.019	0.072	0.069
	(−16.281)	(−15.843)	(8.587)	(9.037)
Male	0.013	0.022	0.580	0.547
	(0.403)	(0.625)	(4.547)	(4.434)
Married	0.054	0.041	0.073	0.105
	(1.876)	(1.289)	(0.642)	(0.891)
Income	−0.020	−0.080	0.012	0.056
	(−0.762)	(−2.449)	(0.113)	(0.439)
Pertrochanteric fracture	−0.221	−0.195	0.287	0.301
	(−7.024)	(−5.812)	(2.318)	(2.437)
Other fracture	−0.100	−0.018	0.075	0.041
	(−2.568)	(−0.390)	(0.464)	(0.225)
0 Comorbidities	1.348	1.737	−1.820	−2.129
	(16.615)	(20.892)	(−6.393)	(−6.721)
1 Comorbidity	1.034	1.373	−0.641	−0.891
	(13.493)	(17.704)	(−3.092)	(−4.021)
2 Comorbidities	0.777	1.044	−0.407	−0.634
	(10.422)	(13.758)	(−2.157)	(−3.240)
3 Comorbidities	0.753	0.958	−0.378	−0.606
	(9.963)	(12.562)	(−1.989)	(−3.146)
4–5 Comorbidities	0.324	0.437	−0.132	−0.301
	(4.544)	(6.105)	(−0.845)	(−1.928)
Comorbidity types:				
$p$value[a]	0.000	0.000	0.000	0.000
π	1	1	−2.664	−1.343
			(−3.877)	(−3.911)
ρ	0.0004	0.0003	0.015	0.015
	(8.696)	(8.621)	(3.571)	(4.049)
α	2.699	2.612	1.454	1.513
	(49.910)	(55.556)	(10.989)	(9.901)
Hospital dummies?	No	Yes	No	Yes
p-value[b]	—	0.000	—	0.000

t-Statistics in parentheses. Each regression based on 7383 patient observations at 66 hospitals. Each regression also includes a constant, dummy variables for year in sample and indicators for 10 co-morbidity types. The age and income variables are deviations from their sample means.
[a]p-Value is from a test of the null hypothesis that the coefficients on the 10 comorbidity indicators are jointly zero.
[b]p-Value is from a test of the null hypothesis that the coefficients on the 65 hospital indicators are jointly zero.

between hospitals over the sample period, are jointly strongly statistically significant.

Columns 3 and 4 show that surgical volume does not have a significant effect on the conditional probability of dying in hospital, although the volume coefficient increases in absolute magnitude when the hospital fixed effects are included in the specification. While Hughes *et al.* [14] find a significant hip surgery volume-in-hospital mortality link (not controlling for fixed differences between hospitals), they include only a small set of patient comorbidity indicators; in contrast, our specification in-

corporates variables measuring the number and type of comorbidities, as well as unobserved patient frailty. The hospital fixed effects may capture some of the between-hospital differences in case-mix. When we adopt a specification similar to Hughes *et al.* which does not allow for unobserved patient differences and hospital fixed effects and only includes comorbidity indicators for diabetes and heart disease, we also find that higher volume is associated with significantly lower in-hospital mortality. Consequently, we suspect that the significant volume–mortality link previously found in the literature reflects patient

Table 9.4 Proportional hazard model heterogeneity
parameter estimates (baseline hazard specification: log–logistic)

Variable	Specification	
	No hospital dummies (Table 9.3, columns 1 and 3)	Hospital dummies (Table 9.3, columns 2 and 4)
v_1	— 1.704	0.336
v_2	-2.360	-0.722
	(4.456)	(2.102)
v_3	-2.862	-2.753
	(3.114)	(3.754)
ω_1	0.714	0.796
	(4.518)	(4.369)
ω_3	0.034	0.005
	(1.153)	(0.856)
Log-likelihood	-30711.9	-30223.1

t-Statistics in parentheses. *t*-Statistics on $v_2(v_3)$ is from a test of the hypothesis that $v_1 = v_2 (v_1 = v_3)$.

case-mix differences across hospitals that are correlated with volume. Note that the joint significance of the hospital dummies in column 4 suggests that the conditional probability of in-hospital mortality differs across hospitals, but this does not appear to be related to volume after controlling for observed and unobserved patient heterogeneity.

The final notable finding in Table 9.3 is the significant and negative estimate of π_d in both columns 3 and 4, implying that unobserved patient characteristics leading to declines in the live discharge transition intensity are associated with higher conditional probabilities of in-hospital mortality. Therefore, treating length of stay and mortality as independent outcomes is overly restrictive.

Table 9.4 presents the estimates of the unobserved heterogeneity distribution for the specifications which exclude and include the hospital fixed effects. For convenience, denote a realization of v_k as a 'type k' patient. One interpretation of the $K = 3$ support points is that there are three types of patients. In the specification which includes hospital dummies, approximately 0.5% of the sample are type 3 individuals who experience significantly longer hospital stays and a substantially higher probability of dying in hospital than do type 1 or type 2 patients.

In summary, surgical volume has a significant and positive effect on the conditional probability of a live discharge from the hospital and an insignificant effect on the conditional probability of in-hospital mortality, thus implying that higher volumes are associated with shorter lengths of stay. However, this relationship appears to primarily reflect differences between hospitals. After including hospital-specific fixed effects, period to period

variation in volume within hospitals has no significant impact on the transition intensities. These results appear to be more consistent with explanations for the volume–outcome relationship that emphasize quality differences between hospitals and casts doubt on the practice makes perfect hypothesis. This conclusion is further strengthened if one believes that quality changes substantially over time and is positively correlated with volume as is usually assumed. In this case, the volume coefficients in the fixed effects models would be an upper bound (lower bound in the case of inpatient mortality) on the practice effect, but of course the coefficients are small and insignificant. However, given our short panel, the assumption of relatively constant quality appears reasonable.

DECOMPOSING THE LIVE DISCHARGE OUTCOME

The live discharge outcome encompasses a wide range of possible discharge destinations, including routine discharges to home, discharges to chronic care facilities and discharges to rehabilitation or other hospitals. While we found no effect of volume on the conditional probability of live discharge as a whole after accounting for hospital-specific effects, it may be the case that this result hides a significant effect of volume on a particular subset of live discharges. To address this possibility, we decompose the live discharge outcome into three subcategories: exits to home (h), comprising 45% of total discharges; exits to a chronic care facility (c), comprising 12% of discharges; and exits to a rehabilitation (or other) hospital (b), comprising 35% of discharges. The impact of volume on the transition intensities is then estimated using a likelihood function similar to Equation 9.6, where the set of mutually exclusive and exhaustive discharge destinations is now $r = h, c, b, d$.

The model was re-estimated for the expanded set of exit destinations including the set of patient characteristics X_{iht} used previously, accounting for unobserved patient heterogeneity as above. The first row of Table 9.5 presents the coefficient estimate on the natural logarithm of surgical volume for each of the four transition intensities when the hospital indicators are excluded from the model. Since our focus is on the volume–outcome relationship, the parameter estimates for the other variables are not presented. The results indicate that the strong positive relationship between surgical volume and live discharge shown in column 1 of Table 9.3 primarily reflects the fact that increases in volume increase the conditional probability of discharge to a rehabilitation hospital. There is little evidence to suggest that higher volumes lead to

Table 9.5   Proportional hazard estimates of log(HVOL$_{ht}$) for expanded set of outcomes, excluding and including hospital indicators

Includes hospital dummies?	Exit destination			
	Home (h)	Chronic care facility (c)	Rehabilitation hospital[a] (b)	Died in hospital (d)
(1) No	0.010	−0.091	0.750)	0.011
	(0.270)	(−1.171)	(16.033)	(0.123)
(2) Yes	−0.140	0.010	−0.013	−0.333
	(−1.061)	(0.075)	(−0.043)	(−1.178)
Fraction discharged to destination	0.45	0.12	0.35	0.08

t-Statistics in parentheses. Each regression based on 7383 patient observations at 66 hospitals. Each regression includes all of the variables shown in Table 9.3, and accounts for unobserved patient heterogeneity.
[a]Rehabilitation hospital includes other hospital.

speedier discharges to home, or have a significant impact on the conditional probability of discharge to a chronic care facility.

The second row of Table 9.5 presents the estimates of the volume variable when hospital fixed effects are included in the specification. The results are similar to those presented in Table 9.3. When the hospital indicators are included in the specification, the effect of surgical volume on the conditional probability of discharge to a rehabilitation hospital becomes small and insignificant, implying that fluctuations in volume within hospitals do not have a substantial effect on this or any of the other transition intensities. Consequently, these results suggest that low and high volume hospitals differ in their propensity to discharge patients to rehabilitation facilities. It may be the case that larger hospitals have developed working relationships with rehabilitation centres, which facilitate placement in these institutions. Overall, the main thrust of our results do not change when live discharges are decomposed into subsets of destinations. The volume–outcome relationship reflects differences between hospitals, rather than within hospitals, for hip fracture patients in Quebec.

CONCLUSIONS

This paper documents a significant relationship between surgical volume and length of stay among hip fracture patients at Quebec hospitals in the early 1990s. This result is similar to those found for American patients undergoing hip fracture surgery as well as surgery for a variety of other procedures. However, in contrast to these studies, which rely on cross-sectional samples of hospital volume and outcomes, we utilize longitudinal data to decompose the volume–outcome relationship into a 'within' hospital effect determined by period to period changes in a hospital's volume and a 'between' hospital effect reflecting differences among hospitals. In addition, we allow for potential correlation in live and dead discharges by incorporating unobserved (by the researcher) differences across patients at the time of hospital admission. Finally, we account for case mix differences between hospitals by including a substantial number of comorbidity variables. Our findings show that accounting for both measured and unmeasured patient characteristics, period to period fluctuations in a hospital's volume have no significant effect on length of stay or mortality. The significant volume–outcome relationship found in the data reflects differences between hospitals that are fixed over time. This finding persists when we decompose live discharges into exits to home, chronic care facilities or rehabilitation hospitals.

These results cast doubt on the practice makes perfect hypothesis in the case of hip fracture surgery. The results are more consistent with the hypothesis that higher quality hospitals attract more surgical volume, thus yielding the positive volume–outcome relationship observed in cross-sectional data. The results have important implications for health care providers and policy makers who must make decisions regarding resource allocation across hospitals. If declining budgets necessitate hospital closures or bed reductions, then closure of small, low quality hospitals and regionalization of care at large, high quality hospitals is likely to maintain or perhaps even improve overall patient outcomes. On the other hand, if hospital closures are not politically feasible, then reductions in surgical volume may be distributed amongst all hospitals, with no significant detrimental effect on overall patient outcomes. Of course, further information on the relationship between volume and costs is necessary before making such decisions.

Our results suggest that the volume–outcome relationship reflects fixed differences across hospital, such as quality. Further research is necessary to examine more deeply the determinants of between hospital variation. For example, these differences may reflect the quality of surgeons or the surgical team, treatment protocols or the scale of production at the hospital. Understanding of these issues may be important for making certain types of detailed policy recommendations, such as standardizing protocols. We intend to pursue these areas of investigation in future work.

Finally, our findings do not necessarily generalize to other types of surgery. For example, while hip fracture surgery is relatively routine, many government health authorities and oversight boards require that surgeons and hospitals performing operations such as PTCA must meet a minimum per year surgical volume in order to maintain competence and remain certified. For these types of procedures, practice makes perfect effects are clearly believed to be present [15]. However, it is the case that studies of the volume–outcome relationship for these procedures found in the literature rely on cross-sectional data and are unable to distinguish between the practice makes perfect and selective referral hypotheses [16]. Moreover, these studies have not controlled for the correlation between length of stay and inpatient mortality; nor have they accounted for potential differences in patient frailty. The empirical methodology outlined in this paper may be fruitfully applied to analysing the volume–outcome relationship for these other procedures.

ACKNOWLEDGEMENTS

This research was supported by a grant from the Social Sciences and Humanities Research Council of Canada. We are grateful for helpful comments from two referees, Rob Manning and participants in the Fifth European Workshop on Econometrics and Health Economics held at Pompeu Fabra University, Barcelona, Spain.

APPENDIX

Summary statistics and patient characteristics are given in Table 9.A1.

Table 9.A1 Summary statistics, patient characteristics

Variable	Mean (SD)
Length of stay (m)	24.7 (29.7)
Died in hospital	0.077 (0.267)
Age	76.1 (13.9)
Male	0.27 (0.45)
Married	0.39 (0.49)
Income (median in postal code)	21 691 (5260)
Pertrochanteric fracture	0.49 (0.50)
Other fracture	0.18 (0.38)
Number of surgeries (HVOL)	70.1 (31.6)
Admitted to university-affiliated hospital	0.54 (0.50)
0 Comorbidities	0.26 (0.44)
1 Comorbidity	0.21 (0.41)
2 Comorbidities	0.17 (0.38)
3 Comorbidities	0.13 (0.34)
4 or 5 Comorbidities	0.14 (0.35)
Charlson index	0.55 (1.1)
N	7383

REFERENCES

1. Luft, H.S., Garnick, D.W., Mark, D.H. and McPhee, S.J. *Hospital Volume, Physician Volume and Patient Outcomes: Assessing the Evidence.* Ann Arbor, MI: Health Administration Press Perspectives, 1990.
2. Luft, H.S., Bunker, J. and Enthoven, A. Should operations be regionalized? An empirical study of the relation between surgical volume and mortality. *New England Journal of Medicine* 1979; **301**: 1364–1369.
3. Hannan, E.L., Kilburn, H., Jr., Bernard, H., O'Donnell, J.F., Lukacic, G. and Shields, E.P. Coronary artery bypass surgery: the relationship between in hospital mortality rate and surgical volume after controlling for clinical risk factors. *Medical Care* 1991; **29**: 1094–1107.
4. Baker, S.P., O'Neill, B. and Karpf, R.S. *The Injury Fact Book.* Lexington, MA: D.C. Heath, 1984.
5. Roos, L.L., Cageorge, S.M., Roose, N.P. and Danziger, R. Centralization, certification and monitoring: Readmission and complications after surgery. *Medical Care* 1986; **24**: 1044–1066.
6. Roos, L.L., Roos, N.P. and Sharp, S.M. Monitoring adverse outcomes of surgery using administrative data. *Health Care Financing Review* 1987; Annual Supplement: 5–16.
7. Wennberg, J.E., Roos, N.P., Sola, L., Schori, A. and Jaffe, R. Use of claims data systems to evaluate health care outcomes: Mortality and reoperation following prostatectomy. *Journal of the American Medical Association* 1987; **257**: 933–936.
8. Farley, D.E. and Ozminkowski, R.J. Volume–outcome relationships and in hospital mortality: The effect of changes in volume over time. *Medical Care* 1992; **30**: 77–94.
9. Heckman, J. and Singer, B. A method for minimizing the impact of distributional assumptions in econometric models for duration data. *Econometrica* 1984; **52**: 271–320.
10. Charlson, M.E., Pompei, P., Ales, K. and MacKenzie, C.R. A new method of classifying prognostic comorbidity in longitudinal studies: development and validation. *Journal of Chronic Diseases* 1987; **40**: 373–383.
11. Romano, P.S., Roos, L.L. and Jolles, J.G. Adapting a clinical comorbidity index for use with ICD-9-CM administrative data: differing perspectives. *Journal of Clinical Epidemiology* 1993; **46**: 1075–1079.
12. Lancaster, T. *The Econometric Analysis of Transition Data.* Cambridge: Cambridge University Press, 1990.
13. Pickles, A. and Crouchley, R. A comparison of frailty models

for multivariate survival data. *Statistics in Medicine* 1995; **14**: 1447–1461.

14. Hughes, R.G., Garnick, D.W., Luft, H.S., McPhee, S.J. and Hunt, S.S. Hospital volume and patient outcomes: the case of hip fracture patients. *Medical Care* 1988; **26**: 1057–1067.

15. Phillips, K.A., Luft, H.S. and Ritchie, J.L. The association of hospital volumes of percutaneous transluminal coronary angioplasty with adverse outcomes, length of stay and charges in California. *Medical Care* 1995; **33**: 502–514.

16. Jollis, J.G., Peterson, E.D., DeLong, E.R. *et al.* The relation between the volume of coronary angioplasty procedures at hospitals treating medicare beneficiaries and short-term mortality. *New England Journal of Medicine* 1994; **334**: 1625–1629.

Flexible and Semiparametric Estimators

10

Individual Cigarette Consumption and Addiction: A Flexible Limited Dependent Variable Approach

STEVEN T. YEN[1] AND ANDREW M. JONES[2]

[1]*Department of Agricultural Economics, University of Tennessee, USA and* [2]*Department of Economics and Related Studies, University of York, York, UK*

Several recent studies have shown the relevance of the double-hurdle approach for microeconomic analysis of cigarette smoking [1–9]. At the same time, Becker and Murphy's [10] model of rational addiction has stimulated research on the role of addiction in empirical analysis of survey data on smoking [11–13]. Here we develop a model of the simultaneous decisions of how many cigarettes to smoke and whether to quit. This incorporates the trade-off between the fixed costs of quitting, associated with nicotine dependence, and the expected future benefits of quitting in terms of health, wealth and self-esteem. Unlike previous work on cigarette consumption [11–13], the model identifies the separate influence of addiction on consumption and participation.

Survey data, whether for individuals or households, and whether based on expenditure or number of cigarettes, invariably contain a high proportion of non-smokers, and appropriate limited dependent variable techniques are required to avoid biased and inconsistent estimates. The special feature of the double hurdle approach is that, unlike the standard Tobit model, the determinants of participation (whether to start or quit smoking) and the determinants of consumption (how many cigarettes to smoke) are allowed to differ. However, a limitation of the standard double hurdle specification is that it is based on the assumption of bivariate normality for the error distribution. Empirical results will be sensitive to misspecification, and ML estimates will be inconsistent if the normality assumption is violated [14,15]. This may be particularly relevant if the model is applied to a dependent variable that has a highly skewed distribu-

tion, as is often the case with survey data on cigarette consumption. In this paper we use a flexible generalization of the model, the Box–Cox double hurdle model introduced by Jones and Yen [16].

The Box–Cox double hurdle model provides a common framework that nests standard versions of the double hurdle model and also includes the generalized Tobit model and 'two-part' dependent variable, as special cases [2,7,9,17,18]. This allows us to make explicit comparisons of a wide range of specifications that have been used in the microeconometric literature on smoking. Our results are based on a sample of 3801 British adults from the 1984–85 Health and Lifestyle Survey (HALS).

A MODEL OF SMOKING AND QUITTING*

This section develops an empirical model of the simultaneous decisions of how many cigarettes to smoke and whether to quit smoking. This model is based on the trade-off between the expected benefits of quitting for the smoker's health, wealth and self-esteem and the fixed costs of quitting associated with nicotine dependence and withdrawal. For similar models of participation based on the expected utility of smoking versus quitting, see Ippolito and Ippolito [19], Jones [20], Mullahy and Portney [21], Viscusi [22] and Blaylock and Blisard [7]. Other studies of addiction based on survey data have concentrated on the impact of addiction on the level of cigarette consumption [11–13]. But because our data set

Econometric Analysis of Health Data. Edited by Andrew M. Jones and Owen O'Donnell
© 2002 John Wiley & Sons Ltd. Previously published in *Health Economics*, Vol. 5; pp. 105–117 (1996). © John Wiley & Sons Ltd

contains information on individuals' history of smoking, irrespective of whether they are current smokers, we are able to analyse the separate influence of addiction on quitting as well as on consumption.

As our empirical application uses cross-section survey data we use a stylized model of addiction that is essentially a static framework. However the specification is intended to include the expected future benefits of quitting and could be interpreted in terms of intertemporal models of rational addiction. Our cross-section data has no price variation (either inter-temporal or inter-regional), so we are not able to investigate the impact of past, current and future cigarette prices. These cross-price effects play a key role in the Becker–Murphy framework for distinguishing between myopic and rational behaviour.

The development of nicotine dependence is often defined in terms of tolerance, reinforcement and withdrawal effects (see e.g. Ashton and Stepney [23], Becker and Murphy [10]). In particular, Ashton and Stepney describe the onset of withdrawal effects as follows:

. . . an important stage in the development of drug dependence is the move from taking the drug in order to feel better to taking it in order to avoid feeling worse.
[Ashton and Stepney [23], p. 58]

Two stylised features of withdrawal effects stand out. Firstly, the effects are asymmetric and only occur when smokers try to cut down or quit. Secondly, once a threshold has been passed, the role of consumption is not simply to provide satisfaction but also to ward off the consequences of withdrawal. In this respect withdrawal can be interpreted as increasing the 'efficiency' of consumption (see Jones [20]).

The influence of nicotine dependence and the associated withdrawl effects can be modelled as a 'fixed cost' of quitting. In line with the literature on the economics of addiction we assume that these expected fixed costs (A_i) will depend on the individual's past consumption. In our empirical application we use a measure of previous peak cigarette consumption (Chaloupka [12], uses a similar measure). However addition is not simply a function of the individual's past behaviour and an individual's degree of dependence will depend on their characteristics and circumstances. Assume that,

$$A_i = x_{0i}\alpha_0 + \varepsilon_{0i}$$

where x_0 is a vector of variables, including past consumption, that affect the expected fixed costs of quitting, α_0 is the corresponding vector of parameters, and ε_{0i} is a random disturbance reflecting unobservable individual heterogeneity.

The expected benefits of quitting are likely to reflect the health, financial and social consequences of the habit. For example, Marsh and Matheson [24] suggest that the decision to quit is typically based on the perceived benefits of abstinence rather than the perceived harm of continuing smoking:

. . . More positive attitudes towards the benefits of giving up smoking lead more smokers first to resolve and then to attempt to give up. The attitudes most effective in this process concern the likelihood of positive health benefits from giving up smoking. Those concerned with money and greater self-esteem are also effective, those with aesthetic and social aspects less so unless linked to self-esteem.
[Marsh and Matheson [24], p. 132]

The 1990 British Social Attitudes Survey has a module on attitudes to smoking. Its findings show that 87% of current and ex-smokers cite health as being a 'very or fairly' important reason for wanting to give up smoking, 51% say that it costs too much to continue smoking, and 43% cite family pressure. In the Health and Lifestyle Survey 34% of men and 26% of women mention ill-health at the time of the decision as the reason for stopping smoking. Fear of future ill-health is mentioned 30% of men and 23% of women, and the expense is mentioned by 28% of men and 27% of women. Other reasons all have less than 13% responses [26].

It is reasonable to assume that the expected benefits of quitting, in terms of health, wealth and self-esteem will depend on how much the individual would have smoked otherwise. In particular it is likely that the benefits will be increasing in the individual's level of cigarette consumption. The financial burden of heavier smoking is clear. As regards the benefits of quitting for current and future health, there is extensive evidence that the health risks of smoking are perceived to be greater for heavy smokers [24]. Also, the social pressures and associated stigma may be greater for heavy smokers than for occasional or 'social' smokers. This is likely to be exacerbated by increasing restrictions on smoking in public places and attitudes towards the risks of passive smoking [25].

We assume that there is a latent variable (y_{2i}^*), which characterizes the individual's demand for cigarettes, such that,

$$y_{2i}^* = g(y_i) \text{ or } g^{-1}(y_{2i}^*)$$

where y_i is their observed level of consumption, and $g(.)$ is an increasing transformation. Then assume that the expected benefits of quitting are given by,

$$B_i = B^*(y_{2i}^*) = B(g^{-1}(y_{2i}^*)) = B(y_i)$$

with $B'(.) > 0$, so that the benefits of quitting are increasing in the level of desired and observed consumption. In our empirical application we use the Box–Cox transformation for $g(.)$; this introduces greater flexibility into the standard double hurdle specification of cigarette consumption.

The decision to attempt to quit smoking will depend on the expected net benefit of quitting $B - A$. In other words, on whether the benefits outweigh the fixed costs caused by nicotine dependence. So the condition for an individual *not* attempting to quit can be written,

$$y_{1i}^* = A_i - B_i = 0.$$

Now let

$$y_{2i}^* = x_{2i}\alpha_2 + \varepsilon_{2i}$$

where x_2 are variables that determine the demand for cigarettes, which may include the addiction effects of tolerance and reinforcement on the level of consumption, α_2 is the corresponding vector of parameters, and ε_{2i} is a random disturbance. For tractability, let $B^*(.)$ be the identity, then,

$$y_{1i}^* = x_{0i}\alpha_0 + \varepsilon_{0i} - x_{2i}\alpha_2 - \varepsilon_{2i}$$

or

$$y_{1i}^* = x_{1i}\alpha_1 + \varepsilon_{1i} \tag{10.1}$$

where x, is the union of x_0 and x_2. α_1 is the corresponding parameter vector, where for variables that appear in both x_0 and x_2 the elements of $\alpha_1 = \alpha_0 - \alpha_2$, and $\varepsilon_{1i} = \varepsilon_{0i} - \varepsilon_{2i}$.

Equation 10.1 gives the first hurdle that the individual must pass to be observed with a positive level of cigarette consumption. But, in line with the double hurdle specification, we also allow for the latent variable y_{2i}^* to generate zero observations. Then, the observed level of cigarette consumption is,

$$y_i = g^{-1}(y_{2i}^*)$$

$$\text{if } y_{1i}^* > 0 \text{ and } g^{-1}(y_{2i}^*) = g^{-1}(x_{2i}\alpha_2 + \varepsilon_{2i}) > 0 \tag{10.2}$$

Notice that for variables that have no (or small) influence on the fixed costs of quitting ($\alpha_0 \cong 0$) we would expect equal and opposite effects on the two decisions ($\alpha_1 \cong -\alpha_2$). This reflects the intuition that, *conditional* on overcoming the fixed costs of quitting (A), it is the heavier smokers who have the greatest incentive to quit.

Given the specification in Equation 10.1 and Equation 10.2 and assuming that ε_{0i} and ε_{2i} have zero mean, con-

stant variances ($\sigma_{\varepsilon0}^2$ and $\sigma_{\varepsilon2}^2$), and covariance $\sigma_{\varepsilon02}$, the covariance matrix for ε_{1i} and ε_{2i} is,

$$\begin{vmatrix} \sigma_{\varepsilon0}^2 + \sigma_{\varepsilon2}^2 - 2\sigma_{\varepsilon02} & \sigma_{\varepsilon02} - \sigma_{\varepsilon2}^2 \\ \sigma_{\varepsilon02} - \sigma_{\varepsilon2}^2 & \sigma_{\varepsilon2}^2 \end{vmatrix}$$

This gives a correlation coefficient,

$$\rho_\varepsilon = \frac{\sigma_{\varepsilon02} - \sigma_{\varepsilon2}^2}{\sigma_{\varepsilon2}\sqrt{\sigma_{\varepsilon0}^2 + \sigma_{\varepsilon2}^2 - 2\sigma_{\varepsilon02}}}$$

which will depend on the degree of correlation between the unobservable elements of the fixed costs of quitting (A_i) and the desire to smoke (y_{2i}^*). In the limit, if $\sigma_{\varepsilon02} = 0$,

$$\rho_\varepsilon = -\frac{\sigma_{\varepsilon2}}{\sqrt{\sigma_{\varepsilon0}^2 + \sigma_{\varepsilon2}^2}}$$

which implies a high degree of negative correlation between the two error terms. When $\sigma_{\varepsilon0}^2$ is small relative to $\sigma_{\varepsilon2}^2$ this expression will tend towards -1. To summarize, this specification suggests that it would not be appropriate to assume independence of the error terms in the double hurdle model, if the benefits of quitting are associated with the individual's level of smoking.

THE ECONOMETRIC SPECIFICATION

To estimate the model we normalize the error distribution so that $\sigma_{21} = 1$, and assume bivariate normality. Then the empirical model corresponds to the Box–Cox double hurdle model of Jones and Yen [16]. Which can be written as (the parameter vectors α_1 and α_2 are replaced by β_1 and β_2, to reflect the normalization of the variance),

$$y_{1i}^* = x_{1i}\beta_1 + u_{1i} \tag{10.3}$$
$$y_{2i}^* = x_{2i}\beta_2 + u_{2i} \tag{10.4}$$

where

$$(u_{1i}, u_{2i}) \sim \text{BVN}(0, \Sigma)$$

and

$$\Sigma = \begin{bmatrix} 1 & \sigma_{12} \\ \sigma_{12} & \sigma^2 \end{bmatrix}$$

In other words, the conditional distribution of the latent variables is assumed to be bivariate normal.

For the function $g(.)$ we use a Box–Cox transformation. Then, the censoring mechanism implies that the observed dependent variable (cigarette consumption, y_i) is such that,

$$y_{2i}^* = (y_i^\lambda - 1)/\lambda \quad \lambda > 0$$

$$\text{if } y_{2i}^* > -1/\lambda \text{ and } y_{1i}^* > 0$$

$$= \log(y_i) \quad \lambda = 0$$

$$y_i = 0 \quad \text{otherwise} \quad\quad (10.5)$$

This specification allows participation to depend on both sets of regressors x_{1i} and x_{2i} and permits stochastic dependence between the two error terms, as predicted by our model. In addition the use of the Box–Cox transformation relaxes the normality assumption on the conditional distribution of y_i. In Jones and Yen [16] we show that the likelihood function for a sample of independent observations is,

$$L = \Pi_i \left[1 - \Phi\left(x_{1i}, \frac{x_{2i}\beta_2 + 1/\lambda}{\sigma}, \rho \right) \right]^{(1-D_i)}$$

$$\times \left[\Phi\left(\frac{x_{1i}\beta_1 + (\rho/\sigma)\{(y_i^\lambda - 1)/\lambda - x_{2i}\beta_2\}}{\sqrt{1-\rho^2}} \right) \right.$$

$$\left. \times y_i^{(\lambda-1)} \frac{1}{\sigma} \phi\left(\frac{(y_i^\lambda - 1)/\lambda - x_{2i}\beta_2}{\sigma} \right) \right]^{D_i} \quad (10.6)$$

where Φ denotes a, univariate or bivariate, standard normal CDF, ϕ denotes the univariate standard normal PDF, $\rho = \sigma_{12}/\sigma$, and D_i is an indicator such that $D_i = 1$ if $y_i > 0$ and 0 otherwise. The advantage of this approach is that it encompasses a wide range of standard limited dependent variable models. The general model Equation 10.6 can be restricted to give various special cases (see Jones and Yen [16] for full details):

(i) $\sigma_{12} = 0$

This gives the Box–Cox double hurdle with independent errors.

$$L = \Pi_i \left[1 - \Phi(x_{1i}\beta_1)\Phi\left(\frac{x_{2i}\beta_2 + 1/\lambda}{\sigma} \right) \right]^{(1-D_i)}$$

$$\times \left[\Phi(x_{1i}\beta_1)y_i^{(\lambda-1)} \frac{1}{\sigma}\phi\left(\frac{(y_i^\lambda - 1)/\lambda - x_{2i}\beta_2}{\sigma} \right) \right]^{D_i} \quad (10.7)$$

(ii) $\lambda = 1$

This gives the standard double hurdle with dependence,

$$L = \Pi_i \left[1 - \Phi\left(x_{1i}\beta_1, \frac{x_{2i}\beta_2 + 1}{\sigma}, \rho \right) \right]^{-(1-D_i)}$$

$$\times \left[\Phi\left(\frac{x_{1i}\beta_1 + (\rho/\sigma)\{y_i - x_{2i}\beta_2 - 1\}}{\sqrt{1-\rho^2}} \right) \right.$$

$$\left. \times \frac{1}{\sigma}\phi\left(\frac{y_i - x_{2i}\beta_2 - 1}{\sigma} \right) \right]^{D_i} \quad (10.8)$$

This model is applied to UK data on household tobacco expenditure from the 1984 Family Expenditure Survey (FES) in Jones [5], and to Spanish Family Expenditure Survey data for 1980–81 in Garcia and Labeaga [6]. The special case in which the error terms are assumed to be independent ($\sigma_{12} = 0$) is applied to FES data on household tobacco expenditure in Atkinson, Gomulka and Stern [1], UK data on individual cigarette consumption from the 1980 General Household Survey (GHS) in Jones [3], and to US data on wine consumption in Blaylock and Blisard [27].

(iii) $\lambda = 0$

In this case the likelihood function reduces to,

$$L = \prod_i \left[1 - \Phi(x_{1i}\beta_1) \right]^{(1-D_i)}$$

$$\times \left[\Phi\left(\frac{x_{1i}\beta_1 + (\rho/\sigma)\{\log(y_i) - x_{2i}\beta_2\}}{\sqrt{1-\rho^2}} \right) \right.$$

$$\left. \times \frac{1}{\sigma}\phi\left(\frac{\log(y_i) - x_{2i}\beta_2}{\sigma} \right)y_i^{-1} \right]^{D_i} \quad (10.9)$$

This corresponds to the Type II or generalized Tobit model with $\log(y_i)$ as dependent variable in the regression part of the model [28,29]. A variant on this specification is used by Fry and Pashardes [9] model UK household tobacco expenditure with pooled FES data. They use a logit equation for participation and the Heckman two-step estimator for the regression equation, with household budget shares as the dependent variable, and their estimation is carried out in the context of a full demand system.

Setting $\sigma_{12} = 0$ gives the so-called 'two-part' model. This has been applied widely and is estimated as a probit equation for participation, based on the regressors x_{1i}, and conditional OLS of $\log(y_i)$ on x_{2i} for the positive observations. Studies of smoking based on the two-part model include Lewit, Coate and Grossman [17], Mullahy [2], Wasserman, Manning, Newhouse and Winkler [18], and Blaylock and Blisard [7]. The issue of choosing between the two-part specification and the Heckman two-stage sample selection model has also provoked considerable debate in the literature on health care utilization (see Hunt-McCool, Kiker and Ng [30] for a recent contribution). The Box–Cox specification makes it clear that the two-part model is a potentially restrictive special case, which requires independence between the unobservable factors underlying participation and consumption ($\sigma_{12} = 0$), and the correct distributional assumption for the conditional level of consumption ($\lambda = 0$).

THE DATA

THE HEALTH AND LIFESTYLE SURVEY

The focus of this study is on individual smoking behaviour and, in particular, on the determinants of the joint decisions of how many cigarettes to smoke and whether to quit. Our model emphasizes the role of addiction in the decision to quit and, to apply it, we need data on past consumption for both current and ex-smokers. Our dataset is the 1984–85 Health and Lifestyle Survey (HALS). The HALS is a large representative cross-section sample of British adults. The survey was conducted by the Office of the Regius Professor of Physics and the Department of Psychiatry at the Cambridge University School of Clinical Medicine, and the sample selection and fieldwork was carried out by Social and Community Planning Research. The data were collected between autumn 1984 and summer 1985 at two home visits; a one hour interview, followed by a nurse visit to collect physiological measurements and tests of cognitive functions. The nurse also gave out questionnaires to assess personality and psychiatric status.

The response rate of 73.5% gives a usable sample of 9003 individuals, aged 18 and over, living in private households. When information from the nurse visit and questionnaire is included the response rate falls to 53.7%. The survey was compared to the 1981 Census of population to gauge its representativeness. There is a slight excess of women, particularly elderly women, and some under-representation of those with low incomes and less education among respondents who completed all three stages of the survey. Overall it was concluded that 'the study appears to offer a good and representative sample of the population' [26].

PRINCIPAL VARIABLES

Microeconomic studies of cigarette consumption that use household expenditure data typically estimate a single participation equation for whether or not individuals or households are 'smokers' or 'non-smokers' [1,5,6,9]. In contrast the HALS provides information that separates non-smokers into those who have never smoked and those who class themselves as ex-smokers. This allows the analysis to be extended to distinguish between starting and quitting. To estimate the double hurdle models the sample is restricted to current and ex-smokers, so that participation corresponds to the decision whether or not to quit smoking. This follows the approach of Jones [3,31]. The final sample consists of 3801 individuals. Of these, 57 per cent are current smokers.

The dependent variable is the number of cigarettes smoked per day (CIGDAY). This volume based dependent variable is typical of health interview surveys and, unlike an expenditure variable, does not control for differences in the price or quality of cigarettes smoked. However, as a measure of 'typical' consumption, it is less likely to suffer from the problems of infrequency of expenditure and recall and response bias that are likely to arise in expenditure surveys. It can also be argued that the typical number of cigarettes is better suited for analysis of the interaction between smoking and health (Jones [3]). It should be stressed that HALS1 is a single cross-section and that the participation variable measures the prevalence rather than the incidence of smoking and therefore reflects the number of individuals who have quit up to the time of the survey. The results should be interpreted in terms of the stock of individuals who have quit rather than the flow of new quits over a specific period.

The independent variables are intended to encompass the determinants of the decision to quit smoking and the level of cigarette consumption. Along with addiction, they include measuring of social interaction, health and health knowledge, and socio-economic status, all of which are thought to be important influences on smoking.

The HALS is a rich source of data to examine addiction effects as it contains a number of variables that describe an individual's past behaviour. We use a measure of previous peak consumption to proxy the 'addictive stock' it gives *the most you have smoked regularly per day* in numbers of cigarettes, and is available for both current and ex-smokers (ADDICTION). Previous studies based on UK survey data have not been able to analyse the effect of lagged consumption, for example the 1980 GHS data used in Jones [3] includes information on past smoking, but only for those who were ex-smokers at the time of the survey. The panel data studies by Chaloupka [12] for the US and Labeaga [13] for Spain do allow analysis of consumption dynamics.

The economic literature on social interaction and consumer behaviour is rather sparse. The standard approach is to introduce social interaction as a form of externality. We adopt the externality approach, and assume that other people's smoking has a direct influence on an individual's decision to quit. The appropriate HALS variable is OTHER-SMOKERS, a dummy variable that equals 1 if there are other smokers in the individual's household. A similar variable proved to be important in Jones [3,31].

The HALS is a single cross-section and it is not possible to identify the impact of price, and hence tobacco taxes, on consumption. Similarly it is not possible to identify the impact of advertising and restrictions on advertising, another policy instrument that has received considerable attention in the time series literature on the demand for cigarettes [32]. However our data does provide indirect evidence on a third area of anti-smoking policy, the impact of health promotion and anti-smoking advice. The HALS includes information on whether or not an individual has received advice to quit smoking. The survey asks: '*Did anyone say that you should stop smoking cigarettes completely?*' the list of possible responses is doctor, spouse, relative, and friend/workmate. Only the highest response on the list is coded. We use a dummy variable (ADVICE) that equals 1 if any advice to quit was received. It should be stressed that this variable is based on retrospective cross-section data and uses the individual's subjective response. With respect to the medical advice to quit, this is a self-reported and unverifiable measure of exposure to a medical intervention, and no allowance can be made for the nature and quality of the advice, it could range from enrolment in a smoking cessation programme to advice given during a routine medical check-up.

As Kenkel [33] points out, the acquisition of health knowledge, which may include the decision to seek out and assimilate anti-smoking advice, is itself a choice. It may also be subject to cognitive dissonance, in that the individual may only seek or recall advice that is consistent with their current behaviour. In addition the individuals who are most likely to receive advice, particularly where that entails the need to visit a doctor, may be those who are most dependent on cigarettes and hence least able to quit or cut-down. This kind of cross-section dataset is not suitable to test hypotheses about the (clinical) effectiveness of medical advice to quit smoking, and is not a substitute for controlled intervention studies. Our evidence simply provides a description of the prevalence of smoking among those who have and have not received advice to quit.

Unfortunately the HALS data for individual income are based on a rather crude categorical scale and are hampered by missing values. Instead, economic status is measured by the Registrar General's classification of socio-economic group. This still allows us to make inferences about the distributional implications of the prevalence of smoking and levels of cigarette consumption, and hence about the possible distribution of the burden of tobacco taxes. Inevitably the use of proxy variables for income will lead to measurement errors that may be correlated with other variables, such as education, and the results for the socio-demographic variables should be viewed with caution.

There are three types of indicator of the individual's current health. Their self-assessed health is based on a standard excellent/good/fair/poor scale. We are a binary variable that equals 1 if the individual's self-rating is fair or poor (HEALTH). Measures of self-reported health include reports of specific symptoms and experience of specific illnesses. We use a binary variable for whether the individual has a disability or long-standing illness (DISABILITY). Finally there are clinical measures of health. We use three of these; lung function is measured by forced expiratory volume in one second (HYFEV1), cardio-vascular condition by the lowest pulse rate (LOWPULSE), and general physique by Quetelet's body mass index (BMI). A full listing of the other socio-demographic variables used in the model is given in Table 10.1, these are primarily indicators of education, marital status and household composition.

EMPIRICAL METHODS AND RESULTS

ESTIMATION AND TESTING

Estimation of the Box–Cox double hurdle model was done by maximizing the log-likelihood function corresponding to Equation 10.6. To avoid evaluations of the bivariate CDF's, the Box–Cox double hurdle model with independence and the generalized Tobit model were estimated using Equations 10.7 and 10.9 respectively. All other restricted models were estimated by imposing the relevant restrictions on model Equation 10.6 (see Table 10.2). The likelihood-ratio tests of the nested models are presented in Table 10.2. All restricted models were rejected, each with a p-value of less than 0.0001. It should be noted that the validity of the LR tests rests on the assumption that the general model is not misspecified, in particular that the assumptions of normality and homoscedasticity are not violated. We performed a RESET-type misspecification test on the general model using the second, third and fourth powers of the fitted values for the consumption equation as extra regressors, the corresponding LR statistic is less than 0.001 providing no evidence of misspecification.

In estimating the full model we selected from a list of explanatory variables in explaining the participation and consumption decisions. This started with a specification that included all the variables in both hurdles, relying on

Table 10.1 Variable definitions and sample statistics ($n = 3801$)

Variable	Full sample	Positive Mean	Std. dev.	Mean	Std. dev.
D	1 if a smoker (0 otherwise)	0.569	0.495		
CIGDAY	Number of cigarettes per day	9.357	10.593	16.565	8.902
ADDICTION	Most smoked regularly per day	22.606	15.151	24.154	14.119
OTHER-SMOKERS	1 if other smokers in household	0.542	0.498	0.678	0.467
ADVICE	1 if received any advice to quit	0.388	0.487	0.480	0.500
AGESTART	Age started smoking	16.900	5.494	16.657	5.436
HEALTH	1 if self-rated health is poor/fair	0.316	0.465	0.362	0.481
FEV1	Forced expiratory volume in 1 sec.	2.652	0.924	2.662	0.907
PULSE	Lowest pulse rate	71.440	11.345	73.099	11.147
DISABILITY	1 if disabled or long standing illness	0.319	0.466	0.279	0.448
BMI	Quetelet's body mass index (wt/ht^2)	24.473	3.949	23.839	3.893
PROFESSIONAL	Registrar General's social class 1	0.047	0.212	0.028	0.165
MANAGERIAL	Registrar General's social class 2	0.209	0.407	0.176	0.381
OTHER NON-MANUAL	Registrar General's social class 3	0.118	0.323	0.113	0.317
SEMI-SKILLED	Registrar General's social class 5	0.174	0.379	0.196	0.397
UNSKILLED	Registrar General's social class 6	0.061	0.239	0.073	0.260
ARMY	Registrar General's social class 11	0.008	0.090	0.007	0.086
WIDOW	1 if widow/widower	0.070	0.254	0.055	0.229
DIVORCED	1 if divorced	0.045	0.207	0.059	0.236
SEPARATED	1 if separated	0.026	0.158	0.032	0.175
SINGLE	1 if single	0.133	0.340	0.173	0.379
AGE	Age in years	46.128	16.455	42.271	15.552
LONDON	1 if resident in Greater London	0.102	0.302	0.125	0.331
DEGREE	1 if individual has a degree	0.042	0.200	0.029	0.169

non-linearity for identification of the model. Insignificant variables were gradually dropped from the list, with the exclusion restrictions putting identification on firmer ground (the likelihood ratio statistic for these restrictions is 0.001). Our search concluded with a homoscedastic specification. For comparisons, the same configuration of variables was used in all restricted models. ML estimates of the Box–Cox double hurdle model are presented in Table 10.3. the parameter σ_{12} is significant at the 0.01 level, rejecting independence of errors. As suggested by the fixed costs model, there is evidence of strong negative correlation between the error terms.

The Box–Cox parameter (λ) equals 0.562 which is significantly different from both zero and one at the 0.01 level. Thus, both the standard double hurdle model and generalized Tobit model are rejected. The value of 0.562 is close to a square root transformation (although the estimate is significantly different from 0.5). The square root is a variance stabilizing transformation for Poisson data [34]. This suggests that it may be more appropriate to interpret the typical number of cigarettes as a count variable rather than as a continuous dependent variable. For example, the model could be estimated by the Negbin

hurdle model used by Pohlmeier and Ulrich [35]. The problem with this approach is that these models do not allow for dependence between the participation and consumption equations, and hence for the selection bias implied by the fixed cost model of addiction. Interestingly, Wasserman et al. [18] estimate a two-part model using the logarithm of cigarette consumption and they interpret the model as a 'pseudo-Poisson' specification. However their model does not allow for selection bias and therefore contradicts the fixed cost model.

In the full Box–Cox double hurdle model the predicted impact of the individual regressors in x_1 and x_2 on the probability of quitting and on the observed level of cigarette consumption are complicated by the dependence between the two hurdles and by the nonlinear transformation between y_2^* and y. As a result the magnitude of the coefficients β_1 and β_2 are difficult to interpret. To give a more intuitive interpretation the marginal effects of the continuous explanatory variables on participation and consumption are explored by calculating elasticities. Table 10.4 gives the elasticities of participation, the conditional level of consumption, and the unconditional level of consumption evaluated at sample means (see Jones and

Table 10.2   LR tests for nested models[a]

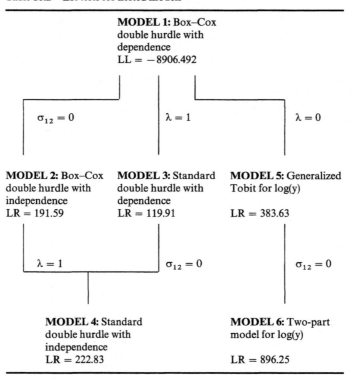

[a]LL, value of log-likelihood function.
LR, likelihood ratio statistic.

Yen [16] for details of the computation of these elasticities, standard errors are computed by the delta method). For the discrete regressors Table 10.5 presents average effects, calculated as the value of the relevant variable changes from zero to one.

INTERPRETATION OF THE RESULTS

The influence of addiction, measured by previous peak consumption, has a positive effect on both the probability of smoking and the level of consumption. The variable ADDICTION is strongly significant in both equations, the LR statistic for excluding the variable from the model is $\chi^2(2) = 1181.53$. A Smith and Blundell [36] type test does not reject the exogeneity of ADDICTION, this is calculated by including the residuals from a reduced form equation for ADDICTION in both hurdles which gives an LR statistic of 3.047 (p-value = 0.2179). This can only be an imperfect test as our cross-section dataset does not include a full set of appropriate lagged values to instrument past consumption. Previous UK studies based on microdata have not analysed the influence of lagged consumption, but the positive effect on consumption is consistent with the evidence from panel data in Chaloupka [12] and Labeaga [13]. However these studies do not identify the separate effect of past smoking on the probability of smoking or quitting. The evidence in Table 10.4 indicates that, on average, a 10 per cent increase in previous peak consumption will increase the probability of remaining a smoker by around 3 per cent and increase the level of current cigarette consumption by around 4 per cent. This suggests that smoking habits persist and that addiction does constrain individuals' ability to quit. The last result complements the finding in Jones [31] that past consumption does not influence the desire to quit, as measured by the individual reporting a 'serious attempt' to quit smoking, but does influence their success in quitting.

In model 1, all of the other regressors show different qualitative effects on participation and on consumption. This is something that is consistent with the behavioural model Equations 10.1 and 10.2, which suggests that the parameters for variables that appear in both equations

Table 10.3 Maximum likelihood estimates of the Box–Cox double hurdle model[a]

Variable	Probability	Level
Constant	0.589**	3.129***
	(0.247)	(0.603)
ADDICTION	0.019***	0.123***
	(0.002)	(0.013)
OTHER-SMOKERS	0.641***	−0.966***
	(0.046)	(0.141)
ADVICE	0.486***	−0.690***
	(0.046)	(0.125)
AGESTART	0.012***	−0.033***
	(0.004)	(0.011)
HEALTH	0.185***	−0.179*
	(0.047)	(0.113)
FEV1	−0.158***	0.312***
	(0.030)	(0.081)
PULSE	0.013***	−0.017***
	(0.002)	(0.005)
DISABILITY	−0.105***	—
	(0.036)	—
BMI	−0.046***	0.087***
	(0.006)	(0.016)
PROFESSIONAL	−0.481***	0.670**
	(0.109)	(0.298)
MANAGERIAL	−0.173***	0.474***
	(0.055)	(0.142)
OTHER NON-MANUAL	−0.120**	—
	(0.047)	—
SEMI-SKILLED	−0.008	—
	(0.042)	—
SKILLED	0.116*	—
	(0.065)	—
ARMY	−0.129	—
	(0.156)	—
AGE	−0.022***	0.040***
	(0.002)	(0.006)
LONDON	0.214***	—
	(0.054)	—
WIDOW	−0.082	—
	(0.061)	—
DIVORCED	0.359***	−0.640***
	(0.102)	(0.242)
SEPARATED	0.127	—
	(0.094)	—
SINGLE	0.096	−0.425***
	(0.067)	(0.164)
DEGREE	−0.239***	—
	(0.082)	—
σ	2.726***	—
	(0.257)	—
σ_{12}	−2.627***	—
	(0.242)	—
λ	0.562***	—
	(0.036)	—
Log-likelihood	−8906.492	—

[a]Asymptotic standard errors in parentheses. Asterisks indicate levels of significance: *** = 0.01, ** = 0.05 and * = 0.10.

Table 10.4 Estimated elasticities[a]

Variable	Probability	Cond. level	Uncond. level
ADDICTION	0.298***	0.435***	0.733***
	(0.027)	(0.033)	(0.020)
AGESTART	0.144***	−0.200***	−0.057**
	(0.049)	(0.060)	(0.028)
FEV1	−0.295***	0.345***	0.050
	(0.057)	(0.072)	(0.038)
PULSE	0.657***	−0.633***	0.023
	(0.096)	(0.123)	(0.073)
BMI	−0.782***	0.901***	0.118**
	(0.095)	(0.125)	(0.072)
AGE	−0.697***	0.796***	0.100
	(0.061)	(0.085)	(0.062)

[a]Asymptotic standard errors in parentheses. Asterisks indicate levels of significance: *** = 0.01, ** = 0.05 and * = 0.10.

Table 10.5 Estimated average effects

Variable	Probability	Cond. level	Uncond. level
OTHER-SMOKERS	0.249	−6.801	−0.089
ADVICE	0.188	−4.388	−0.019
HEALTH	0.072	−1.448	0.132
DISABILITY	−0.041	0.584	−0.243
PROFESSIONAL	−0.190	6.302	−0.072
MANAGERIAL	−0.068	2.509	0.373
OTHER NON-MANUAL	−0.047	0.662	−0.276
SEMI-SKILLED	−0.003	0.041	−0.019
UNSKILLED	0.045	−0.518	0.271
ARMY	−0.051	0.716	−0.296
LONDON	0.083	−0.992	0.502
WIDOW	−0.033	0.472	−0.191
DIVORCED	0.135	−3.067	−0.257
SEPARATED	0.049	−0.612	0.296
SINGLE	0.038	−1.673	−0.476
DEGREE	−0.095	1.565	−0.549

will tend to have opposite signs. The implication is that, after controlling for the fixed costs associated with addiction, the more someone smokes the more likely they are to try to quit, as the potential benefits of quitting are greater. Hence the model predicts that variables which increase the level of smoking will decrease the likelihood of remaining a smoker.

To investigate this result further, we compare the estimates for each of the models (Equations 10.1–10.6) for both the 'addiction' and 'non-addiction' specifications (i.e. where ADDICTION is omitted from both equations). For all of the twelve models the sign of the β_1's are the same for virtually all of the regressors, indicating that the participation part of the model is highly robust. In the other two addiction models that allow for dependence between the error terms (Equations 10.3 and 10.5), the signs of the β_2's are the same as model 1. However, for the models that assured independence (Equations 10.2, 10.4 and 10.6) and for all of the models that omit ADDICTION the β_2's are not consistent with Equation 10.1 and show no clear pattern of opposing signs. To summarize, controlling for addiction and the selection bias associated with the decision to quit does influence the estimates of the demand for cigarettes.

One striking feature of Tables 10.4 and 10.5 is that due to the offsetting effects on participation and consumption the net effect of most of the variables on the unconditional level of consumption is very small. From a policy perspective attention would probably focus on the size of the effects on quitting, as this is of most relevance for public health objectives.

Jones [3,31] shows that those with smokers in their households are less likely to have quit. This result is confirmed here, but the double hurdle specification reveals that, conditional on participation, the variable has the opposite effect on the level of smoking. A similar pattern emerges with the impact of advice to quit (ADVICE). This variable has a positive effect on participation, a counter-intuitive result which can be attributed to the problems of self-selection and heterogeneity bias described above. But the double hurdle model shows that, conditional on remaining a smoker rather than quitting, those who have received advice to quit tend to smoke fewer cigarettes. This result does not hold in the models that assume independence and do not control for the selection bias. We experimented with a dummy variable for whether individuals have received a doctor's advice to quit, but the variable was found to be statistically insignificant.

The indicators of the individual's current health suggest that those with poorer current health, measured by HEALTH, FEVI and PULSE are more likely to smoke, but tend to smoke fewer cigarettes. The opposite effect is revealed with respect to the individual's physique (BMI) and whether they suffer from a disability or long-standing illness (DISABILITY). It should be emphasized that the approach adopted here is to condition current health-related behaviour (in this case smoking) on measures of current health in order to control for individual heterogeneity in health status. The objective of this study is not to analyse the impact of current smoking on future health. With appropriate longitudinal data it would be possible to explore the interactions between an individual's demand for health, their measured health, and their health-related behaviour, including smoking.

For socio-economic group, those in higher groups are more likely to have quit but, conditional on smoking, they smoke more. This is similar to the pattern of income

effects revealed in Jones [3]. One interpretation is that there is a conventional income effect on the level of consumption, but that differences in participation are associated with differences in attitudes towards health, and risk and time preference across socio-economic groups. Alternatively the pattern of consumption may be a cohort effect, reflecting the fact that a higher proportion of smokers have quit in the more affluent groups, and those that remain tend to be confirmed heavy smokers.

CONCLUSIONS

Becker and Murphy's [10] model of rational addiction has stimulated empirical analysis of survey data on smoking habits. But survey data on smoking invariably contains a high proportion of zero observations, and the use of limited dependent variable models is often required. Misspecification in functional form, parameterization and distributional assumptions in the LDV models can lead to inconsistent estimates. We propose a model of the simultaneous decisions of whether to quit and how much to smoke which incorporates the 'fixed costs' of addiction associated with withdrawal effects. This leads to an empirical model that allows more flexible parameterization and distributional assumptions than previous studies.

The Box–Cox double hurdle model nests the standard double hurdle, as well as the logarithmic generalized Tobit model and the 'two-part' model. The model is applied to data on smoking from the 1984–85 UK Health and Lifestyle Survey, and the Box–Cox specification is shown to out-perform all the nested models that have been used extensively in the empirical literature.

Addiction, measured by previous peak consumption, is shown to have a significant effect on both the probability of quitting and the level of smoking. The results for the impact of social interaction, anti-smoking advice, health and socio-economic status are consistent with our model which suggests that, after controlling for the effects of addiction and the interaction between quitting and the level of consumption, there will be an inverse relationship between the determinants of participation and consumption.

ACKNOWLEDGEMENTS

Seniority of authorship is not assigned. We are grateful for comments from Michael Grossman, Don Kenkel, Willard Manning, John Mullahy, Simon Peters, Carol Propper and an anonymous referee, along with seminar participants at Bristol, Erasmus, Kent, Louvain, and Perugia Universities, the 1994 Royal Economic Society

Conference, and the Fourth European Workshop on Econometrics and Health Economics.

REFERENCES

1. Atkinson, A.B., Gomulka, J. and Stern, N.H. *Household expenditure on tobacco 1970–1980: evidence from the Family Expenditure Survey, ESRC Programme on Taxation, Incentives and the Distribution of Income*, London School of Economics, Discussion Paper no. 60, 1984.
2. Mullahy, J. *Cigarette smoking: habits, health concerns, and heterogeneous unobservables in a microeconometric analysis of consumer demand*, PhD dissertation, University of Virginia, 1985.
3. Jones, A.M. A double-hurdle model of cigarette consumption. *Journal of Applied Econometrics* 1989a; **4**: 23–39.
4. Jones, A.M. The UK demand for cigarettes 1954–1986: a double-hurdle approach. *Journal of Health Economics* 1989b; **8**: 133–141.
5. Jones, A.M. A note on computation of the double-hurdle model with dependence. With an application to tobacco expenditure. *Bulletin of Economic Research* 1992; **4**: 67–74.
6. Garcia, J. and Labeaga, J.M. A microeconometric analysis of the demand for tobacco in Spain using cross-section data, mimeo, Universitat Pompeu Fabra, 1991.
7. Blaylock J.R. and Blisard, W.N. Self-evaluated health status and smoking behaviour. *Applied Economics* 1992; **24**: 429–435.
8. Labeaga, J.M. A dynamic panel data model with limited dependent variables: an application to the demand for tobacco, Documento de Trabajo 9201, Fundacion Empresa Publica, Madrid, 1992.
9. Fry, V. and Pashardes, P. Abstention and aggregation in consumer demand: zero tobacco expenditures. *Oxford Economic Papers* 1994; **46**: 502–518.
10. Becker, G.S. and Murphy, K.M. A theory of rational addiction. *Journal of Political Economy* 1988; **96**: 675–700.
11. Chaloupka, F.J. *Men, women, and addition.* NBER Working Paper No. 3267, February 1990.
12. Chaloupka, F.J. Rational addictive behaviour and cigarette smoking. *Journal of Political Economy* 1991; **99**: 722–742.
13. Labeaga, J.M. Individual behaviour and tobacco consumption: a panel data approach. *Health Economics* 1993; **2**: 103–112.
14. Arabmazard, A. and Schmidt, P. An investigation of the robustness of the Tobit estimator to non-normality. *Econometrica* 1982; **50**: 1055–1063.
15. Robinson, P. On the asymptotic properties of estimators of models containing limited dependent variables. *Econometrica* 1982; **50**: 27–41.
16. Jones, A.M. and Yen, S.T. *A Box–Cox double hurdle model.* Institute for Fiscal Studies, Working Paper, W94/6, 1994.
17. Lewit, E.M., Coate, D. and Grossman, M. The effects of government regulation on teenage smoking. *Journal of Law and Economics* 1981; **24**: 545–570.
18. Wasserman, J., Manning, W.G., Newhouse, J.P. and Winkler, J.D. The effects of excise taxes and regulations on cigarette smoking. *Journal of Health Economics* 1991; **10**: 43–64.
19. Ippolito, P.M. and Ippolito, R.A. Measuring the value of life saving from consumer reactions to new information. *Journal of Public Economics* 1985; **25**: 53–81.
20. Jones, A.M. *A theoretical and empirical investigation of the demand for addictive goods*, unpublished D.Phil. thesis. University of York, 1987.
21. Mullahy, J. and Portney, P.R. Air pollution, cigarette smoking, and the production of respiratory health. *Journal of Health Economics* 1990; **9**: 193–205.
22. Viscusi, W.K. Do smokers underestimate risks? *Journal of Political Economy* 1990; **98**: 1253–1269.
23. Ashton, H. and Stepney, R. *Smoking, psychology and pharmacology.* London: Tavistock Publications, 1982.
24. Marsh, A. and Matheson, J. *Smoking attitudes and behaviour: an enquiry on behalf of the Department of Health and Social Security.* London: HMSO, 1983.
25. Ben-Shlomo, Y., Sheiham, A. and Marmot, M. Smoking and health in Jowell, R., Brook, L. Taylor, B. and Prior, G., eds, *British social attitudes, the 8th Report.* Aldershot: Dartmouth, 1991.
26. Cox, B.D. *et al. The health and lifestyle survey.* London: Health Promotion Research Trust, 1987.
27. Blaylock, J.R. and Blisard, W.N. (1993). Wine consumption by US men. *Applied Economics* 1993; **25**: 645–651.
28. Amemiya, T. *Advanced econometrics.* Oxford: Basil Blackwell, 1985.
29. Heckman, J.J. Sample selection bias as a specification error. *Econometrica* 1979; **47**: 153–161.
30. Hunt-McCool, J., Kiker, B.F. and Ying Chu Ng. Estimates of the demand for medical care under different functional forms. *Journal of Applied Econometrics* 1994; **9**: 201–218.
31. Jones, A.M. Health, addiction, social interaction and the decision to quit smoking. *Journal of Health Economics* 1994; **13**: 93–110.
32. Godfrey, C. Banning tobacco advertising: can health economists contribute to the debate? *Health Economics* 1993; **2**: 1–5.
33. Kenkel, D. Health behavior, health knowledge, and schooling. *Journal of Political Economy* 1991; **99**: 287–305.
34. McCullagh, P. and Nelder, J.A. *Generalized linear models, second edition.* London: Chapman and Hall, 1989.
35. Pohlmeier, W. and Ulrich, V. An econometric model of the two-part decision making process in the demand for health care. *Journal of Human Resources* 1995; **30**: 339–361.
36. Smith, R.J. and Blundell, R. An exogeneity test for a simultaneous equation Tobit model with an application to labour supply. *Econometrica* 1986; **54**: 679–685.

11

Identifying Demand for Health Resources Using Waiting Times Information

RICHARD BLUNDELL[1] AND FRANK WINDMEIJER[2]

[1]*University College London, London, UK and* [2]*Institute for Fiscal Studies, London, UK*

INTRODUCTION

The aim of this paper is to consider the specification and estimation of a statistical model for health care utilization. Our model draws on the recent literature which relates waiting times to the demand and supply of services (see, for example, Lindsay and Feigenbaum [1], Gravelle [2] and Goddard *et al.* [3]). In this model, waiting time acts as a hassle cost to treatment and in equilibrium, the waiting time costs will be just sufficient to reduce demand to equal the supply of services. For example, suppose there is an increase in demand, waiting times will increase. Some individuals already on the list will drop out and others who had thought of joining will not join. Similarly for a change in supply. Waiting time essentially plays the role of a price, with people looking for alternative care, possibly private, or no care at all when the waiting time becomes too long. Provided waiting times adjust fairly rapidly, then this equilibrium framework seems reasonable. Martin and Smith [4] use this model to estimate demand and supply models for elective surgery in the UK and find that waiting time is indeed negatively correlated with demand.

The standard equilibrium waiting time approach rests on two assumptions: (1) the observed data are in equilibrium; (2) waiting times accurately measure waiting time costs. Both assumptions may be strong and are not necessary for the central approach taken in this paper. If there is a higher than expected demand then we still observe supply, but demand and waiting times may not have adjusted to equilibrium. This is equivalent to the min{demand, supply} condition in standard disequilibrium models (see Gourieroux *et al.* [5]). Our approach is to select areas in which the waiting times are reasonably low and use these to estimate the determinants of demand. This approach is, therefore, robust to disequilibrium in high waiting time areas and reduces the sensitivity to systematic measurement error in the tails of the waiting time distribution. Our aim is limited: simply to recover characteristics that influence demand for health services at low waiting time costs. The objective is not to estimate a model of both demand and supply but rather to examine the determinants of demands, or needs, abstracting from distortions caused by supply side constraints in health care provision. We use the determinants of supply as instruments for the waiting time to correct for the potentially endogenous selection of low waiting times areas in which services may be more likely to reflect demand. However, we do contrast our results with those for the standard equilibrium specification for demand.

The model we use is based on a regression specification for normalized level of health care utilization. It is precisely this kind of model that is used in the allocation of NHS funds in the UK (see Smith *et al.* [6]); and our application is to the demand for acute hospital care at the local (ward) level in the UK. We introduce the idea that some wards may be supply constrained, so that a regression on needs variables alone on the whole sample will not correctly identify demand parameters. Instead we suggest the use of average waiting time by ward as an indicator of supply rationing. We use wards with relatively low waiting times to capture demand when the time costs of waiting are low. Even within the equilibrium waiting time framework of Lindsay and Feigenbaum [1] this still seems a good idea, since at high waiting times, the waiting time variable will surely interact in quite a complicated way with needs variables. For example, suppose at low waiting times, richer young people place a high demand on resources

Econometric Analysis of Health Data. Edited by Andrew M. Jones and Owen O'Donnell
© 2002 John Wiley & Sons Ltd. Previously published in *Health Economics*, Vol. 9; pp. 465–474 (2000). © John Wiley & Sons Ltd

but drop out if there are high time costs, then at high waiting times, the income and age effects will be different.

Our choice of areas with low waiting times implies that there will be few people who came on the list from the past and who thus reflect demands from earlier periods. Added to this we are worried about systematic reporting bias in the waiting time variable, as there are obvious incentives for providers to underreport high waiting times, and that this variable may not be a good measure of waiting time costs. Also, if individual demands are non-linear in waiting time, then the aggregate demand in a ward will not depend only on the average waiting time (as Martin and Smith [4] point out, there are many measures of waiting time). However, we do also estimate a simple parametric model, which includes the waiting time variable as an endogenous determinant of demand, and show that, when selecting wards with reasonable low levels of waiting times, this variable does not appear to influence demand. This contrasts dramatically with the results for higher waiting time areas, where waiting time is found to be a strongly significant determinant of demand.

The central specification we estimate is a selection model that estimates needs variables for wards that have an average waiting time below some specified cut-off. Since the model estimates are likely to be sensitive to parametric distributional assumptions we check the robustness of our results using semi-parametric selection methods in estimation (see Newey *et al.* [7]). The fact that we have a number of excluded supply side variables that strongly determine waiting times and have a wide variation across the data makes this application well suited to the use of semi-parametric selection methods.

The rest of the paper is organized as follows. In the next section we develop the model. The third section presents the data and estimation results. As the important outcome of the demand model is the actual resource allocations over the regions, we also look at the impact of the various estimation procedures on the estimated regional need indices. Some conclusions appear in the fourth section.

MODEL AND ESTIMATION

AN EMPIRICAL SPECIFICATION OF THE DEMAND FOR SERVICES

Let O_i represent the outflow rate from a particular medical service in ward i and I_i represent the corresponding inflow rate onto the service register for that ward. In any given ward in a given time period, the waiting time, W_i, will be a function of current and past net inflow rates.

There may exist a waiting time, W_i^*, at which the two rates are equilibrated

$$I_i = O_i \Leftrightarrow W_i = W_i^*.$$

In this framework, the waiting time acts like a price of services, reducing demand as W_i rises. Demand for services will depend on characteristics of the local population $\mathbf{x}_i^d$ (needs variables), the waiting time level W_i and unobservables u_i^d

$$y_i^d = f(\mathbf{x}_i^d, W_i) + u_i^d. \tag{11.1}$$

The inflow rate will be directly related to y_i^d. Therefore, W_i and y_i^d will be simultaneously determined.

Two approaches are available for estimation. One could assume a parametric form for Equation 11.1, for example

$$y_i^d = \boldsymbol{\beta}' \mathbf{x}_i^d + \gamma W_i + u_i^d \tag{11.2}$$

and estimate directly. However, note that since W_i is endogenous to demand, a suitable instrument will be required. An obvious choice of instrument would be some determinant of supply. However, current fluctuations in supply could be correlated with unobservables in demand. A safer instrument would be a lagged supply variable or lagged waiting times. We discuss particular choices in the empirical application below. Martin and Smith [4] estimate demand Equation 11.2 within a full equilibrium model.

A number of potential difficulties arise with this approach. First, it is likely that reported waiting time levels W_i, especially at the upper end of the distribution, are likely to be systematically biased. Secondly, it is likely that when waiting times are long, the waiting time variable will interact in quite a complicated way with the needs variables. Thirdly, at low waiting time levels, say below W^m, it is less likely that W_i will influence demand. Given that the aim of this paper is rather modest – to evaluate the importance of different needs variables, not to estimate the impact of W_i on demand directly – we take a slightly different, and hopefully more robust, approach. We specify that demand for services takes the form

$$y_i^d = \boldsymbol{\beta}' \mathbf{x}_i^d + u_i^d \text{ for } W_i < W^m, \tag{11.3}$$

where W^m will be in the lower quantiles of the observed waiting time distribution. To check whether W_i does indeed not influence demand at low levels of waiting times, we also estimate Equation 11.3 with W_i included in the model. We further check the robustness of our results to different choices of cut-off point W^m.

Even in this approach endogeneity arises in estimating Equation 11.3. In particular, there is endogenous selection on W_i, which in turn depends on demand for services through the net inflow rate. Therefore, using this framework, the demand parameters β can be identified from the wards with low average waiting time, while taking care of the endogenous selection rule. If W^m is known, standard (semi-)parametric techniques can be applied, utilizing limited information on the average waiting times in the sense that only the information whether W_i is larger or smaller than W^m is used. As we argued above, the waiting time information is likely to be subject to systematic measurement error especially towards the upper tail. Consequently, the use of the limited information will reduce the impact of this measurement problem.

AN APPROACH TO ESTIMATION

The estimators we utilize in this paper for the standard selection model are a parametric two-step estimator (Heckman [8]), and a semi-parametric estimator as proposed by Robinson [9]. The first step in estimation is to specify a binary indicator for the average waiting time:

$w_i = 1$ if $W_i \geq W^m$

$w_i = 0$ if $W_i < W^m$.

This is assumed to follow some simple linear index probability model

$Pr[w_i = 1] = Pr[\pi' z_i + \varepsilon_i \geq 0].$

Under normality, the parameters π/σ_ε, where σ_ε is the standard deviation of ε, can be consistently estimated by the standard Probit maximum likelihood estimator. The standard Heckman [8] two-step estimator specifies the model of demand for services in wards with low waiting times as

$$y_i^d = \beta' x_i^d + E[u_i^d | W_i < W_i^m] + \eta_i^d$$
$$= \beta' x_i^d + \lambda \frac{\phi(\pi' z_i / \sigma_\varepsilon)}{1 - \Phi(\pi' z_i / \sigma_\varepsilon)} + \eta_i^d,$$

where $\lambda = -\sigma_{u^d \varepsilon}/\sigma_\varepsilon$, and $\sigma_{u^d \varepsilon}$ is the covariance of u^d and ε, which are assumed to be jointly normally distributed. The two-step procedure then amounts to substituting the probit estimate $\widehat{\pi/\sigma_\varepsilon}$ for π/σ_ε, and estimating the parameters β and λ by ordinary least-squares (OLS).

Given the initial estimate for π/σ_ε, the semi-parametric estimator of Robinson [9] proceeds as follows. Let $v_i = \pi' z_i / \sigma_\varepsilon$, then the conditional model can be written as

$$y_i^d = \beta' x_i^d + g(v_i) + \xi_i^d$$

where $g(.)$ is some unknown function. Subtracting the conditional expectation of y_i^d given v_i results in

$$y_i^d - E[y_i^d | v_i] = \beta'(x_i^d - E[x_i^d | v_i]) + \xi_i^d, \tag{11.4}$$

which is no longer a function of $g(v_i)$, and OLS estimation of Equation 11.4 gives consistent and asymptotically normal estimates for β (excluding the constant). The conditional means $E[y_i^d | v_i]$ and $E[x_i^d | v_i]$ are estimated nonparametrically using kernel regressions. The kernel estimator of $E[x | v = c]$ is a weighted average of x for v in the neighbourhood of c, given by (see e.g. Härdle and Linton [10])

$$\hat{E}_h[x | v = c] = \frac{\frac{1}{N} \sum_{i=1}^{N} K_h(c - v_i) x_i}{\frac{1}{N} \sum_{i=1}^{N} K_h(c - v_i)},$$

where

$$K_h(c - v_i) = \frac{1}{h} K\left(\frac{c - v_i}{h}\right),$$

K is a *kernel* function, which is continuous, bounded and symmetric and which integrates to 1, and h is a bandwidth parameter decreasing with sample size N. In estimating Equation 11.4 using kernel regressions to estimate the conditional mean terms, some trimming may be required to remove areas of the data where the density of v is too sparse.

DATA AND ESTIMATION RESULTS

The data for the estimation of the models as described in the second section are the same data as have been used by Smith et al. [6] for the construction of the allocation formula of NHS revenues. In their work, the final needs regression results are based on the hospital utilization of all wards. The waiting times data are the same as in Martin and Smith [4].

The dependent utilization variable is the standardized estimated costs of acute care in 1991–1992 (ACCOS91). The waiting time data are the average numbers of days waited for routine surgery in 1991–1992 (WT91). Supply and demand variables are measured in 1990–1991. In the timing of the utilization we differ from the approach of Smith et al. [6]. In their study, the utilization variable was the average utilization per ward in the years 1990–1991

Table 11.1 Descriptive statistics

Variable	Description	All wards N = 4955		WT91 < 100 N = 1296	
		Mean	SD	Mean	SD
WT91	Average waiting time routine surgery in days	117.08	26.18	85.74	11.10
ACCOS91	Standardized estimated costs 1991–1992 acute care	100.63	23.01	102.07	23.09
ACCNHS	NHS hospital accessibility	2.34	0.75	2.34	0.76
ACCGPS	GP accessibility	0.53	0.13	0.53	0.12
HOMES*	1-proportion of 75+ in nursing and residential homes	0.94	0.06	0.95	0.05
ACCPRI	Private hospital accessibility	0.17	0.13	0.18	0.18
SMR074	Standardized mortality ratio ages 0–74	99.46	23.16	101.52	23.16
HSIR074	Standardized illness ratio ages 0–74, for residents in households only	99.01	30.59	104.15	31.99
MANUAL	Proportion of persons with head in manual class	0.46	0.15	0.49	0.14
OLDALONE	Proportion of those of pensionable age living alone	0.33	0.06	0.33	0.05
S_CARER	Proportion of dependants in single carer households	0.19	0.06	0.20	0.06
UNEMP	Proportion of the economically active that is unemployed	0.09	0.05	0.10	0.05
NOCAR	Proportion of residents in households with no car	0.24	0.14	0.25	0.14

Note: in the regressions, natural logarithms are taken of all variables.

and 1991–1992, and the supply variables had to be instrumented. We avoid the problem of endogeneity by using lagged values of the supply measures.

Table 11.1 gives descriptions and summary statistics of the variables we use in this study. For a further description and guide to the construction of these variables, see Martin and Smith [4], Martin [11] and Carr-Hill et al. [12]. As can be seen from the table, the average waiting time for routine surgery in 1991–1992 was 117 days. There are four supply variables, namely NHS hospital accessibility (ACCNHS), general practitioner accessibility (ACCGP), the proportion of the 75 years and older *not* in nursing and residential homes (HOMES*) and private hospital accessibility (ACCPRI). The needs variables considered are the standardized mortality ratio ages 0–74 (SMR074), a standardized illness ratio ages 0–74 (HSIR074), the proportion of persons in manual class (MANUAL), the proportion of persons of pensionable age living alone (OLDALONE), the proportion of dependants in single carer households (S__CARER), the proportion of the economically active that are unemployed (UNEMP) and the proportion of residents in households with no car (NOCAR). Table 11.1 also reports summary statistics for those wards that have waiting times less than 100 days, and that will be used in our estimation of the demand Equation 11.3 below. The average waiting time in these wards is 86 days. The summary statistics of the other variables in the selected sample are all very similar to those in the full sample.

Table 11.2 presents the probit estimates of the waiting time model with a cut-off point of 100 days, utilizing the

Table 11.2 Results for probit regression

Weighted regression; dependent variable WT91 > 100	N = 4955	R² = 0.14	
Variable	B	SE B	T
ACCNHS	−0.1651	0.1027	−1.6074
ACCGPS	0.1901	0.1212	1.5687
ACCPRI	−0.2361	0.0625	−3.7784
HOMES*	−0.0130	0.3267	−0.0398
OLDALONE	0.3400	0.1784	1.9059
S_CARER	−0.2461	0.1466	−1.6784
UNEMP	0.2912	0.1070	2.7217
HSIR074	−0.3113	0.2078	−1.4979
SMR074	−0.2106	0.1730	−1.2174

LR test for supply variables: 34.51, p value = 0.0000.
Dummies included for RHA.
Observations weighted by ward population.

same supply and needs variables as identified by Smith et al. [6] to determine utilization. After consulting health experts at the King's Fund, we chose 100 days as the cut-off point, as we were advised that this length of waiting time is seen by health care providers as a reasonable time to go through the system. It is clear from the likelihood ratio test that the supply variables are informative for waiting times. Better access to NHS and private hospitals decreases the average waiting time for routine surgery, whereas more GPs in the area has the effect of increasing the average waiting time.

Table 11.3 Results for needs regressions

Weighted regression; dependent variable ACCOS91

Variable	OLS full sample		OLS selected sample		Two-step estimator		Semi-parametric estimator	
N	4955		1296		1296		1296	
R^2	0.50		0.57		0.57		0.53	
Variable	B	SE B	B	SE B	B	SE* B	B	SE* B
OLDALONE	0.1191	0.0190	0.1391	0.0369	0.1670	0.0426	0.1532	0.0409
S_CARER	0.0036	0.0180	0.0755	0.0393	0.0468	0.0301	0.0431	0.0306
UNEMP	0.0248	0.0114	0.0227	0.0202	0.0593	0.0391	0.0490	0.0425
HSIR074	0.2848	0.0241	0.2053	0.0399	0.1595	0.0411	0.1734	0.0449
SMR074	0.1342	0.0219	0.1135	0.0384	0.0831	0.0437	0.1097	0.0469
λ					−0.1865	0.0650		

Dummies included for RHA.
SE*: Standard deviation of 100 bootstrap estimates.
Observations weighted by ward population.

Table 11.4 Population weighted need indices

Cluster summaries	Full sample OLS	Selected sample OLS (%)	Selected two-step (%)	Selected semi-parametric (%)
Inner London	112.3	1.10	1.68	1.28
Mixed status London	100.3	0.76	1.66	1.25
Outer London	94.3	1.10	2.01	1.62
Inner city deprived	113.2	−0.80	−1.30	−1.11
Urban areas	107.9	−1.22	−2.10	−1.72
Resort and retirement areas	96.0	1.07	1.23	0.96
High-status suburban	93.5	0.62	1.14	0.97
High-status rural	88.5	0.29	1.29	1.08
High-status urban	98.0	−0.30	−0.37	−0.25
Rural areas	95.9	0.26	0.09	0.11
Dormitory towns	106.2	1.32	1.55	1.34

Table 11.3 presents four sets of results for the demand equation as specified in Equation 11.3. The first column presents OLS results based on the full sample. The second column gives OLS results on the subsample of wards with an average waiting time less than 100 days. In the third column, the two-step estimation results are presented, and finally in the fourth column, the semi-parametric estimates using the Robinson method are presented. In the Robinson method, the kernel function is specified as the standard normal and the bandwidth is set equal to $N^{-2/5}$. For the OLS estimators, the reported standard errors are robust to general heteroscedasticity. For the two-step and semi-parametric estimators, the standard errors are estimated using bootstrap resampling methods. The estimators, including the probit, are calculated for 100 bootstrap samples, and the reported standard errors are the standard deviations of these estimates. The results of the two-step estimator indicates that the selection is indeed endogenous, as the coefficient on the correction term is significant. It is furthermore negative, indicating

that the unobservables u^d in the demand equation and the unobservables ε in the waiting times model are positively correlated, which is as expected. The coefficient estimates from the two-step estimator are quite different from the OLS results based on the full sample, especially the coefficient on HSIR074 is significantly smaller. The results of the semi-parametric selection estimator are very similar to those of the two-step estimator, indicating that the normality assumption is not violated.

Table 11.4 gives the impact of the four different results for the allocation of resources to the regions. The first column gives the population weighted need indices for a selected clustering of wards, based on the simple OLS regression results of the demand equation using the full sample of wards. Deprived inner city areas and wards in inner London have the highest need indices, whereas rural areas have the lowest. The next columns in Table 11.4 give the percentage change in need indices based on the other three estimation results and show some marked differences. Using the two-step and semi-parametric esti-

Table 11.5   Results for probit regression

Weighted regression; dependent variable WT91 > 100	$N = 4955$	$R^2 = 0.14$	
Variable	B	SE B	T
ACCNHS	−0.1530	0.1073	−1.4264
ACCGPS	0.1743	0.1288	1.3529
ACCPRI	−0.2325	0.0626	−3.7137
HOMES*	−0.1034	0.3370	−0.3066
OLDALONE	0.2274	0.2104	1.0810
NOCAR	0.1192	0.1055	1.1295
MANUAL	−0.0222	0.1003	−0.2210
HSIR074	−0.2377	0.2032	−1.1699
SMR074	−0.1581	0.1734	−1.9118

LR test for supply variables: 30.24, p value = 0.0000.
Dummies included for RHA.
Observations weighted by ward population.

mation results, the wards in greater London have a higher needs index than before, whereas primarily the inner city and urban areas have a lower index. Note that the actual allocation formula that is currently in use is based on multi-level model estimates that take account of 186 District Health Authorities (DHA). As we believe that these district effects are correlated with the explanatory variables, they should be modelled as fixed effects dummy variables (see Blundell and Windmeijer [13]). This is complicated for the non-linear probit model, and we do not pursue it in this paper. The allocation results as presented here are, therefore, not a direct comparison with current practice.

The results presented above were based on the model specification of Smith et al. [6], which were selected without using multi-level modelling procedures. Our results are different for various reasons. Firstly, we used a different dependent variable, the utilization in 1991–1992, and not the average of the years 1990–1991 and 1991–1992. Secondly, we estimated the demand equation using only those wards with low waiting times, correcting for the endogenous selection. As is clear from the results as presented in Table 11.3, not all demand variables have a significant impact on utilization using our modelling approach. We therefore performed a specification search, selecting needs variables using the two-step selection method. The need variables identified in this way are very similar as before, but the variables S_CARER and UNEMP are replaced by NOCAR and MANUAL. Tables 11.5–11.7 present the set of results for this model. Again the sample selection term in the two-step estimator is significant with the expected sign, and the parametric and semi-parametric estimates are very similar. In comparison with the first model, however, the needs indices for London are substantially lower, whereas those for the rural areas are higher.

As stated in the previous section, our modelling strategy assumes that waiting times do not affect demand when they are smaller than W^m. In Table 11.8 we present instrumental variables estimation results for the demand equation that includes the (log of) the waiting times linearly in the model, as specified in Equation 11.2. The endogenous waiting times are instrumented by the four lagged supply variables. The first column presents results for the full sample, and the waiting time has a significant negative effect on demand. The second column presents the results for the selected sample including the Heckman sample selection correction. In this case, the effect of

Table 11.6   Results for needs regressions

Weighted regression; dependent variable ACCOS91								
	OLS full sample		OLS selected sample		Two-step estimator		Semi-parametric estimator	
N	4955		1296		1296		1296	
R^2	0.51		0.57		0.58		0.49	
Variable	B	SE B	B	SE B	B	SE* B	B	SE* B
OLDALONE	0.0916	0.0235	0.0979	0.0423	0.1258	0.0499	0.1224	0.0464
NOCAR	0.0475	0.0101	0.0629	0.0185	0.0775	0.0232	0.0630	0.0214
MANUAL	0.0371	0.0106	0.0433	0.0227	0.0565	0.0237	0.0541	0.0219
HSIR074	0.2166	0.0226	0.1722	0.0390	0.1192	0.0518	0.1482	0.0504
SMR074	0.1259	0.0216	0.1049	0.0379	0.0752	0.0456	0.0996	0.0435
λ					−0.2256	0.0621		

Dummies included for RHA.
SE*, standard deviation of 100 bootstrap estimates.
Observations weighted by ward population.

Table 11.7 Population weighted need indices, as compared with first model, Table 11.4, columns 3 and 4

Cluster summaries	Selected two-step (%)	Selected semi-parametric (%)
Inner London	−2.36	−2.18
Mixed status London	−1.19	−1.18
Outer London	−0.65	−0.79
Inner city deprived	−0.59	−0.40
Urban areas	0.42	0.55
Resort and retirement area	−0.11	−0.14
High-status suburban	−0.05	−0.13
High-status rural	0.69	0.47
High-status urban	0.20	0.19
Rural areas	0.93	0.82
Dormitory towns	−2.36	−2.33

waiting time is small and insignificant, supporting our initial assumptions. The latter model is identified as there are four instrumental variables that instrument both the selection correction term and the waiting times variable.

We have chosen the cut-off point of 100 days as that is seen by health care providers as a reasonable time to go through the system. When we repeat the instrumental variables regression, including waiting times but for different selected samples for different values of W^m, we find that the waiting time variable is significantly negative for values of W^m of 117 and higher, and insignificant for values of W^m lower than 117. In the light of this, it appears that the cut-off point of 100 days is appropriate. However, to check robustness of the results, we present in Table 11.9 estimation results for a selected sample with a cut-off point of 110 days waiting. The sample size in this case is

much larger. The results, however, are very similar to those as presented in Table 11.6.

CONCLUSIONS

The aim of this paper was to recover the determinants of demand for hospital services in a framework that acknowledges the importance of supply constraints in the public sector provision of health care. Waiting times are assumed to act as a hassle cost that chokes off demand when resources are constrained. In the full equilibrium model, waiting times act like a price that maintains full equilibrium. Because our interest has been in the determinants of demand we do not fully model supply but simply use the determinants of supply as instruments for waiting time in our specification of demand.

To measure the determinants of demand we chose, as our central specification, a model that selects only those areas with low waiting times. Our results are then corrected for this endogenous selection. We argue that the focus on demand at low waiting times avoids systematic measurement error at high waiting times and also avoids the specification of the interactions between needs variables at higher waiting times. In estimation, we compare our specification to alternative models.

We have applied our approach to a sample of ward level data from the UK and study the demand for acute care. We contrast our model estimates, and their implications for health services resource allocations in the UK, to more standard allocation models. We find that correcting for supply constraints through the selection of low waiting time areas changes allocation formulae in important ways.

Allocation formulae that are based on models relating

Table 11.8 Results for IV estimator with WT91 included

Weighted regression; dependent variable ACCOS91	Full sample, $N = 4955$		Selected sample, $N = 1296$	
Variable	B	SE B	B	SE* B
OLDALONE	0.2381	0.0846	0.1025	0.0701
NOCAR	0.0773	0.0356	0.0765	0.0271
MANUAL	0.0922	0.0355	0.0568	0.0282
HSIR074	−0.0017	0.0958	0.0736	0.0739
SMR074	0.1350	0.0611	0.1225	0.0758
WT91	−2.4851	0.6750	−0.7449	0.8128
λ			−0.1863	0.0921

Instrumented by lagged supply variables.
Dummies included for RHA.
SE*, standard deviation of 100 bootstrap estimates.
Observations weighted by ward population.

Table 11.9   Results for needs regressions; selected sample, WT91 < 110

Weighted regression; dependent variable ACCOS91	Two-step estimator		Semi-parametric estimator	
N	2016		2016	
R^2	0.57		0.54	
Variable	B	SE* B	B	SE* B
OLDALONE	0.1056	0.0487	0.1094	0.0515
NOCAR	0.0868	0.0223	0.0859	0.0248
MANUAL	0.0574	0.0250	0.0616	0.0257
HSIR074	0.1296	0.0502	0.1288	0.0551
SMR074	0.0740	0.0457	0.0766	0.0484
λ	−0.3505	0.1216		

Dummies included for RHA.
SE*, standard deviation of 100 bootstrap estimates.
Observations weighted by ward population.

needs to use require the explicit modelling of the process by which use is determined. In the case of the NHS, identifying needs from acute hospital care utilization data should take into account the method of rationing by waiting times.

ACKNOWLEDGEMENTS

The authors are grateful to two anonymous referees, participants of the Health Economics Seminars at IFS and the Eighth European Workshop on Econometrics and Health Economics, in particular Hugh Gravelle and Owen O'Donnell for helpful comments, and to Peter Smith and Stephen Martin for providing the data on the health care utilization used in this study. The authors further thank Séan Boyle for stimulating discussions and for the calculations of the resource allocations. This research is part of the programme of the ESRC Centre for the Micro-Economic Analysis of Fiscal Policy at IFS. The financial support of the ESRC is gratefully acknowledged. The usual disclaimer applies.

REFERENCES

1. Lindsay, C.M. and Feigenbaum, B. Rationing by waiting lists. *Am. Econ. Rev.* 1984; **74**: 404–417.

2. Gravelle, H.S.E. Rationing trials by waiting: welfare implications. *Int. Rev. Law Econ.* 1990; **10**: 255–270.
3. Goddard, J.A., Malek, M. and Tavakoli, M. An economic model of the market for hospital treatment for non-urgent conditions. *Health Econ.* 1995; **4**: 41–55.
4. Martin, S. and Smith, P.C. Rationing by waiting lists: an empirical investigation. *J. Public Econ.* 1999; **71**: 141–164.
5. Gourieroux, C., Laffont, J.J. and Monfort, A. Disequilibrium econometrics in simultaneous equations systems. *Econometrica* 1980; **48**: 75–96.
6. Smith, P.C., Sheldon, T.A., Carr-Hill, R.A., Martin, S. and Hardman, G. Allocating resources to health authorities: results and policy implications of small area analysis of use of inpatient services. *Br. Med. J.* 1994; **309**: 1050–1054.
7. Newey, W.K., Powell, J.L. and Walker J.R. Semiparametric estimation of selection models: some empirical results. *Am. Econ. Rev.* 1990; **80**: 324–328.
8. Heckman, J. Sample selection bias as a specification error. *Econometrica* 1979; **47**: 153–161.
9. Robinson, P.M. Root-N-consistent semiparametric regression. *Econometrica* 1988; **56**: 931–954.
10. Härdle, W. and Linton, O. Applied nonparametric methods. In *Handbook of Econometrics,* vol. 4, R.F. Engle and D.L. McFadden (eds). Elsevier: Amsterdam, 1994, 2295–2339.
11. Martin, S. *Data Manual, Version 1.0, Small Area Analysis of Hospital Utilisation.* Institute for Research in the Social Sciences: University of York, 1994.
12. Carr-Hill, R.A., Hardman, G., Martin, S., Peacock, S., Sheldon, T.A. and Smith, P.C. *A Formula for Distributing NHS Revenues Based on Small Area Use of Hospital Beds.* Centre for Health Economics: University of York, 1994.
13. Blundell, R. and Windmeijer, F. Cluster effects and simultaneity in multilevel models. *Health Econ.* 1997; **6**: 439–443.

12

Non- and Semi-parametric Estimation of Age and Time Heterogeneity in Repeated Cross-sections: an Application to Self-reported Morbidity and General Practitioner Utilization

DAVID PARKIN[1], NIGEL RICE[2] AND MATTHEW SUTTON[3]

[1]*Department of Economics, City University, London, UK,* [2]*Centre for Health Economics, University of York, York, UK and* [3]*Department of General Practice, University of Glasgow, Glasgow, UK*

INTRODUCTION

Many population health and health care related indicators vary over time and across age and sex groups. Aggregate measures of health service use and population health status observed at a particular time may differ by year-of-age (an age effect), year-of-observation (a time effect) and year-of-birth (a birth-cohort effect). The patterns of these variations are complex and highly non-linear, such that modelling them requires methods which are flexible. This paper examines a set of non-parametric and semi-parametric techniques which are of value in revealing underlying patterns and trends in repeated cross-sectional health and health care data.

The value of an in-depth appreciation of the patterns of variation of such variables is in creating tools to guide public health policy, direct future planning of services, develop management strategies and allocate resources fairly. It is not uncommon in, for example, explorations of age and sex effects on health service utilization to see crude calculations such as mean utilization rates within arbitrarily defined age–sex groupings compared for different years. More sophisticated analyses rely on parametric specifications of the underlying relationships using, for example, a dummy variable to specify a sex effect and a quadratic or cubic term for age. However, such methods provide, at best, summaries of currently observed heterogeneity, but cannot identify subtle nuances within the underlying patterns and trends. Their value is, therefore, limited.

A problem with such population data is that they are subject to special kinds of 'noise' which may mask the underlying relationships. In particular, there may be considerable year-to-year fluctuations, both over time and over ages, which may obscure patterns and trends. Such 'roughness' in the data requires 'smoothing' before the underlying relationships of interest can be properly understood. The non-parametric estimation technique used in this paper is based on ordinary least squares but includes a roughness penalty to incorporate the desired level of smoothing across age and time. The technique can also be extended to analyse the class of generalized linear models proposed by Nelder and Wedderburn [1]. This paper also explores a semi-parametric equivalent estimator permitting both smoothing over age and time and estimation of the relationship between smoothed variables.

The methods are illustrated using data from successive years of the British General Household Survey (GHS). Non-parametric estimation is used to explore age and sex heterogeneity for the use of general practitioner (GP) services and self-reported morbidity. Semi-parametric

Econometric Analysis of Health Data. Edited by Andrew M. Jones and Owen O'Donnell
© 2002 John Wiley & Sons Ltd. Previously published in *Health Economics,* Vol. 8; pp. 429–440 (1999). © John Wiley & Sons Ltd

estimation includes the morbidity variables as independent predictors in a regression of GP utilization, permitting analysis of how the specification of age and time heterogeneity influences the estimated effects of morbidity on health care use.

DATA

The data are taken from 12 waves of the GHS, covering the period 1984–1995/6 inclusive. The GHS is an annual, nationally-representative survey of over 20 000 individuals living in private households in Great Britain. Respondents are interviewed in their own homes and provide information on demographic and socioeconomic characteristics, health status, health care utilization and lifestyle.

Two self-reported health measures are used: whether or not an individual has a limiting long-standing illness (LS); and whether or not an individual believes that they have had good health in general in the 12 months prior to the interview. The measure of utilization relates to the number of contacts with a GP under the National Health Service (NHS) over the fortnight prior to the interview.

The analysis is undertaken on cell means rather than individual-level data, with each cell representing a particular year-of-age in a particular survey year. In addition, analyses are restricted to those aged 16–80 years and the data for women and men are analysed separately. The data were weighted to reflect the different sizes of survey year and year-of-age cells in the GHS. This is an approximation based on the assumption that data within a particular cell, from which a cell mean is calculated, is drawn from a distribution with the same variance as data within other cells.

The reason cell means were used is that the methods adopted are computationally extremely demanding. Dummy variables are required for each year-of-age and survey year combination, requiring the estimation of a large number of parameters. For these data, analysis of individual-level data would involve over 130 000 data points and estimation of a large vector of parameters. The methods applied also require numerous complex matrix manipulations as well as repeated estimations to implement search procedures. In addition, limited dependent variable models would be required since utilization is measured on a count scale and self-reported morbidity on a categorical scale. Together, these requirements make the analysis of individual-level data computationally infeasible.

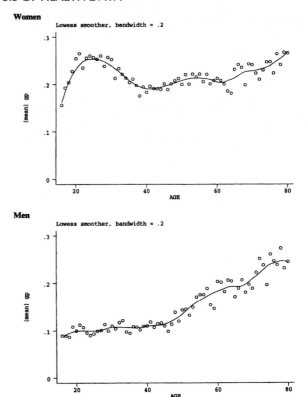

Figure 12.1. Use of GP services per year averaged over 1984–1995/6 by age for women and men with lowess smoothers

METHODS

The rationale for the adopted method can be seen by reference to Figure 12.1, which plots separately mean utilization rates against years of age for women and men. A model based solely on goodness-of-fit criteria would simply join the various points in succession, which would add nothing to our understanding of the underlying trends and fail to summarize the data adequately. Superimposed upon this is a plot of a lowess estimator [2] which incorporates a degree of smoothing. Clearly, these lines offer a summary of the data, but one that is flexible enough to detect subtle perturbations in underlying trends across age. Simple parametric specifications would not offer the degree of flexibility required to track these data.

Lowess is one of a wide range of smoothing techniques available. However, this paper follows Chesher [3,4] in employing a bivariate thin spline smoother, using a discretized version of roughness penalized least squares (RPLS). The advantage of RPLS is that it has the ability to extend data analyses to the class of generalized linear models, including additional predictor variables which may be specified either non-parametrically or parametrically.

The non-parametric analysis has three main elements: estimation of smoothed functions for the utilization and morbidity measures using RPLS; testing of the appropriate degree of smoothing through cross-validation; and testing of restrictions on the estimated parameters. An extension to the non-parametric approach applied to GP utilization by incorporating parametric specifications of self-reported morbidity measures is also considered. The resulting estimator is semi-parametric, but retains the same general properties of the non-parametric approach.

ROUGHNESS PENALIZED LEAST SQUARES (RPLS)

A thorough account of RPLS estimation as an approach to non-parametric regression, together with descriptions of alternative approaches, can be found in literature such as Green and Silverman [5], Hardle [6] and Bowman and Azzalini [7]. The classic RPLS approach is, for the univariate case, based on a general model:

$$y = g(x) + \varepsilon, \tag{12.1}$$

where y is the variable to be smoothed, x is the variable across which smoothing is to take place, g is an undefined curve function, and ε is an error term. Given any twice-differentiable function g, defined in the interval $[a, b]$, a penalized weighted sum of squares can be defined as:

$$\Omega_W(g) = \sum_{i=1}^{n} w_i \{y_i - g(x_i)\}^2 + \alpha \int_a^b \{g''(x)\}^2 \, dx, \tag{12.2}$$

where w_i are weights attached to each observation and α is a parameter representing the degree of smoothing required. The weights are defined as the number of observations on which each cell mean is estimated and is directly analogous to weighting an OLS model by multiplying both sides of the equation by $\sqrt{w_i}$. The penalized least squares estimator, $\hat{g}$, is the minimizer of $\Omega_W(g)$ over all twice-differentiable functions g.

The cost $\Omega_W(g)$ of a particular curve is, therefore, determined not only by its goodness-of-fit, defined by the conventional weighted residual sum of squares, but also by its roughness, defined by summed squared second derivatives. The smoothing parameter α determines the relative importance attached to residual error and local variation. If α is infinitely large, then the dominating expression in Equation 12.3 is the roughness term, and

hence the minimizer of $\Omega_W(g)$ will display very little curvature and will approach a linear regression fit. As α tends to zero, $\hat{g}$ will approach the interpolation curve that simply joins consecutive data points. Formally, this is the amount of smoothing afforded by binning into annual age and time groups.

Applying this approach in practice gives a specific form to the general model in Equation 12.1. It is necessary for the model to be bivariate, because it is necessary to smooth over both age and time, and also discrete, because of the nature of the data employed. For all of the variables of interest the aim is to estimate the generic model:

$$y_{at} = \sum_{t=1}^{l} \sum_{a=1}^{m} \beta_{at} X_{at} + \varepsilon_{at}, \tag{12.3}$$

where y is the variable of interest, a = year-of-age, t = year-of-observation, X_{at} = age and survey year binary indicators, ε = random errors with conditional mean of zero, and β is the parameter to be estimated. (Since we have 12 survey years (1984–1995/6) and 65 years-of-age (16–80), the analysis is undertaken on 780 (12 × 65) observations and the same number of independent (dummy) variables.)

The discretized bivariate roughness penalty is

$$\Omega_W(g)$$
$$= \sum_{t=1}^{l} \sum_{a=1}^{m} w_{at} \{y_{at} - g(x_{at})\}^2 + \alpha^2 \sum_{t=1}^{l} \sum_{a=1}^{m} g_{aa}(x_{at})^2$$
$$+ 2\alpha^2 \sum_{t=1}^{l} \sum_{a=1}^{m} g_{at}(x_{at})^2 + \alpha^2 \sum_{t=1}^{l} \sum_{a=1}^{m} g_{tt}(x_{at})^2, \tag{12.4}$$

where g_{aa}, g_{at} and g_{tt} are own and cross second-differences:

$$g_{aa} = \beta_{a+1,t} - 2\beta_{a,t} + \beta_{a-1,t}$$
$$g_{at} = \beta_{a+1,t} - 2\beta_{a,t} - \beta_{a+1,t-1} + \beta_{a,t-1}$$
$$g_{tt} = \beta_{a,t+1} - 2\beta_{a,t} + \beta_{a,t-1}.$$

The actual estimation method was to apply weighted least squares (WLS) to a data set augmented by a 'smoothing matrix' of dummy observations. Full details of this are given in the Appendix. The weights for the data are, as stated, cell sizes; the weights for the set of augmented dummy observations are set to one.

CROSS-VALIDATION

A free choice may be exercised over the size of parameter α and it is, therefore, necessary to define criteria for choosing a particular value. A non-statistical method is to use an 'eyeball test' according to the appearance of the smoothed data when plotted. However, it is also possible to estimate α using Green and Silverman's [5] method of cross-validation (CV). Essentially, CV is based upon a 'jack-knife' procedure whereby the predicted value of each observation from a particular model is compared with the predicted value derived from an estimation omitting that observation from the data set. Such a procedure would be computationally extremely cumbersome, but a shortcut is available making use of the 'hat' or projection matrix, P, which has the property that when multiplied by observed values results in predicted values, that is $YP = \hat{Y}$. The method, therefore, involves choosing the value for α which minimizes CV(α) as given by:

$$CV(\alpha) = \sum_{t=1}^{l} \sum_{a=1}^{m} w_{at} \left(\frac{y_{at} - \hat{g}(x_{at})}{\{I - A_W(\alpha)\}_{nn}} \right)^2, \qquad (12.5)$$

where I is the identity matrix of size $n \times n$ (where $n = l \times m$) and $A_W(\alpha)$ is the $n \times n$ projection matrix for weighted smoothing. The term $\{I - A_W(\alpha)\}_{nn}$ represents the elements on the leading diagonal of the square matrix $I - A_W(\alpha)$, such that when $t = 1$ and $a = 1$, $n = 1$; when $t = 1$ and $a = 2$, $n = 2$; when $t = 1$ and $a = m, n = m$; when $t = 2$ and $a = 1, n = m + 1$, etc. until $n = m + n$ when $t = 1$ and $a = m$. The CV-minimizing value for α is located using a grid search in increments of 50 for α^2.

Estimates are obtained using OLS on the weighted data:

$$\hat{\beta} = \hat{g} = (X'X + \alpha^2 S'S)^{-1} X'y^*, \qquad (12.6)$$

in which y^* is the vector of observations weighted for sample size, such that $y_{at}^* = \sqrt{w_{at}} \times y_{at}$. X represents the vector of age–year dummy variables, again weighted appropriately for sample size. The roughness penalty term in Equation 12.3 above can be represented by a matrix S which is shown in the Appendix.

The variance of $\hat{\beta}$ is given by

$$\text{var}(\hat{\beta})$$
$$= (X'X + \alpha^2 S'S)^{-1} X' \sum X (X'X + \alpha^2 S'S)^{-1}, \qquad (12.7)$$

where $\Sigma = diag(\varepsilon_{at} | x)$. The corresponding projection matrix that transforms the matrix of actual observations into a matrix of predictions is:

$$A_W(\alpha) = X(X'X + \alpha^2 S'S)^{-1} X'. \qquad (12.8)$$

Connections with classical regression allow us to define equivalent df for the penalized least squares estimator.

This measure provides an indication of the effective number of parameters that are fitted for any particular value of the smoothing parameter α. If we consider a parametric regression with two explanatory variables and a constant term, then the number of df for the residual sum of squares is simply $n - k$, where n is the number of observations and $k = 3$. Assuming the parameters are identifiable on the basis of available observations, the hat matrix A is then the projection onto a space of dimension k, the number of parameters fitted, and hence its trace is also equal to k. Therefore, the model df k, are equal to the trace of the hat or projection matrix, whilst the residual df are equal to $tr(I - A)$ (tr representing the trace). By analogy to the simple regression case, we define the equivalent df for the non-parametric penalized least squares model considered here as:

$$EDF = tr\{I - A_W(\alpha)\} \qquad (12.9)$$

$$\Rightarrow EDF = tr(I) - tr(X(X'X + \alpha^2 S'S)^{-1} X'). \qquad (12.10)$$

TESTING RESTRICTIONS

Three types of restrictions were tested relating to age, time and cohort effects.

Age effects

The functional form for age heterogeneity was tested using four functional forms: linear, quadratic, cubic and 4th order polynomial. The tests are a form of the Chow test [8] with the switch-point in the middle of the age interval.

In the linear case the first derivative of the dependent variable with respect to age is constant. This can be tested using the following restriction on the estimated $\hat{\beta}$ parameters.

$$\sum_{a=16}^{47} [\hat{\beta}_{a+1,t} - \hat{\beta}_{a,t}] - \sum_{a=48}^{79} [\hat{\beta}_{a+1,t} - \hat{\beta}_{a,t}] = 0 \qquad (12.11)$$

which simplifies to

$$\hat{\beta}_{16,t} - 2\hat{\beta}_{48,t} + \hat{\beta}_{80,t} = 0. \qquad (12.11a)$$

The quadratic functional form assumes the second derivative with respect to age is constant and can be tested using the following restriction:

$$\sum_{a=16}^{46} [\hat{\beta}_{a+2,t} - 2\hat{\beta}_{a+1,t} + \hat{\beta}_{a,t}]$$

$$-\sum_{a=47}^{77} [\hat{\beta}_{a+2,t} - 2\hat{\beta}_{a+1,t} + \hat{\beta}_{a,t}] = 0 \qquad (12.12)$$

which simplifies to

$$\hat{\beta}_{16,t} - \hat{\beta}_{17,t} - 2\hat{\beta}_{47,t} + 2\hat{\beta}_{48,t} + \hat{\beta}_{78,t} - \hat{\beta}_{80,t} = 0. \qquad (12.12a)$$

The cubic functional form is rested using the following restriction on the following discrete approximations to the third derivative:

$$\sum_{a=16}^{45} [\hat{\beta}_{a+4,t} - 2\hat{\beta}_{a+3,t} + 2\hat{\beta}_{a+1,t} - \hat{\beta}_{a,t}]$$

$$-\sum_{a=46}^{75} [\hat{\beta}_{a+4,t} - 2\hat{\beta}_{a+3,t} + 2\hat{\beta}_{a+1,t} - \hat{\beta}_{a,t}] = 0 \qquad (12.13)$$

which is equivalent to

$$\hat{\beta}_{16,t} - \hat{\beta}_{17,t} - \hat{\beta}_{18,t} + \hat{\beta}_{19,t} - 2\hat{\beta}_{46,t} + 2\hat{\beta}_{47,t}$$

$$+ 2\hat{\beta}_{48,t} - 2\hat{\beta}_{49,t} + \hat{\beta}_{76,t} - \hat{\beta}_{77,t} - \hat{\beta}_{78,t} + \hat{\beta}_{79,t} = 0. \qquad (12.13a)$$

Finally, the age-polynomial of order four is tested using the following restriction on the estimated parameters:

$$\sum_{a=16}^{43} [\hat{\beta}_{a+8,t} - 2\hat{\beta}_{a+7,t} + \hat{\beta}_{a+5,t} - 2\hat{\beta}_{a+4,t}$$

$$+ 2\hat{\beta}_{a+3,t} - 2\hat{\beta}_{a+1,t} + \hat{\beta}_{a,t}]$$

$$-\sum_{a=44}^{71} [\hat{\beta}_{a+8,t} - 2\hat{\beta}_{a+7,t} + 2\hat{\beta}_{a+5,t} - 2\hat{\beta}_{a+4,t}$$

$$+ 2\hat{\beta}_{a+3,t} - 2\hat{\beta}_{a+1,t} + \hat{\beta}_{a,t}] = 0, \qquad (12.14)$$

which simplifies to an expression involving 24 of the $\hat{\beta}$ parameters. The age restrictions can be undertaken for any combination of the survey years. The results presented in Table 12.1 represent simultaneous testing of these restrictions across all 12 survey years (1984–1995/6 inclusive).

Time effects

Time effects were investigated by comparing the values for particular ages in the first and second 6 survey years:

$$\sum_{t=1984}^{1989} \hat{\beta}_{at} - \sum_{t=1990}^{1995} \hat{\beta}_{at} = 0. \qquad (12.15)$$

The restriction can be imposed for any combination of ages. The results in Table 12.1 relate to a joint-test for ages 16–80.

Cohort effects

In a matrix with rows representing ages and columns representing survey years, cohorts can be followed by moving diagonally through the matrix. For example, a cohort aged 16 years in the 1984 survey is aged 17 in 1985, 18 in 1986 and so on. A cohort effect can be investigated

Table 12.1 Non-parametric analysis of general practitioner (GP) utilization and morbidity measures: smoothing parameters, equivalent df and F-test statistics for age, time and cohort restrictions

	Women			Men		
	LS	GH	GP	LS	GH	GP
α	41.8	33.2	94.9	42.4	24.5	186.7
EDF	731	720	755	733	704	765
Age effect – linear	21.81	11.00	1.77	9.85	12.13	7.39
	($p < 0.001$)	($p < 0.001$)	($p = 0.049$)	($p < 0.001$)	($p < 0.001$)	($p < 0.001$)
Age effect – quadratic	0.84	0.67	2.23	1.34	0.98	0.45
	($p = 0.612$)	($p = 0.781$)	($p = 0.009$)	($p = 0.192$)	($p = 0.465$)	($p = 0.943$)
Age effect – cubic	0.62	1.61	0.95	1.01	0.46	2.46
	($p = 0.825$)	($p = 0.084$)	($p = 0.495$)	($p = 0.438$)	($p = 0.935$)	($p = 0.004$)
Age effect – 4th order polynomial	0.81	0.50	1.11	0.99	0.48	0.87
	($p = 0.637$)	($p = 0.914$)	($p = 0.348$)	($p = 0.453$)	($p = 0.926$)	($p = 0.575$)
Time effect	1.44	1.16	1.38	1.39	0.99	1.74
	($p = 0.015$)	($p = 0.186$)	($p < 0.001$)	($p = 0.027$)	($p = 0.506$)	($p < 0.001$)
Cohort effect	1.17	1.11	0.83	0.86	1.19	0.88
	($p = 0.190$)	($p = 0.284$)	($p = 0.796$)	($p = 0.755$)	($p = 0.175$)	($p = 0.721$)

LS = limiting long-standing illness; GH = general health.

by comparison with terms adjacent to the diagonal.

In a comparison of 2 survey years, a birth-year cohort effect is represented by rejection of the following restriction:

$$\hat{\beta}_{a+1,t+1} + \hat{\beta}_{a,t} - \hat{\beta}_{a+1,t} - \hat{\beta}_{a,t+1} = 0. \qquad (12.16)$$

We undertake tests for cohort effects following birth-years through all 12 survey years. The results in Table 12.1 relate to a joint-test for each age 16–68 in 1984. Note, however, that this test is rather weak and is conditional on finding age and/or time effects since Equation 12.16 can be re-expressed as the difference between two age effects $((\hat{\beta}_{a,t} - \hat{\beta}_{a+1,t}) - (\hat{\beta}_{a,t+1} - \hat{\beta}_{a+1,t+1}))$, or the difference between two time effects $((\hat{\beta}_{a+1,t+1} - \hat{\beta}_{a+1,t}) - (\hat{\beta}_{a,t+1} - \hat{\beta}_{a,t}))$. If there are no age or time effects, or if the effects of time and age are independent of one another, then Equation 12.16 will not detect evidence of cohort effects.

Semi-parametric analysis

The method of RPLS can be easily extended to enable estimation of a model in which a response variable has a linear relationship with some explanatory variables and a non-parametric (smoothing) relationship with others. The underlying model is

$$y_{at} = Z_{at}\beta + g(X_{at}) + \varepsilon, \qquad (12.17)$$

where y_{at}, X_{at}, g and ε are as defined earlier, Z_{at} is a vector of explanatory variables and β is a vector of linear parameters to be estimated. The penalized sum of squares (cf. Equation 12.2) is, therefore, defined as:

$$\Omega_W(\beta, g)$$

$$= \sum_{t=1}^{l} \sum_{a=1}^{m} w_{at}\{y_{at} - Z_{at}\beta - g(x_{at})\}^2$$

$$+ \alpha \int_a^b \{g''(x)\}^2 \, dx. \qquad (12.18)$$

The response variable y_{at} was defined to be the number of GP consultations. The 'splined' explanatory variables a and t are age and time as before, and the 'linear' explanatory variables Z_{at} are the two self-reported morbidity variables.

The weighted ROLS estimation used the CV-minimizing value for α obtained in the non-parametric analysis. For comparison, three different specifications for an ordinary linear model using WLS were estimated. One ex-

cluded age and time effects entirely. The others included age effects, using two different functional forms.

RESULTS

NON-PARAMETRIC ANALYSIS OF AGE AND TIME VARIATIONS

Figure 12.2 shows an example of the effect of bivariate smoothing on the data when the extent of smoothing is guided by visual inspection of the predicted values. However, the main focus of this paper is on the derivation of the smoothing parameter α and the testing of the estimated effects rather than the output from the smoothing procedure itself. It is noticeable that in all cases the extent of smoothing indicated by the CV-minimizing approach is less than is suggested by eye-balling the resulting plots. This result was also found by others using these techniques [4].

Table 12.1 shows the results of the non-parametric analysis for self-reported limiting LS, self-reported general health (GH) and consultations with a GP. For each variable, the value of the smoothing parameter α and the estimated equivalent df are given. The CV procedure suggests that, for both women and men, the GP variable can be smoothed the most and the GH variable the least. Correspondingly, for both women and men, the equivalent df are greatest for the GP variable.

Table 12.1 also shows F-test statistics for the various functional form restrictions on age and time heterogeneity. For the age effects, only the linear functional form can be rejected. This result is surprising because the period-averaged data shown in Figure 12.1 suggest complex non-linearities which could not be represented by parametric functional forms. Our restrictions may suffer from the familiar problem with this type of test that the choice of the wrong switch-point does not affect the validity of the tests under the null but can have serious consequences for the power of the test [9]. This is particularly the case for the GP variable for women, since there seems to be substantial non-linearity within the lower age range.

For both women and men, significant changes over time are observed for LS and the number of consultations, but not for the reporting of 'not-good' GH. For both women and men, LS and GP utilization have increased over time. No evidence of cohort effects in any of the variables is apparent. However, our comparisons involved adjacent birth-years and it may be that cohort effects are manifest for broader age groups, suggesting that there may be some value in comparing birth-years which are further apart.

Table 12.2 General practitioner (GP) consultations by women regressed on limiting long-standing illness (LH), 'not-good' general health (GH) and different specifications for age and time heterogeneity

Dependent variable: average number of consultations	Model (1) WLS – no age		Model (2) WLS – quadratic age		Model (3) WLS – 4th order polynomial in age		Model (4) WRPLS – $\alpha = 94.9$	
	Coefficient	t value	Coefficient	t value	Coefficient	t value	Coefficient	t value
Constant	0.180	19.197	0.216	12.155	−0.387	−5.339	—	—
LS	−0.124	−2.760	0.109	2.008	0.187	3.551	0.146	2.921
GH	0.165	3.724	0.213	4.678	0.192	4.307	0.218	5.183
Age			−0.0027	−4.594	0.058	7.681	—	—
Age^2			5.71e^{-6}	0.729	−0.0020	−7.553	—	—
Age^3					0.00003	7.031	—	—
Age^4					−1.38e^{-7}	−6.497	—	—
Test of joint significance of age terms								
$F(2, 775)$			36.69	$p < 0.01$				
$F(4, 773)$					41.45	$p < 0.01$		

WLS = weighted least squares.

Table 12.3 General practitioner (GP) consultations by men regressed on limiting long-standing illness (LS), 'not-good' general health (GH) and different specifications for age and time heterogeneity

Dependent variable: average number of consultations	Model (1) WLS – no age		Model (2) WLS – quadratic age		Model (3) WLS – 4th order polynomial in age		Model (4) WRPLS – $\alpha = 186.7$	
	Coefficient	t value	Coefficient	t value	Coefficient	t value	Coefficient	t value
Constant	0.049	10.612	0.091	8.043	0.032	0.545	—	—
LS	0.195	5.734	0.164	4.331	0.172	4.286	0.179	4.565
GH	0.144	4.688	0.084	2.412	0.091	2.561	0.042	1.212
Age			−0.0017	−3.664	0.0037	0.594	—	—
Age^2			0.00003	4.309	−0.00014	−0.619	—	—
Age^3					2.04e^{-6}	0.587	—	—
Age^4					−8.57e^{-9}	−0.460	—	—
Test of joint significance of age terms								
$F(2, 775)$			9.31	$p < 0.01$				
$F(4, 773)$					5.22	$p < 0.01$		

WLS = weighted least squares.

SEMI-PARAMETRIC ANALYSIS OF MORBIDITY EFFECTS ON GP UTILIZATION

Table 12.2 presents parametric and semi-parametric estimates for women. When we do not allow for age heterogeneity, LS is estimated to reduce GP utilization. The incorporation of age terms reverses this effect but the coefficient on LS remains more sensitive to the functional form which is chosen for time and age variations than is 'not-good' GH.

Table 12.3 shows a similar set of results for me. Both self-reported morbidity variables are estimated to increase GP utilization. However, in this case it is the coefficient on 'not-good' GH which is sensitive to the allowance made for age and time heterogeneity. In the weighted RPLS regression, the coefficient on 'not-good'

Unsmoothed

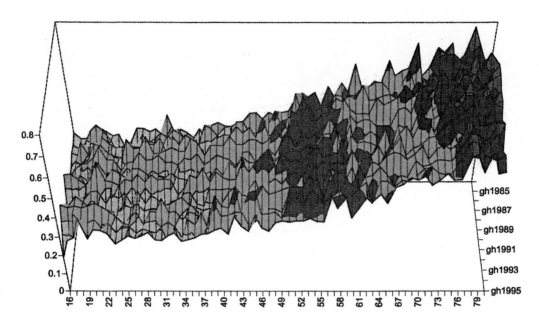

Smoothed

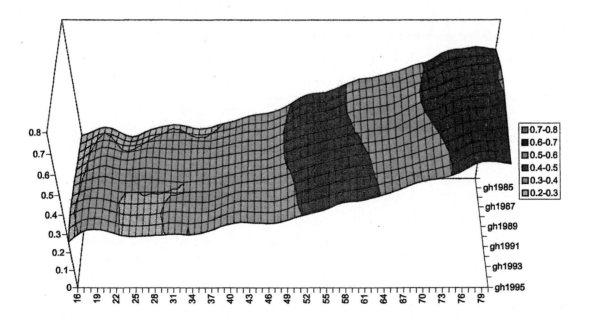

Figure 12.2. The effect of bivariate smoothing on the predicted proportion of women reporting 'not-good' general health

GH is not significantly different from zero. The coefficient on LS changes very little across the various specifications and the weighted RPLS value is similar to that for women. The estimated effect of 'not-good' general health is quite different for men and women.

DISCUSSION

Non- and semi-parametric methods have a number of advantages in analysing time series data from pseudo-panels such as those used throughout this paper, whose variables reflect non-random variations over time, age and cohort in ways unlikely to be modelled well by imposed parametric functional forms. The added flexibility afforded by the lack of imposition of a more simple parametric formulation is valuable. Their results might simply be used to inspire an informed parametric formulation, which may have some purpose or advantages for inference. However, where complex relationships unfold, calls for simplicity will largely be fruitless and the non- or semi-parametric estimates will remain the best way to summarize patterns in the data.

Many different non- and semi-parametric techniques are available, for example, alternative spline methods or kernel smoothing estimators. However, broadly speaking all of these methods are equivalent, and the roughness penalty approach appeals because of its simplicity and intuitiveness. More importantly it has the desirable property that it can be applied in the broader context of generalized linear models in a straightforward manner.

Although flexibility of functional form is a virtue of the analysis, it is necessary to maintain a framework within which competing forms can be judged. In this paper, two of these were examined – the method of cross-validation to structure the otherwise arbitrarily-chosen smoothing parameter, and the testing of restrictions on the parameter estimates to investigate the nature of time and age heterogeneity.

In general, the CV method proved valuable, albeit computationally time-consuming. However, the 'optimal' level of smoothing selected using CV did not coincide with what an 'eyeball test' of smoothness would produce. This appears to be a reasonably consistent finding in the applied literature [4] and a degree of subjectivity in selecting the appropriate level of smoothing seems sensible. The restriction testing was, however, less successful, since the age effect analysis did not pick up the clear non-linearities in the data. This is likely to be due to the weak power of the tests resulting from the chosen switch-point. In future work it may be better to compare the estimated year-of-age coefficients with those estimated using par-

ametric functional forms or undertake a randomly selected series of year-of-age comparisons. Silverman [9] has described a number of alternative methodological approaches to making confidence statements about quantities of interest such as cohort effects, for example, making inferences based on a Bayesian framework, possibly through the use of Markov Chain Monte Carlo methods.

Although theoretical literature on smoothing estimation has existed for a number of years, few applications in health care have been reported. However, the methods are accessible and are particularly suited to problems where complex relationships requiring flexible functional forms are being interrogated. Analyses of relationships between health experience, demands for health care and utilization of health services and age could benefit greatly from these methods. Smoothing is essential if complex age and time profiles are to be retrieved from what may otherwise appear as extremely noisy, heterogenous data, and the analyses reported in this paper suggest that roughness penalty-based methods are well-suited to this task. In particular, they may permit the analysis of repeated cross-sectional population surveys such as the GHS by regarding them as pseudo-panels defined on birth-year [10].

ACKNOWLEDGEMENTS

We thank Paul Grootendorst, Andrew Jones, other participants in the workshop, Peter Smith and Hugh Gravelle for comments. The work began during a visit by David Parkin to the Centre of Health Economics at York, and thanks are due to the Universities of York and Newcastle upon Tyne for making that possible. GHS data were supplied by the ESRC Data Archive at Essex. STATA do files to perform non-parametric and semi-parametric estimation are available upon request from NR. Funding from the Department of Health through NPCRDC is acknowledged.

APPENDIX: CONSTRUCTION OF SMOOTHING MATRIX

The data contain l survey years, and m years-of-age and are ordered as an $(l \times m)$ by $(l \times m + 1)$ matrix of the form

$$[\mathbf{y} \quad \mathbf{D} \quad \mathbf{w}],$$

where $\mathbf{y}$ is a vector of observations consisting of elements y_{at}, ordered from $a = 1$ to l and $t = 1$ to m; $\mathbf{w}$ is an identically ordered vector of weights; and $\mathbf{D}$ is an $(l \times m)$ by $(l \times m)$ dummy variable matrix of the form

$$\begin{bmatrix} \mathbf{I} & \mathbf{0} & \cdots & \mathbf{0} \\ \mathbf{0} & \mathbf{I} & \cdots & \mathbf{0} \\ : & : & & : \\ \mathbf{0} & \mathbf{0} & \cdots & \mathbf{I} \end{bmatrix},$$

where $\mathbf{I}$ is an identity matrix and $\mathbf{0}$ is a null matrix, both of size $m \times m$.

To these data is appended a matrix of dummy observations of the form

$$[\mathbf{0} \quad \mathbf{S} \quad \mathbf{I}],$$

where $\mathbf{S}$ is a *smoothing matrix* consisting of three stacked matrices:

$$\mathbf{S} = \begin{bmatrix} \mathbf{S_1} \\ \mathbf{S_2} \\ \mathbf{S_3} \end{bmatrix}.$$

$\mathbf{S_1}$ is a second-difference matrix of size $(l \times m - 2)$ by m which penalizes differences between the estimated parameters for adjacent years-of-age within each survey year:

$$\mathbf{S_1} = \begin{bmatrix} \mathbf{Q} & \mathbf{0} & \cdots & \mathbf{0} \\ \mathbf{0} & \mathbf{Q} & \cdots & \mathbf{0} \\ : & : & & : \\ \mathbf{0} & \mathbf{0} & \cdots & \mathbf{Q} \end{bmatrix}.$$

$\mathbf{Q}$ and $\mathbf{0}$ are sub-matrices of size $m \times m - 2$. $\mathbf{0}$ is a null matrix and $\mathbf{Q}$ is a second-difference matrix with the following structure:

$$Q = \begin{bmatrix} 1 & -2 & 1 & 0 & \cdots & 0 & 0 & 0 \\ 0 & 1 & -2 & 1 & \cdots & 0 & 0 & 0 \\ : & & & & & & & : \\ 0 & 0 & 0 & 0 & \cdots & 1 & -2 & 1 \end{bmatrix}.$$

$\mathbf{S_2}$ is a second-difference matrix of size $[(l \times m) + 1][m \times (l - 2)]$, which penalizes differences between the estimated parameters for adjacent survey years within each year-of-age:

$$\mathbf{S_2} = \begin{bmatrix} \mathbf{I} & -2\mathbf{I} & \mathbf{I} & \mathbf{0} & \cdots & \mathbf{0} & \mathbf{0} & \mathbf{0} & \mathbf{0} \\ \mathbf{0} & \mathbf{I} & -2\mathbf{I} & \mathbf{0} & \cdots & \mathbf{0} & \mathbf{0} & \mathbf{0} & \mathbf{0} \\ : & : & : & : & & : & : & : & : \\ \mathbf{0} & \mathbf{0} & \mathbf{0} & \mathbf{0} & \cdots & \mathbf{I} & -2\mathbf{I} & \mathbf{I} & \mathbf{0} \\ \mathbf{0} & \mathbf{0} & \mathbf{0} & \mathbf{0} & \cdots & \mathbf{0} & \mathbf{I} & -2\mathbf{I} & \mathbf{I} \end{bmatrix},$$

where $\mathbf{I}$ is an identity matrix and $\mathbf{0}$ is a null matrix, both of size $m \times m$.

$\mathbf{S_3}$ is a first-difference matrix of size $[(l \times m) + 1][(m - 1)(l - 1)]$ which penalizes differences between the estimated parameters for adjacent years-of-age in adjacent survey years and, therefore, smoothes across birth-year cohort:

$$\mathbf{S_3} = \begin{bmatrix} \mathbf{F} & -\mathbf{F} & \mathbf{0} & \cdots & \mathbf{0} & \mathbf{0} & \mathbf{0} \\ \mathbf{0} & \mathbf{F} & -\mathbf{F} & \cdots & \mathbf{0} & \mathbf{0} & \mathbf{0} \\ : & : & : & & : & : & : \\ \mathbf{0} & \mathbf{0} & \mathbf{0} & \cdots & \mathbf{F} & -\mathbf{F} & \mathbf{0} \\ \mathbf{0} & \mathbf{0} & \mathbf{0} & \cdots & \mathbf{0} & \mathbf{F} & -\mathbf{F} \end{bmatrix},$$

where $\mathbf{F}$ and $\mathbf{0}$ are sub-matrices of size $(m)(m - 1)$. $\mathbf{0}$ is a null matrix and $\mathbf{F}$ is a first-difference matrix with the following structure:

$$\mathbf{F} = \begin{bmatrix} 1 & -1 & 0 & \cdots & 0 & 0 \\ 0 & 1 & -1 & \cdots & 0 & 0 \\ : & & & & & : \\ 0 & 0 & 0 & 0 & 1 & -1 \end{bmatrix}.$$

REFERENCES

1. Nelder, J.A. and Wedderburn, R.W.M. Generalized linear models. *Journal of the Royal Statistical Society, Series A* 1972; **135**: 370–384.
2. Cleveland, W.S. *Visualizing Data*. Summit, NJ: Hobart Press, 1993.
3. Chesher, A. Individual demands from household aggregates: time and age variation in the composition of diet. *Presented to IFS Seminars on Health Economics*, 1996.
4. Chesher, A. Diet revealed?: Semiparametric estimation of nutrient intake–age relationships (with discussion). *Journal of the Royal Statistical Society, Series A* 1997; **160**: 389–420.
5. Green, P.J. and Silverman, B.W. *Nonparametric Regression and Generalized Linear Models: a Roughness Penalty Approach*. London: Chapman Hall, 1994.
6. Hardle, W. *Applied Nonparametric Regression*. Economic Society Monographs. Cambridge: Cambridge University Press, 1989.
7. Bowman, A.W. and Azzalini, A. *Applied smoothing techniques for data analysis: the Kernel approach with S-Plus illustrations*. Oxford: Clarendon Press, 1997.
8. Godfrey, L.G. Misspecification tests in economics: the

Lagrange Multiplier principle and other approaches. *Econometric Society Monographs No. 16.* Cambridge: Cambridge University Press, 1988.

9. Silverman, B.W. Some aspects of the spline smoothing approach to nonparametric regression curve fitting (with discussion). *Journal of the Royal Statistical Society, Series B* 1995; **47**: 1–52.

10. Browning, M., Deaton, A. and Irish, M. A profitable approach to labour supply and commodity demands over the life-cycle. *Econometrics* 1985; **53**: 503–544.

Classical and Simulation Methods for Panel Data

13

Unobserved Heterogeneity and Censoring in the Demand for Health Care

ANGEL LÓPEZ-NICOLÁS

Departament d'Economia i Empresa, Universitat Pompeu Fabra, Barcelona, Spain

INTRODUCTION

Health care takes one of the largest shares of the public budget in countries such as Spain, where citizens have access to subsidized assistance in both publicly and privately owned centres, enjoy several copayment schedules in the purchase of medicines and are also able to claim a 15% tax deduction for all expenses on health care. Recently, measures such as the exclusion of a substantive range of medicines from the list of products within the copayment schedules have been implemented in order to curb public expenditure. The concern about the distributional effects of this and related potential policy changes on the population has brought the debate on fiscal matters associated with health care to the attention of both academics and decision-makers. In particular, the effects of the tax expenditure associated with the deductions mentioned above are worth analyzing. Who do these deductions benefit? Could they be replaced by some kind of tax expenditure related to demographic structure?

In this paper we provide an empirical account of the consumption of one of the components in the vector of health care inputs of Spanish households: privately purchased medical services. This category of consumption includes all expenditure on visits to practitioners, specialists or surgery related to all types of treatments except dental care. The study of the patterns of consumption for this component of private health care is partly motivated by the fact that these services are available in the public network at no monetary cost. The data shows clearly that only a portion of the population participates in the purchase of these services, and it is conceivable that the benefits of greater promptness of delivery [1] and/or perceived quality are enjoyed by households in the upper part of the income distribution. This raises the question of whether the associated tax deduction is regressive. In parallel, it is interesting to assess how price sensitive this type of demand is, for a withdrawal of the tax expenditures can lead to substantial reductions in usage, part of which might have to be absorbed by the public sector.

In order to shed some light on the questions posed above, we estimate a demand for private medical services equation based on the tradition of Grossman's [2] demand for health model. This model motivates not only the choice of the variables that we use in order to explain the variation in demand but also the incorporation of unobserved heterogeneity in the econometric specification. A second econometric issue arises due to the fact that the category of expenditure that we examine is (i) not universally consumed and (ii) is purchased infrequently. As is well-known, standard estimators for limited dependent variable models such as the tobit are not appropriate in these circumstances.

In the second section we briefly comment upon the economic model on which our empirical analysis will be based and highlight the fact that Grossman's formulation leads naturally to an econometric model with unobserved heterogeneity. In the third section we discuss the data on which we estimate the model and describe the nature of the censuring processes before proposing an estimator related to the family of multivariate models analyzed by Blundell and Meghir [3] that deals simultaneously with the possibility of no participation and the noise induced by infrequent purchases. In this section we also describe the way in which the LDV estimates are used in order to deal with the unobserved heterogeneity problem. The fourth section presents the empirical results and the fifth section concludes.

Econometric Analysis of Health Data. Edited by Andrew M. Jones and Owen O'Donnell
© 2002 John Wiley & Sons Ltd. Previously published in *Health Economics*, Vol. 7; pp. 429–437 (1998). © John Wiley & Sons Ltd

THE DEMAND FOR PRIVATE MEDICAL SERVICES AS A HEALTH CARE INPUT

The demand for private medical services we are about to specify is related to the demand for health care in Grossman's model. Recall that, according to the latter, agents maximize the life-cycle discounted sum of utilities defined over sick time and consumption subject to an asset accumulation constraint and a particular technology in the production of health capital. The first order conditions for the desired stock of health in this intertemporal problem equate the marginal benefits (both pecuniary and non-pecuniary) of health capital to its marginal cost. In order to fulfil this condition over the life-cycle, agents use time and medical care to generate health capital. Under the pure investment version of the model, and assuming a Cobb–Douglas production function for the health stock, an operational [4] representation of the reduced form of the demand for health care equation implied by the model is given by

$$\ln M(t) = \alpha_1 + \alpha_2 \ln w(t) + \alpha_3 \ln P^m + \alpha_4 E + \alpha_5 X$$

$$+ \alpha_6 t + \ln\left[1 + \frac{\tilde{H}(t)}{\delta(t)\mu}\right] \qquad (13.1)$$

where $w(t)$ is the wage rate, P^m is the price of medical services, E is education, t is a time index and X is a vector of conditioning variables picking up environmental conditions. The terms involving the stock of health, H, are (i) its relative change over time $\tilde{H}(t) = \dot{H}(t)/H(t)$, (ii) its rate of depreciation δ and (iii) μ, a partial adjustment parameter reflecting the potential inability of individuals to adjust to their desired health capital stock instantaneously. Although we follow Wagstaff [5] in the introduction of partial adjustment, we retain the log-linearization of the investment schedule originally proposed by Grossman in order to arrive at the demand for health care equation.

Equation 13.1 forms the basis of the econometric model that we estimate in this paper, as private medical services are a component of health care in general. To the extent that the rate of change of the health stock relative to the depreciation rate is not available to the researcher, and more so if no information whatsoever on health state can be used as a proxy, the model above will have to be estimated in the presence of unobserved heterogeneity.

DATA AND ECONOMETRIC SPECIFICATION

THE CENSORING PROBLEM

The data we use is taken from the Spanish Continuous Family Expenditure Survey (CFES). This is a quarterly expenditure survey where a (stratified) random sample of 3200 households is rotated 1/8 every quarter. This allows the construction of panels with information on households covering up to 8 quarters. In particular we use a balanced panel of 6100 households observed during 8 time periods. The time periods range from the first quarter of 1986 to the last of 1987 for the first households that entered the survey and the third quarter of 1992 to the second quarter of 1994 for the most recent entrants in our sample.

Apart from detailed demographic information, the survey contains records on 11 categories of health related expenditures, namely medicines with and without prescription, other pharmaceutical products, therapeutical material with and without subsidy, medical services, dental services, nursing services, hospital services, insurance premia and a residual category. The quality of the information contained in these records varies according to the monitoring period (the length of time over which the household is asked to report expenditures, which in this survey can be either 1 week, 1 month or 1 quarter). In some cases, such as prescribed medicines, it is just 1 week and we find that 70% of households are not observed spending on this category in any of the 8 periods. To some extent this is due to the fact that the copayment for prescriptions is zero for a substantial part of the population. But the problem of infrequent purchases is pervasive: even if all households have to face the full cost of self prescriptions, only 43% report a positive expenditure over any other 8 periods. Further, more than half of these (23% of the total) have one positive record only.

The situation improves when the monitoring period is 1 month, as is the case with our object of study. In Table 13.1 we present the pattern of observed positive expenditures on private medical services and the mean and median of the purchases by number of observed purchases. The table shows that 42.7% of the 6100 households are never observed purchasing this category of health care. The rest of households are observed incurring positive purchases at least once and roughly one-third of the total are observed purchasing more than once. The median expenditure is 15 000 pta per quarter and the mean level is around 25 000 pta per quarter.

For the rest of the categories the percentage of households who never report a positive expenditure are 68% (dental services), 91% (nursing services), 98% (hospital services), 96% (therapeutical material with subsidy), 57% (therapeutical material without subsidy), 79% (insurance premia) and 99% (residual category).

The econometrics literature distinguishes three main causes for the existence of zero records in micro-expenditure surveys, namely no participation in the consumption

Table 13.1 Pattern of observed positive expenditures on medical services in estimating sample

Proportion of households reporting positive records in # quarters ($N = 6100$) (%)	# quarters	Median expenditure (pta per quarter)	Mean expenditure (pta per quarter)
42.7	0	—	—
23.78	1	15 000	27 163
15.41	2	15 000	23 809
8.30	3	15 000	24 052
5.51	4	15 000	23 299
3	5	15 000	24 659
0.7	6	15 000	20 647
0.44	7	15 000	27 322
0.16	8	15 000	34 408
57.3	Any quarter	15 000	24 792

of the relevant commodity, corner solutions and infrequent purchases. In many applications it is reasonable to assume from the outset which cause operates. For instance, in studies on the demand for clothing it would be reasonable to assume infrequency of purchase to be the main explanation. Similarly, in the case of the demand for tobacco, abstention (no participation) will explain a substantial proportion of zero records [6,7]. For some goods, however, there is no clear cut cause and, in a cross-section of households, more than one or even the three causes might induce the existence of zero records. The case of expenditures on health care are a paradigmatic example of this type of situation. Even if it can reasonably be argued that all households participate in the consumption of some form of health care (i.e. there are no nonparticipants in the sense applicable to tobacco consumption or labour force participation), the existence of different types of copayment policies, substitutes at zero money cost and the difference between monitoring periods and the period for which information in the survey is supposed to be representative, leads to the existence of a high percentage of zero records when disaggregated categories are examined.

In the particular case of household expenditure on private medical services in Spain, the existence of a free substitute will clearly induce some households to never consume this type of service. This free substitute is the coverage given by the social security contributions, which is provided either through publicly owned outlets – the case for most households – or the private sector – the case for some of the households who are entitled to choose which provider their contributions are directed to (civil servants). Similarly, households who buy private insurance on top of the compulsory scheme will rarely be observed paying for this service unless there exists a copayment contract. Concerning the latter group, only 20% of the households who ever purchase private medi-

cal services are observed ever paying for an insurance premium. However, the survey pools together policies that cover medical assistance with those that provide compensation from death so it is not possible to know whether the latter group of households are really covered for medical assistance. In any case the presumption that a portion of the population does not participate in the consumption of this category is consistent with the evidence shown in Table 13.1, which suggests that there are some households who never purchase private medical services and can be classified as non participants, and, moreover, we are able to identify them. The data also suggest that those who participate in the consumption of this commodity do not do so every month. For these households, a pattern of alternating positive and zero records is observed. This structure for the data generating process implies that, first, a household decides whether to participate in the consumption of this service and then, if the decision is to do so, how often to make the purchases. Finally, the amount of service purchased is decided. In this sense the corresponding econometric model is trivariate: it contains a process for participation, a process for the frequency of purchase and a process for the amount of purchases.

Let us start with the first of the processes, which we assume is ruled by a latent index such as in the standard probit model (individual subscripts are omitted for notational simplicity).

$$H^* = \alpha r + \eta$$
$$H = l(H^* > 0)$$
$$\eta \approx N(0, 1) \tag{13.2}$$

where l is the indicator function.

Focusing now on participating households let $y^* = \exp(\beta x + e)$, where e is a random error, denote latent consumption of private medical services and y its observational expenditure counterpart. Following Blundell and Meghir [3] in assuming that $E(y^*) = E(y)$ and expanding the last expectation, we obtain

$$E(y \mid D = 1)P(D = 1) = E(y^*) \qquad (13.3)$$

where we assume that

$$D^* = \theta z + w$$
$$D = l(D^* > 0)$$
$$w \approx N(0, 1) \qquad (13.4)$$

is a probit type process determining whether a purchase is made during the monitoring period. The relationship between latent consumption and observed expenditure is then given by

$$y = (y^*/P(D = 1))\exp(v)$$
$$v \approx N(0, \sigma_v^2) \qquad (13.5)$$

and taking logarithms

$$\log y = \log y^* - \log P(D = 1) + v$$
$$= \beta x - \log \Phi(\theta z) + u$$
$$u = e + v$$
$$u \approx N(0, \sigma_u^2) \qquad (13.6)$$

Even though the model is trivariate, only two 'hurdles' have to be passed in order to observe a positive expenditure: the participation one and the purchase one. The model does not accommodate standard corner solutions. That is, conditional on being a participant, y^* cannot be zero. This is a model of 'first hurdle dominance' in the terminology of Jones [6]. Given that we allow for a separate participation process, it makes sense to treat zeros in the observed counterpart of consumption as a result of the semidurable nature of this category of consumption only. The use of a logarithmic specification for the consumption equation (which is justified by the skewness of observed expenditures) also rules out values of zero of y^*.

Under independence of the three stochastic errors η, w and u, the sample log likelihood for this data generating process is given by

$$\log L = \sum_{y=0} \log(1 - \Phi(\theta z)\Phi(\alpha r)) + \sum_{y>0} - \log \sigma_u$$
$$+ \log \phi((\log y + \log \Phi(\theta z) - \beta x)/\sigma_u)$$

$$+ \log \Phi(\theta z) + \log \Phi(\alpha r) \qquad (13.7)$$

As discussed above, an important feature of the panel format of the data is that it provides sample separation information: we have identified which households do participate in the consumption of private medical services. Under the assumption of independence this implies that the model can be estimated as a separate probit for participation on the whole sample and an infrequency of purchase model for the subsample of participants [6]. The likelihood function for the latter is easily obtained from Equation 13.7:

$$\log L = \sum_{\substack{y=0 \\ H=1}} \log(1 - \Phi(\theta z)) + \sum_{\substack{y>0 \\ H=1}} - \log \sigma_u$$
$$+ \log \phi((\log y + \log \Phi(\theta z) - \beta x)/\sigma_u)$$
$$+ \log \Phi(\theta z) \qquad (13.8)$$

INDIVIDUAL EFFECTS

From the discussion in the second and third sections, we can conclude that the econometric representation of Equation 13.1 belongs to the general class of models given by

$$\log y_{it}^* = \beta' X_{it} + \gamma_{it} + \varepsilon_{it} \qquad (13.9)$$

where γ_{it} is an unobserved individual effect, y^* is not directly observable and ε_{it} is a purely random error term. Given that the time span during which all households stay in the survey is 2 years, we may treat the individual effect as a fixed unobserved heterogeneity term and drop the time subscript. In previous studies of demand for health care based on Grossman's model, this term has been assumed to be either zero, invariant across individuals or randomly distributed. The latter is the least restrictive of these assumptions and if we interpret this term as an individual effect uncorrelated with the rest of regressors, only problems of efficiency will arise when using a cross-section to retrieve the parameters of interest. However, in the context of a demand for health care model, there are intuitive grounds to expect that these individual effects are correlated with some of the regressors, especially age, education and the environmental variables (in fact, the recognition of the potential correlation of the rate of depreciation and the speed of adjustment with demographic characteristics led Wagstaff [4] to carry out separate analyses for different age groups). In these circumstances, standard cross-sectional estimation techniques will yield biased parameters.

Our aim is to obtain consistent estimates in the presence of both the type of censoring described above and the potential correlation of the individual effects with the regressors. In order to do so we resort to a variation of Chamberlain's [8] Minimum Distance method proposed by Arellano and Bover [9] and applied, in the context of dynamic demand equations, by Labeaga [10]. In particular, Chamberlain explicitly models the relation between individual effects and regressors in the following way:

$$E(\gamma_i \mid X_i, R_i) = \gamma^0 + \gamma_1' X_{i1} + \gamma_2' X_{i2} + \cdots + \gamma_T' X_{iT} + \gamma_R' R_i \tag{13.10}$$

that is, individual effects are a function of lead and lags of all explanatory variables (the vector X) and interactions of the latter with demographics, and nonlinear terms, the vector R.

Our model can then be written as

$$E(\log y_i^* \mid W_i) = \psi' W_i \tag{13.11}$$

where W contains X and R. This is used to obtain a prediction for $\log y_i^*$ in each one of the T periods making up the panel by means of the limited dependent variable estimator discussed in the section on the censoring problem. Once such predictions have been obtained, we can recover the parameters of interest by applying the within-groups estimator to the following equation:

$$\widehat{\log y_{it}^*} = \beta x_{it} + \gamma_i + \tau_{it} \tag{13.12}$$

where $\widehat{\log y_{it}^*}$ is the predicted value of $\log y_{it}^*$ and τ is a purely random term. This estimator is consistent, but less efficient than the minimum distance method originally proposed by Chamberlain.

EMPIRICAL RESULTS

ECONOMETRIC ESTIMATES

In Table 13.2 we present the estimates for the model. The first three columns show the maximum likelihood estimates of: the probability of participation (I), the frequency of purchase process (II) and the consumption equation (III). These estimates are corrected for the censoring problem but not the unobserved heterogeneity problem. Column (IV) presents the estimates for the consumption equation using the within groups estimator with censoring for the full panel. Finally column (V) shows the OLS estimates of the consumption equation for comparison purposes. The results for participation in column (I) are obtained from a probit on the cross section

of 6100 households at their first interview, whereas the results in columns (II) and (III) are obtained from the maximum likelihood estimator (whose likelihood function is given in Equation 13.8) on the subsample of 3494 participating households at first interview. The results in column (IV) are obtained from the full panel of 27 952 participating households and those in (V) from the pool of all households over the eight periods. For the within-group censored panel estimator, we have maximized the likelihood function in Equation 13.8 on each of the 8 waves of the panel including all leads and lags, interactions and power terms (up to the cube) of the regressors in both the frequency of purchase process and the consumption process in a first step. This produces a prediction for $\log y^*$ according to Equation 13.11 for each household, which is then used as the dependent variable in Equation 13.12. The table includes statistics for the null hypothesis of no fit and the relevant measures of goodness of fit.

The specification for participation (column I) includes variables that proxy situations which pose a threat to health such as the risks involved in child bearing and neonatal related diseases and the existence of smokers in the household. Both of these significantly increase the probability of participation with respect to the reference household. A higher level of current household income affects positively the probability of participation for two reasons: higher ability to pay and a higher opportunity cost for the waiting time due to foregone earnings. Employment, in whichever form but more so for white collar workers, increases the probability of participation with respect to the reference households where the head is not active or unemployed. Owner occupiers were expected to be more likely to participate due to the correlation of this characteristic with lifetime wealth and thus ability to pay and the results shows a significant (at the 10% level) positive impact. The observation of a payment for insurance premia is not associated with any significant effect on the probability of participation. As mentioned before, the premia payments that we observe in the survey include life insurance policies and consequently are an imperfect indicator for the existence of coverage for private medical services.

Concerning the process for frequency of purchases (in column II), we have included the size of the household as a proxy for the frequency with which the need to purchase the service arises. The corresponding estimate suggests a positive and significant impact. The presence of babies of less than 1 year of age or a pregnant woman also seem to affect positively the frequency of purchases. Household income (excluding income from capital), the availability of private transport, and the participation of the spouse in the labour market have been included in the specification for the frequency of purchase in order to proxy the oppor-

Table 13.2   Model estimates

	I ML	II ML	III ML	IV WGC	V OLS
Household size		0.043	0.102	0.081	0.090
		(2.73)	(3.51)	(22.57)	(13.92)
Baby or pregnancy*	0.167	0.167	−0.234	−0.064	0.133
	(2.07)	(2.45)	(−1.17)	(−7.82)	(3.34)
Smoking members*	0.121				
	(3.33)				
Head of household has secondary education*	−0.015		0.103	0.195	−0.020
	(−0.37)		(1.82)	(25.36)	(−0.86)
Head of household has university education*	0.117		0.168	0.224	0.139
	(1.89)		(1.36)	(15.59)	(3.91)
Log total household real income	0.118	−0.031	−0.472	0.018	−0.115
	(4.85)	(−0.94)	(−3.68)	(3.04)	(−3.25)
Log total household real income squared			0.048	0.019	0.021
			(4.34)	(30.19)	(6.90)
Log real price of private medical services			1.152	−0.414	0.408
			(2.26)	(−9.21)	(3.17)
Age of head of household	−0.004	−0.003	0.002	0.005	−0.003
	(−2.26)	(−1.61)	(0.65)	(9.32)	(−4.00)
Quarter 1*		0.085	0.083	0.019	0.026
		(1.34)	(0.68)	(6.47)	(0.99)
Quarter 2*		0.087	0.088	0.146	0.096
		(1.37)	(0.72)	(49.15)	(3.67)
Quarter 4*		0.080	0.162	0.062	0.051
		(1.24)	(1.29)	(21.28)	(1.94)
Spouse in employment*		0.056			
		(1.24)			
Car available*		0.027			
		(0.52)			
Head of household is self-employed*	0.191				
	(3.40)				
Head of household is blue collar worker*	0.180				
	(2.79)				
Head of household is white collar worker*	0.247				
	(4.66)				
Owner occupier household*	0.076				
	(1.18)				
Under coverage of private insurance*	0.054				
	(1.32)				
Constant	−0.850	−0.405	4.290	1.979	0.307
	(−4.01)	(−1.31)	(6.41)	(50.84)	(2.26)
N	6100	3494	3494	27 952	48 800
Chi squared (df in parenthesis)	233 (11)	7165 (21)	7165 (21)		
F (111, ∞)				17.90	8.20
Pseudo R^2/R^2	0.02	0.49	0.49	0.23	0.07

*Variables are binary (dummy) indicators.

tunity cost (foregone earnings and/or leisure) of visits, but neither seems to exert a significant effect.

Turning to the consumption equation, note that while OLS estimates suggest that every decade there is a decrease in consumption of 3% and the ML estimator suggest an insignificant effect, the censored panel estimator (column IV) suggests a significant increase of 5%

every decade. Once the effect of participation is netted out, both the ML and the censored panel estimator (the latter in a significant way) show a negative effect associated with the presence of babies or pregnancy on the consumption schedule. It is interesting to note that while the two latter factors affect participation positively, they reduce consumption conditional to participation. This might be caused by the income effect associated with a larger family size. Both categories of education are associated with a greater (and by a sizeable percentage) consumption with respect to households headed by an individual with basic schooling. Note also that both the ML and OLS estimators show a U profile for the effect of household income on consumption. However the profile shown in column IV always has a positive slope, and moreover, this slope is increasing with the level of (log) income. Thus the associated elasticity of expenditure with respect to income increases with the latter. The estimated value at the mean of income is 0.34, which reveals the necessity (conditional upon participation) nature of the service under consideration.

Concerning the estimated price elasticity, note that since our dependent variable is expenditure, it is obtained by subtracting one to the coefficient on the logarithm of prices. The censored panel estimate is -1.41. The price sensitivity that this estimator suggests is very much greater than the one associated with the OLS estimator (-0.6).

It seems clear, therefore, that ignoring the censoring processes and unobserved heterogeneity can lead to substantially different results, apart from ignoring relevant information such as the separate effects on participation and rate of consumption that some factors may have.

IMPLICATIONS FOR HEALTH AND FISCAL POLICIES

The results suggest that the probability of participation in the consumption of private medical care is positively associated with two relevant characteristics from the point of view of fiscal policy, namely wealth (proxied by income, occupational category and home ownership status) and fertility (pregnancy and presence of small children). Conditional on participation, income exerts a positive effect on the rate of consumption too. It would seem, therefore, that the tax deduction associated with the consumption of private medical care is regressive, at least in the sense that the absolute amounts deducted are greater for richer households. Withdrawing or reducing these deductions would penalize households within fertility periods. But the existing deductions for children could be increased to compensate this effect.

As far as second round effects (behavioural responses) are concerned, the estimated elasticity of -1.41 suggests that increases in prices would lead to more than proportional changes in demand for private medical services. A withdrawal or reduction of the deduction is very much equivalent to an increase in prices (even if its effect is not perceived until tax forms are filled), so it would be reason-

able to expect a substantial reduction in demand for private medical services should the government eliminate it completely. Whether a parallel increase in demand at public outlets would ensue is something that our estimated model cannot produce inferences about. The crucial issue here is the extent to which Spanish households perceive private medical services as a close substitute for their public counterparts, and this is an issue which merits further research.

The ability of these results to provide insights into the likely consequences of revisions in the copayment policies of other categories of health care currently provided by the Spanish public health network is also limited. However, in connection with the recent government plans for the withdrawal of the subsidy for a substantial number of medicines, a policy relevant message might be extracted: participation in the consumption of private health care is associated with ability to pay. Thus the maintenance of close substitutes within the subsidized list would cushion the effects of the policy change on households at the bottom of the income distribution.

CONCLUSION

In this paper we have estimated a demand for private medical services equation based in the tradition of Grossman's model of demand for health using data for a panel of Spanish households. We have paid particular attention to the censored nature of the data and the existence of unobserved heterogeneity and our results suggest that ignoring these issues has a significant impact on the size, sign and significance of the parameters of the model. The estimated demand equation offers useful policy evidence on the likely effects of altering expenditure deduction schemes currently applicable in the Spanish tax system.

ACKNOWLEDGEMENTS

I am grateful to Jose Maria Labeaga, Jaume Puig and the participants in the Fifth European Workshop on Econometrics and Health Economics for useful comments. The final version has benefited from the comments of the editor of this journal and two anonymous referees. Financial support from Merck through the Centre de Recerca d'Economia i Salut is gratefully acknowledged. The usual disclaimer applies.

REFERENCES

1. Jofre, M. *Health care interaction between public system and*

private sector. Doctoral Dissertation. Universitat Pompeu Fabra, Department of Economics and Business, 1998.

2. Grossman, M. On the concept of health capital and the demand for health. *Journal of Political Economy* 1972; **80**: 223–255.

3. Blundell, R.W. and Meghir, C. Bivariate alternatives to the tobit model. *Journal of Econometrics* 1987; **34**: 179–200.

4. Wagstaff, A. The demand for health: some new empirical evidence. *Journal of Health Economics* 1986; **5**: 195–233.

5. Wagstaff, A. The demand for health: an empirical reformulation of the Grossman model. *Health Economics* 1993; **2**: 189–198.

6. Jones, A. A double hurdle model of cigarette consumption. *Journal of Applied Econometrics* 1989; **4**: 23–39.

7. Garcia, J. and Labeaga, J.M. Alternative approaches to modelling zero expenditure: an application to Spanish demand for tobacco. *Oxford Bulletin of Economics and Statistics* 1996; **58**: 489–506.

8. Chamberlain, G. Panel data. In: Griliches, Z. and Intriligator, M. (eds) *Handbook of Econometrics*. Amsterdam: North Holland, 1984; **2**: 1247–1318.

9. Arellano, M. and Bover, O. La econometria de datos de panel. *Investigaciones Económicas* 1990; **14**: 3–45.

10. Labeaga, J.M. A dynamic panel data model with limited dependent variables: an application to the demand for tobacco. DT 9201; Departamento de Análisis Económico, Universidad Nacional de Educación a Distancia, Madrid 1996.

14

A Discrete Random Effects Probit Model with Application to the Demand for Preventive Care

PARTHA DEB

Department of Economics, Indiana University-Purdue University Indianapolis, IN, USA

INTRODUCTION

Random effects models in which individuals who belong to a given group share a common intercept have become increasingly popular in applied research. In the case of linear regression, estimation and inference in such models are conducted using the well-established framework for panel data models. In situations involving non-linear models (e.g. for discrete, count and duration data) there is no standard methodology.

The standard random effects probit (REP) model assumes that the random intercept is normally distributed. In the maximum likelihood estimation of this model, numerical integration [1] or stochastic integration [2] methods are typically used to integrate over the distribution of the random intercept in order to calculate the value of the objective function. A two-step method [3] is also available. In this paper, I have developed an alternative REP model in which the true density of the random intercept is approximated by a discrete density. The discrete REP model is appealing for two main reasons. First, it eliminates the need for numerical or stochastic integration, both of which are computationally complex and time consuming. Only summation over the discrete points of support is required. Second, if the random intercept is not normally distributed, the standard model is misspecified. The discrete REP model, which is a special case of finite mixture models, is semiparametric. Under suitable regularity conditions, the discrete density of the random intercept can serve as an approximation to any probability density [4,5].

Although the discrete representation of the density of the random group effect is conservatively framed as an approximation to the underlying continuous density, the discrete formulation itself may be a natural and intuitively attractive representation of heterogeneity. In this representation, groups are drawn from a finite number of latent classes or 'types'. The vast majority of studies using finite mixture models find that two to four latent classes adequately describe the data. A similar finding for the REP model would make this interpretation especially attractive. Moreover, in standard REP analysis, the strength of the group effect is typically summarized by the variance of the distribution of the group effect. Specific group effects are not identified unless a fully Bayesian analysis of the REP is undertaken. In the discrete approach, one can classify each group as a particular type using Bayesian posterior analysis after classical maximum likelihood estimation. Once classified, types may be related to group characteristics.

In this paper, the discrete REP is used to analyse the effects of family characteristics on the demand for preventive care. Because preventive care involves planned visits to a medical facility, characteristics other than health status are more important in determining such demand than medical care demand in illness events. Moreover, family characteristics are likely to play an important role in determining whether or not preventive care is taken. Although some observable family characteristics are controlled for as covariates in typical studies, other important sources of family-level effects are excluded. Random effects models provide an opportunity to test for the existence and strength of such excluded family-level effects after controlling for observable ones.

Econometric Analysis of Health Data. Edited by Andrew M. Jones and Owen O'Donnell

In recent studies of preventive care, Gordon *et al.* [6] and Potosky *et al.* [7] examine the determinants of cancer screening tests. Saag *et al.* [8] examines tertiary prevention in the Medicare population with at least one chronic disease for which specific tertiary prevention measures have been shown to reduce or eliminate disease progression or illness-related dysfunction. In each of these studies, covariates are measured at the individual level; no attempt is made to ascertain whether family characteristics matter. I examine the determinants of blood pressure checks, cholesterol checks, influenza shots and physical examinations with explicit attention to observed family-level covariates and unobserved family-level random effects. The data are obtained from the 1996 Medical Expenditure Panel Survey (MEPS) [9], which provides national representative estimates of health care utilization, expenditures, sources of payment and insurance coverage for the US non-institutionalized population.

Random effects models for discrete data with discretely distributed random intercepts have been recently applied in other areas of research. Pudney *et al.* [10] estimate a discrete random effects logit model in an analysis of farm tenures. Jain *et al.* [11] and Kim *et al.* [12] estimate discrete random effects multinomial logit models to assess features of consumer brand preferences. To the best of my knowledge, there is no published application of a discrete random effects model in health economics. There are numerous potential applications of such models in health economics, however, in contexts where individual decisions are made within families, where individual decisions are made within hospitals, etc.

The discrete REP model is developed in the following section. Although there are a few applications of similar discrete random effects models, their finite sample properties have not been examined in controlled conditions. Therefore, I conduct Monte Carlo experiments to examine the ability of the discrete REP model to provide unbiased estimates when the true source of the unobserved heterogeneity is continuously distributed. These are described in the third section, entitled 'Monte Carlo Experiments'. The empirical analysis of the determinants of preventive care is described in the fourth section, entitled 'Empirical Example'. I conclude in the final section.

THE MODEL

Consider the following latent variable specification of a REP model in which the random effect results from a group-specific error term, i.e.

$$y_{ij}^* = x_{ij}\beta + z_j\gamma + u_j + \varepsilon_{ij} \qquad (14.1)$$

for groups $j = 1, 2, \ldots, J$ and individuals $i = 1, 2, \ldots, N_j$ in

each group for a total of $\Sigma_j N_j = N$ observations. x_{ij} is a vector of individual-specific covariates and z_j is a vector of group-specific covariates. The random effect u_j is assumed to be uncorrelated with x_{ij} and z_j. The ε_{ij} are i.i.d. normal errors and are orthogonal to the group specific errors u_j. As is standard in probit models, I assume that ε_{ij} is drawn from a normal density with unit variance without loss of generality. The sign of the latent variable determines the observed binary outcome variable, i.e. $y_{ij} = 1$ if $y_{ij}^* > 0$; $y_{ij} = 0$ otherwise.

Let f be the density of u. In the standard REP model, f is a normal density. For notational convenience, let $d_{ij} = 2y_{ij} - 1$, i.e. d_{ij} is an indicator variable that takes the value 1 when $y_{ij} = 1$ and -1 when $y_{ij} = 0$. The contribution of the jth group to the log likelihood is given by

$$l_j = \ln\left\{\int_{-\infty}^{\infty}\prod_{i=1}^{N_j}\Phi[d_{ij}(x_{ij}\beta + z_j\gamma + u_j)]f(u_j)\,du\right\} \qquad (14.2)$$

where $\Phi(.)$ denotes the standard normal cumulative density function. Integration over u_j marginalizes the likelihood function with respect to the random group effect. The sample log likelihood is given by

$$l = \sum_{j=1}^{J} l_j \qquad (14.3)$$

In the standard REP, as with many other reasonable choices for f, the integral given in Equation 14.2 does not have a closed form solution. Butler and Moffitt [1] show that this integral can be effectively evaluated using a Gauss–Hermite quadrature; this is the most commonly used procedure. Other numerical integration procedures are also feasible. The integral may also be approximated by stochastic simulation using random draws from $f(u)$ as the underlying basis. Gouriéroux and Monfort [13] show that consistent estimates of model parameters can be obtained by maximizing such a simulated approximation of the log likelihood function.

DISCRETE REP MODEL

In the discrete REP model, $f(u)$ is assumed to be a discrete density. Specifically, u has S points of support with values $u_1, u_2, \ldots, u_S$ and associated probabilities $\pi_1, \pi_2, \ldots, \pi_S$, respectively. Then the contribution of the jth group to the log likelihood is given by

$$l_j = \ln\left\{\sum_{s=1}^{S}\pi_s\prod_{i=1}^{N_j}\Phi[d_{ij}(x_{ij}\beta + z_j\gamma + u_s)]\right\} \qquad (14.4)$$

where $0 < \pi_1, \pi_2, \ldots, \pi_S < 1$ and $\Sigma_{s=1}^{S}\pi_s = 1$. If there is an intercept in the model, i.e. if x_{ij} includes a vector of ones, the mean of u is not identified without a normalization. I chose one point of support u_S such that the mean of u is zero, so

$$u_S = -\frac{1}{\pi_S} \sum_{s=1}^{S-1} \pi_s u_s. \tag{14.5}$$

Note that this normalization gives the typical zero-mean property of errors, but identification may be achieved in other ways.

Post-estimation, one can calculate the variance of the distribution of the group-specific effect as $\mathrm{Var}(u) = \sum_{s=1}^{S} \pi_s u_s^2$. But if one takes the latent class interpretation of the random intercept, each point of support and associated probability describes a latent class. The posterior probability that a particular group, j, belongs to a particular class, c, can be calculated as

$$\Pr[j \in \text{class } c \,|\, x_{ij}, y_{ij}]$$

$$= \frac{\pi_c \prod_{i=1}^{N_j} \Phi[d_{ij}(x_{ij}\beta + z_j\gamma + u_c)]}{\sum_{s=1}^{S} \pi_s \prod_{i=1}^{N_j} \Phi[d_{ij}(x_{ij}\beta + z_j\gamma + u_s)]};$$

$$c = 1, 2, \ldots, S \tag{14.6}$$

These posterior probabilities may be used to classify each group into a latent class in order to study the properties of the classes further (see Deb and Trivedi [14] for an example). Note that, although the random effect itself is uncorrelated with the covariates, the posterior probability of class membership is, in general, a function of the values of the covariates.

The estimation of finite mixture models and REP models raise a number of difficult computational issues. One issue involves the possible existence of multiple local maxima in finite mixture models. The second issue involves computer precision of products of cumulative normals, a necessary calculation in maximum likelihood estimation of random effects probit models. Since parameter estimates of discrete REP models may be sensitive to these issues, strategies to minimize any detrimental effects are discussed in the Appendix.

MONTE CARLO EXPERIMENTS

In this section, I describe Monte Carlo experiments that examine the ability of the discrete REP model to provide unbiased estimates of the model parameters and variance of the random intercept when, in fact, the true source of

the unobserved heterogenity is continuously distributed. In other words, the experiments evaluate the extent to which the discrete REP model with a small number of points of support is able to mimic the underlying continuous distribution of the random intercept.

DESIGN

Consider, once again, the latent variable specification of a REP model,

$$y_{ij}^* = \alpha + x_{ij}\beta + z_j\gamma + u_j + \varepsilon_{ij} \tag{14.7}$$

for groups $j = 1, 2, \ldots, J$ and individuals $i = 1, 2, \ldots, N_j$ in each group, for a total of $\sum_j N_j = N$ observations. I evaluate performance for small ($N_j = 10$) and large ($N_j = 100$) group sizes with $J = 500$ and $J = 50$ respectively. The overall sample size is held fixed ($N = 5000$), rather than the number of groups, because such group size/number trade-offs are typical in data available to empirical researchers. Moreover, I limit the experiments to balanced panel designs for simplicity. Although unbalanced panels are common in practice, the results of these experiments should directly apply to unbalanced panels.

In the data generating process (d.g.p.), both x_{ij} and z_j are drawn from $N(0, \sigma_x^2)$ although z_j takes the same value for each observation within a group. The ε_{ij} are drawn from $N(0, 1)$ and u_j from $f(0, \sigma_u^2)$. In the first set of experiments, f is a normal density; in the second f is a chi-squared density with four degrees of freedom (shifted to have a zero mean). The main model parameters are fixed at $\alpha = 0$, $\beta = 1$, and $\gamma = 1$ throughout the experiment. The ratio of the variance of the group-level random effect, u_j, to the variance of the idiosyncratic noise, ε_{ij}, takes two values (0.4 and 0.8). The signal-to-noise ratio, defined as the ratio of the variances of the observed and unobserved components in Equation 14.7, also takes two values (1 and 2). The values of σ_u^2 and σ_x^2 are chosen accordingly. The parameters of the data generating process for each group size and error density are summarized in Table 14.1. For each design point, 400 replications are used to

Table 14.1 Monte Carlo experiments: data generating processes (d.g.p.)

d.g.p.	α	β	γ	σ_u^2	σ_x^2	S/N
1	0	1	1	0.4	0.7	1
2	0	1	1	0.4	1.4	2
3	0	1	1	0.8	0.9	1
4	0	1	1	0.8	1.8	2

The signal-to-noise (S/N) ratio is calculated as $\mathrm{S/N} = 2\sigma_x^2/(\sigma_u^2 + \sigma_\varepsilon^2)$.

Table 14.2   Monte Carlo experiments: normally distributed random intercept

d.g.p.	$J = 500, N_j = 10$				$J = 50, N_j = 100$			
	α	β	γ	σ_u^2	α	β	γ	σ_u^2
Density with three points of support								
1	−0.001	0.996	0.992	0.385	−0.003	0.979	0.920	0.335
	(0.036)	(0.035)	(0.048)	(0.043)	(0.090)	(0.033)	(0.160)	(0.071)
2	−0.001	0.998	0.995	0.388	−0.004	0.981	0.943	0.341
	(0.038)	(0.031)	(0.042)	(0.048)	(0.090)	(0.030)	(0.130)	(0.074)
3	−0.001	0.984	0.956	0.708	−0.004	0.960	0.858	0.618
	(0.046)	(0.034)	(0.060)	(0.062)	(0.124)	(0.033)	(0.192)	(0.124)
4	−0.001	0.983	0.969	0.722	−0.005	0.960	0.892	0.631
	(0.050)	(0.031)	(0.048)	(0.072)	(0.123)	(0.030)	(0.149)	(0.132)
Density with four points of support								
1	−0.001	1.000	1.001	0.415	−0.006	0.900	0.934	0.411
	(0.037)	(0.035)	(0.047)	(0.083)	(0.091)	(0.034)	(0.163)	(0.285)
2	−0.001	1.002	1.002	0.408	−0.005	0.992	0.949	0.426
	(0.039)	(0.032)	(0.042)	(0.060)	(0.091)	(0.031)	(0.133)	(0.318)
3	0.000	0.998	0.994	0.791	−0.005	0.980	0.903	0.713
	(0.048)	(0.035)	(0.059)	(0.099)	(0.124)	(0.033)	(0.178)	(0.147)
4	−0.001	0.997	0.996	0.792	−0.007	0.982	0.929	0.752
	(0.051)	(0.032)	(0.049)	(0.095)	(0.125)	(0.030)	(0.152)	(0.375)
Density with five points of support								
1	−0.003	1.000	1.002	0.442	−0.009	0.996	0.972	0.537
	(0.038)	(0.036)	(0.048)	(0.265)	(0.090)	(0.034)	(0.153)	(0.614)
2	−0.001	1.002	1.002	0.415	−0.008	0.998	0.977	0.525
	(0.039)	(0.032)	(0.042)	(0.177)	(0.090)	(0.030)	(0.112)	(0.576)
3	−0.001	1.001	1.003	0.870	−0.010	0.991	0.936	0.814
	(0.051)	(0.035)	(0.058)	(0.407)	(0.127)	(0.034)	(0.163)	(0.474)
4	−0.001	1.001	1.002	0.831	−0.008	0.993	0.967	0.843
	(0.052)	(0.032)	(0.048)	(0.270)	(0.127)	(0.031)	(0.130)	(0.526)

evaluate the finite sample properties of the discrete REP estimator.

RESULTS

Results for the normal density are reported in Table 14.2 and results for the chi-squared density are reported in Table 14.3. The results for 500 groups with 10 observations per group are displayed in columns 2–5 of Table 14.2. They show that the parameter estimates of the individual and group-level variables are unbiased throughout. The implied values of the variance of the random effect, σ_u^2, are also unbiased when four or five points of support are used but they appear to be underestimated (although not in a statistically significant way) when three points of support are used. More striking is the fact that the precision of the estimated random effect variance decreases three- to fourfold when five points of support are used for the density of the random effect. It appears that three to four points of support may be sufficient to capture the key characteristics of the underlying normally

distributed random intercept. Models with five points of support may be under-identified in some cases. When the data consist of only 50 large groups with 100 observations per group, displayed in columns 6–9 of Table 14.2, the precision of the estimates of the parameter associated with the group-level covariate decreases considerably. Although the main parameter estimates are not significantly biased, the implied values of the variance of the random effect are too small when three points of support are used in the discrete density. The variance estimates improve when four or five points of support are used but, once again, the estimates from models with five points of support have greater dispersion.

Overall, three to four points of support in the discrete density adequately capture the salient features of the underlying normal density in both cases. As expected, precision of the group-level parameters falls when there are fewer groups in the data. In the case of 50 groups, discrete densities with five points of support seem to be useful more often. If within group sample sizes were held constant, this finding would be counterintuitive. But they

Table 14.3   Monte Carlo Experiments: $\chi^2(4)$ distributed random intercept

d.g.p.	$G = 500, N_g = 10$				$G = 50, N_g = 100$			
	α	β	γ	σ_u^2	α	β	γ	σ_u^2
Density with three points of support								
1	0.000	0.001	0.995	0.393	0.007	0.983	0.949	0.347
	(0.037)	(0.035)	(0.046)	(0.099)	(0.095)	(0.032)	(0.118)	(0.170)
2	−0.000	0.998	0.995	0.393	0.010	0.983	0.960	0.362
	(0.038)	(0.031)	(0.038)	(0.074)	(0.098)	(0.029)	(0.090)	(0.234)
3	−0.004	0.991	0.976	0.710	−0.009	0.961	0.873	0.572
	(0.049)	(0.034)	(0.052)	(0.169)	(0.040)	(0.011)	(0.054)	(0.052)
4	−0.003	0.988	0.979	0.725	0.005	0.967	0.922	0.631
	(0.048)	(0.032)	(0.044)	(0.097)	(0.130)	(0.030)	(0.117)	(0.182)
Density with four points of support								
1	0.005	1.006	1.006	0.452	0.019	0.994	0.963	0.434
	(0.040)	(0.035)	(0.047)	(0.165)	(0.099)	(0.031)	(0.120)	(0.269)
2	0.002	1.004	1.004	0.433	0.017	0.996	0.974	0.425
	(0.038)	(0.032)	(0.040)	(0.104)	(0.100)	(0.030)	(0.090)	(0.245)
3	0.008	1.002	1.000	0.879	0.026	0.985	0.924	0.821
	(0.056)	(0.035)	(0.051)	(0.308)	(0.136)	(0.031)	(0.135)	(0.356)
4	0.003	1.002	1.001	0.843	0.029	0.981	0.944	0.798
	(0.050)	(0.032)	(0.043)	(0.206)	(0.131)	(0.029)	(0.111)	(0.297)
Density with five points of support								
1	0.007	1.006	1.006	0.465	0.017	1.001	0.984	0.454
	(0.041)	(0.035)	(0.046)	(0.232)	(0.101)	(0.032)	(0.129)	(0.209)
2	0.003	1.005	1.004	0.434	0.017	1.000	0.988	0.456
	(0.038)	(0.032)	(0.040)	(0.107)	(0.102)	(0.031)	(0.093)	(0.275)
3	0.008	1.002	1.000	0.879	0.026	0.996	0.950	0.885
	(0.056)	(0.035)	(0.051)	(0.308)	(0.137)	(0.031)	(0.143)	(0.419)
4	0.005	1.005	1.007	0.880	0.024	0.995	0.959	0.871
	(0.050)	(0.033)	(0.045)	(0.325)	(0.139)	(0.029)	(0.105)	(0.392)

are not; instead the experiments with $J = 50$ have many more observations per group. This increases the relative importance, in the likelihood function, of groups located in the tails of the normal density, which manifest in the discrete approximation as the existence of an additional point of support.

Similar results are obtained when the random intercept is generated from a chi-square density with four degrees of freedom. Although the distribution of the random effect is substantially skewed in this case, the parameter estimates are unbiased throughout. Models with three points of support tend to underestimate the variance of the random effect, especially in the cases in which the true underlying density has a relatively large variance (d.g.p.s 3 and 4). Unlike the normal case, there is only a small deterioration in performance, as measured by precision, in going from a discrete density with four points of support to one with five points of support. It appears that densities with five points of support may be necessary in cases where the underlying random effect density is highly skewed.

Overall, the results of the Monte Carlo experiments demonstrate that the estimation of discrete REP models is feasible and provides reliable estimates in a variety of circumstances. Although the true density of the random intercept is specified using a continuous distribution, relatively few points of support are necessary to achieve adequate approximation. Indications are that three to five points of support for the discrete density may be sufficient in many empirical applications.

EMPIRICAL EXAMPLE

In this section, the discrete REP model is used to determine the effects of family and individual characteristics on the demand for preventive care. The discrete REP model is used to test for the existence and strength of excluded family-level effects after controlling for observable characteristics.

Table 14.4 Frequency distribution of family group sizes

Size	Number	Frequency
2	2919	51.71
3	1229	21.77
4	970	17.18
5	360	6.38
6	109	1.93
7	29	0.51
8	21	0.37
9	4	0.07
10	3	0.05
13	1	0.02

DATA

The data for this analysis are taken from the 1996 MEPS [9], henceforth referred to as MEPS, which are publicly available through the Agency for Health Research and Quality (AHRQ). The MEPS is being conducted to provide national representative estimates of health care utilization, expenditures, sources of payment and insurance coverage for the US non-institutionalized population. The first round of the MEPS, conducted in 1996, consists of a sample of 23 230 individuals in 10 639 households. In this paper I consider the subsample of individuals who are at least 16 years of age because the use of preventive care was not ascertained for individuals who were less than 16 years old. There are 12 442 individuals in 5645 families in the sample used for estimation. Table 14.4 reports the frequency distribution of family sizes. Although just over half the families have two members, the largest has 13 adults.

The four general preventive care measures available in the dataset are blood pressure and cholesterol checks, influenza shots and physical exams. Precise definitions and summary statistics of these variables are provided in Table 14.5. Among the individual level covariates are measures of health status given by dummy variables for functional disability (FUNCLIM) and self-perceived levels of health (HLTH_E, HLTH_V, HLTH_F and HLTH_P). The demographic variables include AGE, age squared (AGE2), a dummy variable for whether the person is a child of the head of the family (CHILD), ethnicity (BLACK and HISPANIC), gender (MALE), years of education (EDUC), and whether the person is INSURED. Family-level covariates include urban status (URBAN), family size (FAMSIZE), family income (FAMINC), whether the spouse of the head of the family is present (SPOUSEPR) and the years of education of the family head (HEADEDUC). Definitions and summary statistics for the individual and family-level covariates are also presented in Table 14.5. Given the computational com-

plexity of REP models with exogenous covariates, potential endogeneity of health status and insurance are assumed away to keep the complexity manageable.

ESTIMATES

In order to ascertain the number of components in the discrete density necessary to adequately describe the underlying distribution of the random intercept, I present likelihood ratio (LR) statistics and values of the Akaike information criterion (AIC) in Table 14.6. The distribution of the LR test is non-standard but the usual null $\chi^2(k)$ distribution is likely to under-reject the null hypothesis [15,16]. On the other hand, the use of the AIC for model selection has a formal justification for finite mixture models [17]. Nevertheless, the results of the LR tests using a conservative χ^2 criterion to assess statistical significance dramatically demonstrate the existence of family-level unobserved heterogeneity. There is also significant improvement in going from a model using a density with two points of support to one with three points of support. Adding a fourth point of support provides insufficient improvement to merit further consideration. The AIC provides results that are completely consistent with the LR tests. Consequently, I focus on results from the model with three points of support in subsequent analysis.

Parameter estimates and marginal effects of individual and family-level characteristics are displayed in Table 14.7. In general, the parameters are statistically significant across types of preventive care. Individuals who are insured are substantially more likely to seek each type of preventive care. The effect of health status is monotonic; individuals in poor health are most likely to seek preventive care and those in excellent health are least likely to do so. Although Hispanics and Blacks are just as likely to receive blood pressure checks and influenza shots as individuals of other ethnicities, they are substantially more likely to receive cholesterol checks and physical examinations. Age has u-shaped quadratic effects on the demand for blood pressure checks, influenza shots and physical examinations. The marginal effect of age reaches its minimum between 30 and 34 years and rises steeply thereafter. The effect of age on cholesterol checks, however, is monotonically increasing.

At the family level, the presence of the spouse of the head of the family in the household increases the likelihood of all preventive care services except influenza shots by over three percentage points. Although the individual's education does not seem to matter, the effect of the education of the head of the family is significant and substantial in each case. Preventive care, which is gen-

Table 14.5 Summary statistics

Variable	Definition	Mean	SD
Dependent variables ($N = 12\,442$)			
Blood pressure check	1 if person checked in the past year	0.772	0.419
Cholesterol check	1 if person checked in the past 2 years	0.626	0.484
Influenza shot	1 if person had a shot in the past year	0.277	0.447
Physical exam	1 if person had an exam in the past year	0.506	0.500
Individual-level covariates ($N = 12\,442$)			
AGE	Age in years/10	4.195	1.665
AGE2	Age squared	20.371	15.622
FEMALE	1 if person is female	0.525	0.499
HISPANIC	1 if person is Hispanic	0.196	0.397
BLACK	1 if person is non-Hispanic African American	0.118	0.323
CHILD	1 if the person is a child of the family head	0.147	0.354
EDUC	Years of education	12.198	3.106
HLTH__E	1 if person reports being in excellent health	0.308	0.462
HLTH__V	1 if person reports being in very good health	0.302	0.459
HLTH__F	1 if person reports being in fair health	0.100	0.300
HLTH__P	1 if person reports being in poor health	0.039	0.193
	Good health is the omitted category		
FUNCLIM	1 if the person has difficulty performing an activity of daily living	0.208	0.406
INSURED	1 if the person has health insurance	0.805	0.397
Family-level covariates ($J = 5645$)			
URBAN	1 if the family resides in a metropolitan area	0.781	0.414
SPOUSEPR	1 if the spouse of the family head is present	0.743	0.437
HEADEDUC	Years of education of the family head	12.416	3.190
FAMINC	Family income in $'000	48.111	37.251
FAMSIZE	Family size	2.889	1.162

Table 14.6 Selection criteria for number of support points

	Blood pressure check	Cholesterol check	Influenza shot	Physical exam
LR tests				
REP(2) versus no RE	148.09*	386.62*	457.18*	336.80*
REP(3) versus REP(2)	8.36*	25.50*	81.56*	14.99*
REP(4) versus REP(3)	0.02	0.07	2.35	0.34
AIC				
No RE	6055.62	7429.26	6479.44	8248.44
REP(2)	5983.58	7237.95	6252.85	8082.04
REP(3)	5981.40	7227.20	6214.07	8076.55
REP(4)	5983.38	7229.16	6214.89	8078.38

REP(s) denotes the random effects discrete density.
*Statistically significant at the 0.05 level.

erally a planned activity, is significantly affected by the presence and education of primary adult decision makers. Finally, all else equal, individuals in larger families are less likely to receive preventive care.

The parameters associated with the discrete density of the random effect are generally well determined. The variances of the distributions of the random effect range from 0.452–1.837. These are quite large relative to the

variance of the individual-level idiosyncratic error, which is scaled to have unit variance, thus highlighting the importance of unobserved family-level characteristics in examinations of the demand for preventive care. The implied intra-family correlations are also substantial, ranging from 0.31–0.65.

The characteristics of the latent classes displayed in Table 14.8 provide insight into the types of families

Table 14.7 Parameter estimates and marginal effects

	Blood pressure check		Cholesterol check		Influenza shot		Physical exam	
	π	$\dfrac{\partial \Pr(y=1)}{\partial x}$	π	$\dfrac{\partial \Pr(y=1)}{\partial x}$	π	$\dfrac{\partial \Pr(y=1)}{\partial x}$	π	$\dfrac{\partial \Pr(y=1)}{\partial x}$
Individual-level effects								
AGE	−0.243	−0.056	0.160	0.043	−0.733	−0.159	−0.304	−0.094
	(0.067)		(0.071)		(0.092)		(0.064)	
AGE2	0.039	0.009	0.014	0.004	0.114	0.025	0.046	0.014
	(0.007)		(0.008)		(0.011)		(0.007)	
FEMALE	0.459	0.107	0.116	0.031	0.052	0.011	0.173	0.054
	(0.031)		(0.028)		(0.030)		(0.026)	
HISPANIC	−0.137	−0.032	0.138	0.037	−0.136	−0.030	0.125	0.039
	(0.047)		(0.050)		(0.054)		(0.046)	
BLACK	−0.030	−0.007	0.419	0.112	−0.152	−0.033	0.479	0.148
	(0.054)		(0.060)		(0.061)		(0.053)	
CHILD	0.186	0.043	0.322	0.086	0.593	0.128	0.383	0.119
	(0.060)		(0.063)		(0.071)		(0.060)	
EDUC	0.009	0.002	0.016	0.004	−0.010	−0.002	0.002	0.001
	(0.008)		(0.008)		(0.009)		(0.007)	
HLTH_E	−0.284	−0.066	−0.234	−0.063	−0.066	−0.014	−0.170	−0.053
	(0.043)		(0.043)		(0.048)		(0.040)	
HLTH_VG	−0.117	−0.027	−0.103	−0.028	0.002	0.000	−0.112	−0.035
	(0.042)		(0.041)		(0.047)		(0.038)	
HLTH_F	0.319	0.074	0.222	0.059	0.352	0.076	0.193	0.060
	(0.064)		(0.061)		(0.065)		(0.055)	
HLTH_P	0.470	0.109	0.519	0.139	0.300	0.065	0.346	0.107
	(0.105)		(0.097)		(0.095)		(0.082)	
FUNCLIM	0.119	0.046	0.042	0.011	−0.010	−0.002	0.061	0.019
	(0.047)		(0.044)		(0.048)		(0.040)	
INSURED	0.511	0.119	0.488	0.131	0.306	0.066	0.388	0.120
	(0.043)		(0.043)		(0.051)		(0.042)	
Family-level effects								
URBAN	0.033	0.008	0.263	0.070	−0.030	−0.007	0.120	0.037
	(0.041)		(0.045)		(0.048)		(0.039)	
SPOUSEPR	0.139	0.032	0.314	0.036	0.002	0.000	0.109	0.034
	(0.043)		(0.044)		(0.049)		(0.040)	
HEADEDUC	0.035	0.008	0.024	0.007	0.037	0.008	0.021	0.007
	(0.008)		(0.008)		(0.010)		(0.008)	
FAMINC	0.002	0.000	0.003	0.001	0.000	0.000	0.001	0.000
	(0.001)		(0.001)		(0.001)		(0.000)	
FAMSIZE	−0.084	−0.019	−0.034	−0.009	−0.053	−0.012	−0.042	−0.013
	(0.015)		(0.016)		(0.021)		(0.015)	
Discrete random effect density								
u_1	0.943		1.186		1.982		1.111	
	(0.597)		(0.241)		(0.258)		(0.302)	
u_2	−0.395		−0.184		0.493		−0.033	
	(0.159)		(0.125)		(0.090)		(0.146)	
π_1	0.315		0.244		0.097		0.197	
	(0.200)		(0.074)		(0.036)		(0.103)	
π_2	0.669		0.653		0.685		0.683	
	(0.184)		(0.052)		(0.028)		(0.071)	
Variance	0.452		0.642		1.837		0.565	
Intra-family correlation	0.311		0.391		0.648		0.361	

Numbers in parentheses are asymptotic standard errors.

Table 14.8   Characteristics of latent classes

	Blood pressure check		Cholesterol check		Influenza shot		Physical exam	
	π	$\Pr(y = 1)$	π	$\Pr(y = 1)$	π	$\Pr(y = 1)$	π	$\Pr(y = 1)$
Class 1	0.315	0.955	0.244	0.920	0.097	0.763	0.197	0.848
Class 2	0.669	0.701	0.653	0.591	0.685	0.293	0.683	0.484
Class 3	0.016	0.175	0.103	0.161	0.218	0.006	0.120	0.065

present in the sample. For each of the three points of support in the discrete random effects density, the predicted probability of seeking care, $\Pr(y = 1)$, is calculated as the sample average over all individuals in the sample. Although most families (latent class 2) have average probabilities of seeking care that are close to those calculated by crude relative frequencies (reported in Table 14.5), a number of families (latent class 1) have substantially higher probabilities of seeking preventive care while others (latent class 3) have substantially lower probabilities of seeking care. Therefore, the population can be segregated into three types of families with *low*, *average* and *high* propensities to seek preventive care. In what follows, I use this terminology to describe the latent classes.

These differential propensities probably arise from differences in unobservable risk aversion or taste characteristics of different families. Nevertheless, a posterior analysis of class membership may reveal useful information on observable characteristics of family types. In order to do so, the posterior probability (Equation 14.6) of belonging to each of the three classes was calculated for each family, conditional on observed covariates and outcomes. Next, each family was classified as a high, average or low type on the basis of the maximum posterior probability. Finally, sample averages were calculated for each covariate stratified by family classification. The results show consistent patterns across measures of preventive care for four covariates: AGE, HLTH_E, HLTH_P and FUN-CLIM. Sample averages for each of these covariates by family type are displayed in Figure 14.1. Pairwise differences between the sample means are statistically significant. Families with older members tend to have low propensities to seek preventive care. Healthy families, measured by self-perceived health and the existence of a functional limitation, tend to have high propensities to seek preventive care. In other words, healthy and young families are either more risk averse or have greater preference for preventive care. The effect of health status, at first glance, appears to contradict its effect obtained from the basic model parameters. These parameters, reported in Table 14.7, show that individuals in better health are less likely to seek preventive care. In fact, the findings are not contradictory. Although healthy individuals are less likely to seek preventive care, *ceteris paribus*, they tend to

belong to families who have high unobservable-based propensities to seek such care.

Do these findings contradict the random effects assumption? Specifically, since the random intercept is assumed to be uncorrelated with the covariates, why are the covariate averages significantly different across latent classes? A closer look at the definition of the posterior probability (Equation 14.6) reveals that the random effects assumption is consistent with posterior inferences regarding a relationship between covariates and class membership. The *a priori* assumption regarding the relationship between the random intercept and the covariates is conditional only on the covariates. The posterior relationship, however, is conditional on covariates and outcomes. In other words, armed with only knowledge of an individual's covariates, it is not possible to infer anything about the type of family to which this individual belongs. But once the outcome is known for each family member, this additional information makes it possible to infer features of the type of family.

CONCLUSION

In this paper, I develop a REP model in which the distribution of the random component is approximated by a discrete density. The experimental evidence shows that discrete densities with only three to four points of support mimic normal and chi-squared densities sufficiently well so as to provide unbiased estimates of the structural parameters and the variance of the random effect. This is important because models that use discrete densities can become quite cumbersome to estimate if the number of points of support required to produce adequate approximations is large.

The model is applied to the demand for preventive care. Although individual-level covariates are significant, family-level covariates are also important determinants of the demand for preventive care. Moreover, unobservable family-level effects, captured through the discretely distributed random intercept, are also important. In fact, a substantial portion of the total variance of the unobserved components is due to the family-level unobserved component.

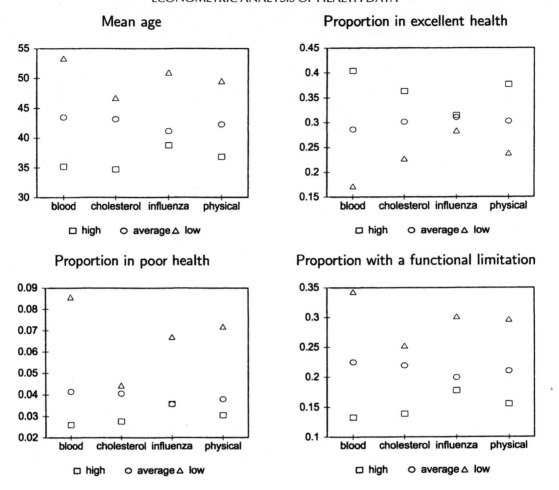

Figure 14.1. Characteristics of individuals by posterior class assignment

Although the model developed in this paper is for binary choice, the general method can easily be extended to discrete formulations of random effects models for multinomial, count and duration data. The computational issues, testing and model selection principles, and finite sample performance described in this paper are likely to be of value to researchers conducting analyses in those related frameworks.

ACKNOWLEDGEMENTS

This paper has benefited from comments by participants at the 2000 European Workshop in Econometrics and Health Economics, and seminars at the University of Chicago, University of New Hampshire and IUPUI. I would like to thank Karen Conway, Daniele Fabbri, Robert Sandy and two anonymous referees for their helpful comments. As usual, all errors are mine.

APPENDIX: COMPUTATIONAL ISSUES

Estimation of finite mixture models is not always straightforward. The likelihood functions of finite mixture models can have multiple local maxima so it is important to ensure that the algorithm converges to the global maximum. In general, random perturbation or grid search techniques, or algorithms such as simulated annealing [18], designed to seek the global optimum, should be utilized. Moreover, if a model with too many points of support is chosen, one or more points of support may be degenerate, i.e. the π_s associated with those densities may be zero. In such cases, the solution to the maximum likelihood problem lies on the boundary of the parameter space. This can cause estimation algorithms to fail, especially if unconstrained maximization algorithms are used. Constrained maximization algorithms are preferred. Such cases are a strong indication that a model with fewer components adequately describes the data. Therefore, a small-to-large model selection approach is recommended, i.e. the number of points of support in the discrete density should be increased one at a time starting with a model with only two points of support. In this paper, I estimate the discrete REP models by maximum likelihood using the Broyden–Fletcher–Goldfarb–Shanno quasi-Newton constrained maximization algorithm in SAS/IML [19]. Models with two, three and four points of support are successively estimated.

The performance of the maximum likelihood estimators of standard and discrete REP models given by Equation 14.2 and Equation 14.4, respectively, may not be satisfactory for large group sizes, N_j, since the log likelihood involves the integration or summation over a term involving the product of cumulative normals for all group members. Borjas and Sueyoshi [3] point out that with 500 observations per group, and assuming a generous likelihood contribution per observation, the product would be well below standard computer precision. They speculate that group sizes over 50 may create significant instabilities if the model has low predictive power. Based on Monte Carlo experiments, they find that such computational problems lead to quite inaccurate statistical inference on the parameters of the model. Lee [20] provides two methods that considerably alleviate this computational problem, both of which involve interchanging the inner product with the outer summation.

In the first method, the likelihood function (Equation 14.4) is evaluated as

$$l_j = \sum_{i=1}^{N_i} \ln\left\{ \sum_{s=1}^{S} \omega_{i-1,js}\Phi[d_{ij}(x_{ij}\beta + z_j\gamma + u_s)]\right\} \quad (14.A1)$$

where

$$\omega_{i,jc} = \frac{\omega_{i-1,jc}\Phi[d_{ij}(x_{ij}\beta + z_j\gamma + u_c)]}{\sum_{s=1}^{S} \omega_{i-1,js}\Phi[d_{ij}(x_{ij}\beta + z_j\gamma + u_s)]},$$

$$i = 1, 2, \ldots, N_j; c = 1, 2, \ldots, S \quad (14.A2)$$

with $\omega_{0,jc} = \pi_c$ for all $j = 1, 2, \ldots, J$. The weights $\omega_{i,jc}$ can be computed recursively. Computational efficiencies can be realized if the computer programming makes use of the fact that the formulation of the log likelihood in Equation 14.A1 contains the denominator term of Equation 14.A2.

In the second method, the likelihood function Equation 14.4 is evaluated as

$$l_j = \ln\left\{ \sum_{s=1}^{S} \exp(h_{js})\right\} \quad (14.A3)$$

where

$$h_{js} = \ln(\pi_s) + \sum_{i=1}^{N_i} \ln\{\Phi[d_{ij}(x_{ij}\beta + z_j\gamma + u_s)]\} \quad (14.A4)$$

for all $s = 1, 2, \ldots, S$ and $j = 1, 2, \ldots, J$. Denote $p_j = \max\{h_{js}: s = 1, 2, \ldots, S\}$. Then

$$l_j = p_j + \ln\left\{ \sum_{s=1}^{S} \exp(h_{js} - p_j)\right\}, \quad j = 1, 2, \ldots, J \quad (14.A5)$$

Note that this formulation requires the calculation of the maximum of h_{js} for each group, but does not involve a recursion.

In a Monte Carlo setting, Lee [20] shows that both methods are numerically stable for large group sizes. The choice, therefore, depends on computational efficiency. Although Lee [20] reports that Equation 14.A1 is computationally quicker than Equation 14.A2, I find the opposite result when the algorithms are programmed in SAS/IML. In Equation 14.A1, the programming complexity arises from the recursion, which requires a loop. In Equation 14.A3, no loops are required but maximal elements of vectors must be calculated. The relative computational speed depends on the efficiency with loops are executed relative to that of calculation of maximal elements in the computer software used. For the estimation in the Monte Carlo and empirical sections of this paper, I used the algorithm in Equation 14.A3.

REFERENCES

1. Butler, J.S. and Moffitt, R. A computationally efficient quadrature procedure for the one-factor multinomial probit model. *Econometrica* 1982; **50**: 761–764.
2. Keane, M.P. Simulation estimation for panel data with limited dependent variables, Chapter 20. In *Handbook of Statistics*, vol. 11, Maddala, G.S., Rao, C.R. and Vinod, H.D. (eds). North Holland: Amsterdam, 1993; 545–572.
3. Borjas, G.J. and Sueyoshi, G.T. A two-stage estimator for probit models with structural group effects. *J. Econom.* 1994; **64**: 165–182.
4. Lindsay, B.J. *Mixture Models: Theory, Geometry, and Applications*, NSF-CBMS Regional Conference Series in Probability and Statistics, vol. 5. Institute of Mathematical Statistics (IMS): California and the American Statistical Association: Virginia, 1995.

5. Heckman, J.J. and Singer, B. A method of minimizing the distributional impact in econometric models for duration data. *Econometrica* 1984; **52**: 271–320.

6. Gordon, N.P., Rundall, T.G. and Parker, L. Types of health coverage and the likelihood of being screened for cancer. *Med. Care* 1998; **36**: 637–643.

7. Potosky, A.L., Breen, N., Graubard, B.I. and Parsons, P.E. The association between health care coverage and the use of cancer screening tests: Results from the 1992 National Health Interview Survey. *Med. Care* 1998; **3**: 257–270.

8. Saag, K.G., Doebbeling, B.N., Rohrer, J.E., Kolluri, S., Peterson, R., Herman, R.E. and Wallace, R.B. Variation of tertiary prevention and health service utilization among the elderly: The role of urban-rural residence and supplemental insurance. *Med. Care* 1998; **36**: 965–976.

9. Cohen, J. Design and methods of the medical expenditure panel survey household component. Agency for Health Research and Quality, MEPS Methodology Report No. 1, 1997.

10. Pudney, S., Galassi, F.L. and Mealli, F. An econometric model of farm tenures in fifteenth-century Florence. *Economica* 1998; **65**: 535–556.

11. Jain, D.C., Vilcassim, N.J. and Chintagunta, P.K. A random-coefficients logit brand-choice model applied to panel data. *J. Bus. Econ. Stat.* 1994; **12**: 317–328.

12. Kim, B.-D., Blattberg, R.C. and Rossi, P.E. Modeling the distribution of price sensitivity and implications for optimal retail pricing. *J. Bus. Econ. Stat.* 1995; **13**: 291–303.

13. Gouriéroux, C. and Monfort, A. *Simulation Based Econometrics Methods.* Oxford University Press: New York, 1996.

14. Deb, P. and Trivedi, P.K. The structure of demand for health care: Latent class versus two-part models. Working Paper, 1999.

15. Böhning, D. A review of reliable maximum likelihood algorithms for semiparametric mixture models. *J. Stat. Plan. Infer.* 1995; **47**: 5–28.

16. Deb, P. and Trivedi, P.K. Demand for medical care by the elderly in the United States: A finite mixture approach. *J. Appl. Econom.* 1997; **12**: 313–336.

17. Leroux, B.G. Consistent estimation of a mixing distribution. *Ann. Stat.* 1992; **20**: 1350–1360.

18. Goffe, W.L., Ferrier, G.D. and Roger, J. Global optimization of statistical functions with simulated annealing. *J. Econom.* 1994; **60**: 65–69.

19. SAS Institute. SAS/IML Software: Changes and Enhancements through Release 6.11. SAS Institute Inc.: North Carolina, 1997.

20. Lee, L.-F. A numerically stable quadrature procedure for the one-factor random-component discrete choice model. *J. Econom.* 2000; **95**: 117–129.

15

The Use of Long-term Care Services by the Dutch Elderly

FRANCE PORTRAIT,[1] MAARTEN LINDEBOOM[2] AND DORLY DEEG[3]

[1]Department of Econometrics, Free University, Amsterdam, Netherlands, [2]Department of Economics, Free University and Tinbergen Institute, Amsterdam, Netherlands and [3]Longitudinal Ageing Study Amsterdam, Faculty of Medicine and Faculty of Social and Cultural Sciences, Free University, Amsterdam, Netherlands

INTRODUCTION

During the past decades, the elderly population of most Organization for Economic Co-operation and Development (OECD) countries has increased both in absolute terms and as a percentage of the full population. In the mid-1950s in the Netherlands, for instance, about 7% of the population consisted of individuals aged 65 and older. Since then, this fraction has doubled, and is expected to rise to about 25% in the year 2040 [3]. This trend towards ageing is expected to have a large impact on many aspects of current society – elements of social security and the health care system being the most prominent ones. With respect to the health care system, expenditures currently add up to 8.2% of the Dutch gross domestic product. This percentage is one of the highest among the European countries. Long-term care is a major component of the health care system, as it currently accounts for approximately 23% of total Dutch health care expenditures [21]. Long-term care is provided when individuals experience disabilities or chronic diseases and is, by consequence, largely reserved for the elderly, and generally provided until the end of life. By consequence and in view of the expected growth of the Dutch elderly population, the needs for long-term care services may greatly increase in the next decades, and largely exceed the available resources. There is already some evidence that the Dutch long-term care system is currently supply constrained. Therefore, the sustainability of the existing long-term care system is questionable. Sensible reforms require insight into the forces that determine the use of these services. The main objective of the present paper is to gain a better understanding of the process underlying the utilization of long-term care services by the Dutch elderly.

A large number of care alternatives is available to the elderly in the Netherlands. In our analyses, three comprehensive categories of long-term care services are considered, namely, informal care, formal care at home, and formal care in institutions for the elderly. Briefly, informal care means 'unpaid, non-organized assistance given to an ill or disabled person offered within the social network' [20], and formal care is professionally organized paid help. The bulk of care assistance is provided informally and, consequently, informal care plays a major role in the support of older populations. Informal care has often been ignored in the economic literature on use of long-term care services, which generally focuses on institutional care, with a few studies concentrating on formal home assistance [4]. However, there is some evidence that some kinds of formal care and informal care are close substitutes [15]. In consequence, informal and formal care should definitely be analyzed jointly in studies on use of long-term care. For an extensive survey of long-term care, see Norton [14].

The main trigger for use of care services is the recognition of a need for care. In a context of supply limitations – waiting lists exist for all types of formal care in the Netherlands – access to care services may be restricted. Observed utilization is thus likely to differ from actual needs. In the present paper, the use of care arrangements is conditional on the perception of a need for care. Only individuals with a need for care are likely to make use of care services, the needs of some of them being unmet as a result of supply restrictions. The utilization of the

Econometric Analysis of Health Data. Edited by Andrew M. Jones and Owen O'Donnell

different care arrangements, measured by discrete variables, is modelled here jointly. Unobserved preferences – such as the wish to maintain familiar surroundings – or general attitudes towards receiving care may affect the individual choices towards these care options, and may cause these to be stochastically related. This specification is, thus, technically speaking, a conditional multiple discrete choice model with correlated unobservables. This model does not have a simple analytical form and its estimation requires the evaluation of higher order integrals. To circumvent this numerical difficulty, estimation methods based on 'simulated maximum likelihood' techniques will be used [7].

Research has often shown that needs for long-term care services – and their use – depend primarily on the health conditions of the elderly population [10,22]. Health status is not a well-defined concept, but it can be safely stated that it is multidimensional and dynamic. Most previous research on determinants of health care utilization at older ages uses a small set of indicators to measure different aspects of health status – the majority of these indicators focusing on physical limitations [10,21]. In addition to the physical dimension, aspects of emotional and cognitive health should simultaneously be considered. Research has indeed often shown significant influences of emotional and/or mental disabilities – such as depressive complaints and loneliness – on long-term care utilization [1,10,25]. In Portrait et al. [16], we discussed methods that summarize the multidimensional and dynamic health status – measured by a large set of indicators – into a limited number of valid and reliable indices. The grades of membership (GoM) approach, introduced by Manton and Woodbury in 1982 is the most suitable candidate for this procedure [11,12]. The method simultaneously identifies all dimensions of the concept of interest and derives individual GoM, i.e. the degree to which an individual belongs to each dimension. In Portrait et al. [16], we applied the GoM method to a set of 21 health indicators from the Longitudinal Ageing Study Amsterdam (LASA) data set [5,6]. Six health dimensions were identified. The degrees to which an individual belongs to these types (i.e. GoM) were derived for both waves of the LASA data set. These GoM characterize the health status of the LASA respondents, and are used in the present analysis to determine which health dimensions are the most predictive of long-term care utilization.

While the health status of the elderly highly influences the utilization of care, this relationship also holds in the opposite direction. Hence, the health status of older individuals at a certain point in time is not independent of their use of care services. This potential endogeneity should be addressed to avoid biased estimates. As far as

we know, this problem has often been ignored in the empirical literature on the utilization of health care services. Major exceptions are the studies based on the theory of production of health originally formulated by Grossman [9]. In our analyses, health status is treated explicitly as an endogenous variable. The potential endogeneity of health status is addressed using a procedure introduced by Mundlak in 1978 [13], in which the correlation between unobservables and the included regressors is captured through the use of instrumental variables.

This analysis is conducted within a longitudinal context, using a unique panel survey of the LASA data set. Panel data analyses indeed control for the presence of individual time-constant unobservables and this is relevant for our study, as unobserved time-constant individual characteristics – such as care preferences, general attitudes towards care, genetic factors or life style – may play an important role in determining the need for care and/or the use of care. However, longitudinal data – especially on the elderly – are likely to suffer from attrition because mortality and exclusion of the deceased respondents may result in non-random selection. As far as we know, recent longitudinal studies on use of care by elderly populations do not correct for this potential sample selection effect. The present paper goes one step further and proposes panel data analyses – corrected for attrition owing to mortality – of the determinants of the utilization of care services at older ages.

The second section briefly describes the Dutch long-term care system. The third section presents the data set and gives some information on the variables used in subsequent sections. The following section is devoted to the development of an appropriate framework to analyse the process of use of informal help, formal care at home, and institutional care by the Dutch elderly. The next section presents the results of our analyses. Special focus is on an analysis of the discrepancies between the need for and the use of care services. The final section discusses the results and concludes the paper.

LONG-TERM CARE IN THE NETHERLANDS

Long-term care consists of informal care and formal care. Briefly described, informal care is unpaid assistance provided from within a person's social network, and formal care is professionally organized help, financed mostly by national insurance systems. Both types of care can be provided either at home or in an institutional setting. However, in institutions for the elderly, informal care is negligible compared with the predominant role of formal help.

Informal care may be supplied by the partner, children,

other family members, neighbours and acquaintances. A substantial part of the Dutch older population – about 30% of the elderly aged 65 and more [25] – receive some kind of informal care. This percentage inceases to 40% for the eldest old, i.e. individuals aged 85 and more. In case of the absence of an adequate social network, or reluctance to ask for help from relatives, disabled elderly individuals may ask for formal care. *Formal care* is generally divided into community and institutional care. Of Dutch individuals above 65 years, close to 30% receive formal care at home and 8.6% live in an institution [25]. Community care consists, for the most part, of home care and nursing care, but is also likely to be provided by the personnel of institutions for the elderly. The bulk of institutional care is provided in residential and nursing homes – geriatric units and general or psychiatric hospitals supplying the remaining part. Residential homes provide living assistance only, whereas nursing homes provide both personal care and living assistance. The health condition of clients in nursing homes is generally much poorer than those of residential home occupants. However, the differences in health status between these two types of intramural care have faded during the last decades – with their client populations, mostly elderly individuals in need of intensive care, overlapping more and more [20].

It is important to mention that the availability of formal long-term care services is cururently highly regulated. The service capacity within a specific region is strongly related to the budget received by local authorities – with the distribution of this budget depending on the number of inhabitants aged 75 and more. During recent decades, national governments have promoted the increase of community help capacity and the decrease of the number of beds in institutional care. However, expansion of community care has been restricted by a shortage of governmental funding and of manpower. Therefore, and given the recent expansion in the elderly populations, the Dutch long-term care system is currently supply constrained, as waiting lists exist for all kinds of care. Accessibility to formal long-term care services is also strongly regulated. The choice of formal care in the Netherlands is free only for those who pay the costs themselves. In all other cases, a person has to apply for formal care to a Municipal Committee on Need Assessment. The applicant may be rejected or, in a context of supply constraint, put on a waiting list. If the request is granted, a (large) share of the costs incurred for formal care utilization is covered by national insurance systems. Individual charges for home care are primarily related to the volume of care received. They also depend on the size of the household and are income-related, with a minimum per week of $2 and a maximum of $113. Since 1997, the regulations regarding costs are very similar for recipients

of nursing or residential care. A part of the elderly's monthly income is protected, but the rest of their income, up to a maximum of $1565, is fully retained by the institution. Since 1997, the costs of living in a nursing home have considerably increased. The costs for institutional care are high, and generally not paid by public and private insurances. Two-thirds of the Dutch elderly population are covered by public insurance, with one-third privately insured. Thus, virtually all the Dutch elderly are health insured. Being privately or publicly insured is income-related, as only individuals with an income below a specific threshold may benefit from public insurance.

DATA

SAMPLE

Our data come from the LASA [5,6]. This interdisciplinary study is intended to lead to policy relevant information on the ageing population in the Netherlands. It follows a representative sample of non-institutionalized and institutionalized adults older than 55 years over an extended period of time. Currently, two waves are available (the 1992–1993 wave and the 1995–1996 wave). Data have been gathered on health status, on factors that are expected to predict changes in health status, and on utilization of care services. Health status is assessed by a broad set of objective and subjective instruments, including clinical assessments. A total of 3107 respondents participated in the first wave of the survey. Of this first wave, we selected all individuals of 65 years and older. Two thousand, one hundred and forty-one respondents remain, 1659 of whom also participated in the second wave. Respondents were given either a complete or a short interview, according to their ability to sustain a lengthy interview. Of interest for our analyses is that the bulk of the sample attrition is caused by the mortality of respondents in the time intervening between the two waves. Seventy-nine percent of the 482 non-respondents to the second wave died in the 3-year time period.

NEED FOR CARE AND ACTUAL UTILIZATION

Need for care

In our model, the utilization of care services is assumed to be driven by the recognition by the elderly of a need for care. The need for care is related to the person's (in)ability to perform some daily tasks. However, the person's general attitude and evaluation of his or her health status also influence the perception of the need for care. In our study, *need for care* is, therefore, measured by a combination of subjective and objective factors.

Elderly individuals who report difficulties in daily activities are considered to be experiencing a need for care. The variable indicating the need for care can take the values 0, if the respondent does not report any difficulties in daily activities, 1, if he or she reports some difficulties, and 2, if he or she reports severe difficulties. However, given the self-reported nature of the variable, it probably measures the respondent's perception of his or her ability to perform daily activities. Therefore, for individuals experiencing no difficulties in daily activities, but with some indication of objective needs, the need variable is constructed as follows.

Clearly, the health status of personal care recipients is generally poor. Therefore, these respondents are considered to suffer from severe difficulties in daily activities. For these individuals, the variable indicating the need for care services matches the score (2). Likewise, elderly individuals with no perceived need for care, but receiving formal housekeeping assistance, are considered in our study to have a need for care[a]. As a matter of fact, in a context of supply restrictions, individuals receiving formal care services may be validly considered as needing care, even if they have a recorded score of 0 for the variable, indicating perceived difficulties in daily activities. Finally, older people receiving domestic assistance from non-household members are also considered as having actual needs for care.

Actual utilization of care

It is worth recalling that, in our analyses, three broad categories of caregivers are considered – namely informal caregivers, formal caregivers at home, and formal caregivers in an institutional setting. Private help is excluded from our analyses. Utilization of long-term care is measured by a set of three binary variables indicating whether respondents make use of these services or not. Information on the volume of care used is only available for respondents with a complete interview, and could, therefore, not be included in our analyses. Elderly individuals may clearly opt for a combination of informal and formal services to more adequately meet their needs for care. It is important to note that about 20% of our respondents with needs for care do not receive any kind of assistance.

Table 15.1 gives some details on the variables indicating need for care and actual utilization.

INDEPENDENT VARIABLES

Health status

Health conditions have repeatedly been shown as the primary determinant of use of care services [14]. A major issue when dealing with health status is how to measure it. The elderly's health status is clearly multidimensional and dynamic. Therefore, a large set of indicators is required to capture all its aspects, and it is difficult to handle all these variables in statistical analyses. The GoM technique, introduced by Woodbury and Manton (1982), is a flexible non-parametric method specifically designed to summarize the multidimensional and dynamic health status – measured by a large set of indicators – into a limited number of valid and reliable indices [11,12]. GoM identifies simultaneously latent multidimensional profiles and the degrees to which the respondent's features fit these profiles. The degrees of similarity between pure types and respondents, viz. GoM, are described by weights constrained to fall in the interval [0, 1] and that sum to unity over all profiles. So the method recognizes that health status of the elderly is a concept of graded participation into several aspects of health status. Several types of health disorders exist and different degrees of impairment in these types are possible, and should be

Table 15.1 Summary statistics for need for care and actual use in wave I of the LASA data set

Need for care	Frequency	No care	Informal care only	Formal care only	Both types of care	Institutional care
No difficulties with daily activities	857	527	330	—	—	—
Some difficulties	385	141	94	114	24	12
Severe difficulties	284	43	79	82	42	38
Recoded	246	5	111	82	24	24
Total respondents needing care	915 (100.0%)	189 (20.6%)	289 (31.6%)	273 (29.8%)	90 (9.8%)	74 (8.1%)
Total	1772	716	330	—	—	—
Missing values	369	—	—	—	—	—

allowed for. In Portrait *et al.* [16], the GoM method is applied to summarize the health information given by the set of 21 health variables from the LASA data set. We refer to this paper for the technical details. The empirical results of this study revealed that the health concept can be described by six underlying health dimensions which can be described as follows.

The *first* group is characterized by the prevalence of two life threatening diseases: chronic obstructive pulmonary diseases and cancer. Group I members are also characterized by physicial limitations, and are more likely to be depressed than other pure types. The functional status of *second* pure types is very good. However, group II is characterized by the presence of 'other chronic diseases': these are mainly diseases which are not specific to the elderly, and generally not too serious. Examples of these are hypertension, back troubles or diseases of the stomach or intestines. The *third* type is physically healthy but has poor cognitive function. The *fourth* type is characterized by the prevalence of serious arthritis (almost all respondents follow a continuous medical treatment). Moreover, the probability of having another chronic disease besides arthritis is very high. Pure type IV is physically impaired and often depressed. The cognitive function of pure type IV is also relatively poor. The presence of cardiovascular diseases (heart diseases, atherosclerosis, stroke and diabetes) characterizes the *fifth* pure type. For this group, vision is much poorer than the mean, likely because of the presence of diabetes and stroke. Finally the *sixth* group is the healthy one.

The degrees to which an individual belongs to these types (i.e. GoM) were successively derived for both waves of the LASA data set. These GoM characterize the health status of the elderly and are used, in the present analysis, to determine which health dimensions are the most predictive of long-term care utilization.

Other independent variables

In addition to the health status of the elderly, the out-of-pocket prices of close substitutes and available economic resources are major factors explaining long-term care utilization [14]. *Monthly maximum individual payments* related to formal home care and institutional care are, therefore, included in the present study. As mentioned in the section 'Long-term care in the Netherlands', Dutch individual payments for long-term care utilization depend on family size, income, and the volume of care received. No information on the volume of care used is available in the data set. Therefore, we calculate the payments as the maximum payable based on family size and income[b]. The means and standard errors equal $152 and

$150, respectively, for home care, and $682 and $516 for institutional care. Information on *income* is also used in our analyses. Respondents were asked to assign their monthly total income – derived from pension, savings, dividends, and other sources – to four categories ($), namely 0–794 (in line with the Dutch minimum income), 795–1134, 1134–1815 and more than 1815. Missing values for income were relatively frequent (14.61%), and were imputed on the basis of the results of regression analyses. Looking only at total incomes may mask the level of economic status experienced by older adults during their lives [19]. The level of economic status is also likely to influence individual decisions towards care arrangements. A categorical variable indicating the *level of education attained* is used as a supplementary measure of socioeconomic status. Education is determined by the following question: 'Which is the highest education level attained?' Nine categories were reported, varying from 'elementary education not completed' to 'university education'.

Utilization of long-term care services is also related to demographic variables – in particular *age* and *gender*. As a consequence, these variables are used in our analyses. The characteristics of household size, as well as the size of the social network, reflecting social conditions related to living arrangements, are also included in the study. *Household size* is represented by the binary variable 'living alone' (1) versus 'not living alone' (0). In the equations modelling utilization of institutional care, this variable is replaced by a variable indicating marital status. Institutional care utilization is indeed likely to be more affected by the marital status of the respondents, than by his or her current living situation. Marital status gives some information on the household size of the elderly before entering the institution, and is represented by the binary variable 'married' (1) versus 'not married' (0). The variable '*network size*' [24] indicates the number of network members – including children, other family members, friends, and neighbours – who have regular contacts with the elderly person. Previous studies indicate that having children is one of the best predictors of formal and informal care [14]. Our network variable includes this. We opted for the variable 'network size' instead of a set of variables measuring the number and gender of children, because 'network size' excludes children with whom elderly individuals do not have any contact, or who do not support their parents.

The presence of special *housing adaptations* – such as lowered doorsteps, an alarm system, handgrips – may allow old persons to remain independent in their own environment for a longer period of time. A categorical variable determining the number of special housing adaptations in the dwelling is included in our study. The degree of urbanization of the area where respondents live is an indicator of the external living conditions, and may influence positively or negatively the use of care services in the elderly population through a variety of mediating factors – such as feelings of insecurity and availability of both formal and informal caregivers. Therefore, a variable reflecting the *degree of urbanization* of the municipality where respondents live is also used in our analyses.

We have already mentioned the presence of possible supply restrictions in the availability of formal care. In the absence of relevant data on waiting lists and to correct for possible differences in availability of care services across municipalities, a set of ten binary variables indicating the municipality in which the respondent lives is included in our analyses.

A MODEL FOR LONG-TERM CARE UTILIZATION

THEORETICAL BACKGROUND

Only elderly individuals with a need for care are actually likely to express a demand for informal care (I), formal care at home (FH), and/or institutional care (FI). Needs for care can be modelled as a function of health status and demographic and socio-economic variables, namely:

$$N_I = f(g, x \mid \beta_I)$$
$$N_{FH} = f(g, x \mid \beta_{FH})$$
$$N_{FI} = f(g, x \mid \beta_{FI}) \qquad (15.1)$$

where N_K is a variable measuring the needs for care services K, $K \in \{I, FH, FI\}$. g is a set of GoM, characterizing the health status of respondents, and x is a set of observed variables. In the Netherlands, needs for care are assessed by governmental experts (see section 'Long-term care in the Netherlands'). Positive recommendations of the state committees are required to make use of any kind of subsidized formal care. Recommendations are exclusively based on the current needs of the applicant – namely his or her health status and social situation – and does not take into account actual supply conditions. More formally, say that recommendations are governed by the constructs R_{FH} and R_{FI}:

$$R_{FH} = g\delta^1_{FH} + x\delta^2_{FH}$$
$$R_{FI} = g\delta^1_{FI} + x\delta^2_{FI} \qquad (15.2)$$

The parameters δ are decided by governmental regulations. Assume that individuals get a positive recommen-

dation for care services K if $R_K \geq 0$ and are not allowed to make use of care services K if $R_K < 0$, for $K \in \{FH, FI\}$.

$\bar{I}$, $\overline{FH}$ and $\overline{FI}$ refer to the total market capacity of informal care, formal care at home, and institutional care, respectively. The volume of formal care services on the market is not left to market forces, but decided by the Dutch cabinet. Therefore, and given the significant delay required by the set-up of new formal care services, the supply of formal care services can be safely considered as fixed in the short-term. Informal care is free care offered within the social network of the elderly. In this paper, the volume of informal care available to elderly individuals is considered as fixed in the short-term – we ignore events like the death or illnesses of caregivers. The modelling of these events goes beyond the scope of this paper. An additional major feature of the long-term care market is that the price paid by consumers is fixed by governmental regulations, and will not vary to clear the market. The supply restrictions can be expressed in terms of the Models (Equations 15.1 and 15.2). Say that demand would exceed current availability of care resources in a given time period:

$$\sum_i N_{iI} > \bar{I}$$

$$\sum_i R_{iFH} > \overline{FH}$$

$$\sum_i R_{iFI} > \overline{FI}$$

Clearly the length of the waiting lists is given by $(\Sigma_i N_i - \bar{I})$ for informal care, $(\Sigma_i R_{iFH} - \overline{FH})$ for formal care at home, and $(\Sigma_i R_{iFI} - \overline{FI})$ for institutional care.

In the context of supply restrictions, where price and supply are fixed, it is likely that only individuals with the most urgent situation actually make use of care. In this case, it is neither the price nor the supply of care services that vary to clear the market, but the standards required to make use of long-term care services. The standards used on the market are actually more severe than the ones used by the governmental committees. More formally, say that utilization is governed by the constructs U_{FH} and U_{FI}:

$$U_{FH} = g\gamma^1_{FH} + x\gamma^2_{FH} + y\gamma^3_{FH}$$
$$U_{FI} = g\gamma^1_{FI} + x\gamma^2_{FI} + y\gamma^3_{FH} \qquad (15.3)$$

where y refers to additional explicative variables indicating, for instance, the current supply conditions. The parameters γ refers to the standards required on the market to make use of care services. Assume that individuals actually use formal care services K if $U_K \geq 0$ and that they make no use of care services K if $U_K < 0$. A comparison of the parameters of the state committees δ with the use parameters γ gives insights into the effects of supply restrictions on the needs for the elderly, with a positive recommendation for care.

EMPIRICAL SPECIFICATION

Need for long-term care

Our variable measuring needs for care (see section 'Data') does not specify the kind of care required. This information is not recorded in our data set. Consequently, the three equations (Equation 15.1) collapse into a unique equation, indicating needs for any kinds of care services. The constructed variable to measure the need for care can take the values 0; no difficulties with daily activities, 1; experiencing some difficulties with daily activities, and 2; suffering from severe difficulties with daily activities. The modelling for the need for care is a longitudinal ordered probit specification, in which the need for care is determined by observed and unobserved characteristics. More specifically:

$$N^{t*} = g^t \beta_N^1 + x^t \beta_N^2 + \alpha_N + u_N^t \qquad (15.4)$$

where N^{t*} is the latent continuous counterpart of the discrete variable N^t and measures the underlying inclination of needing care in period t. t accounts for a specific wave of the data set and can take the values 1 and 2. Currently, we only have access to two waves of the survey and we, therefore, abstract from time effects. N^{t*} is a latent variable and is unobserved. What we do observe is:

$$N^t = 0 \text{ if } N^{t*} \leq 0$$

$$N^t = 1 \text{ if } 0 < N^{t*} \leq l_N$$

$$N^t = 2 \text{ if } l_N < N^{t*}$$

In Equation 15.4, g^t is a set of GoM, characterizing the health status of respondents in wave t. So $N^t = (N_I^t + N_{FH}^t + N_{FI}^t)$. x^t is a set of demographic and socioeconomic variables in wave t. l_N is an unknown parameter and has to be estimated with the other parameters. Unobserved individual effect α_N is assumed to be normally distributed, and to have zero mean. Residuals u_N^t are assumed to be independently and normally distributed with mean zero and unit variance. Individual effect α_N is also assumed to be independent of u_N^t.

Unfortunately, we do not have sufficient information

to estimate parameters of Model 2 (Equation 15.2). We do not observe the recommendation for care given by governmental experts for the LASA respondents. We refer to a forthcoming study by Portrait [18], in which the standards used by the Municipal Committees on Need Assessment are analysed and estimated.

The use of long-term care

A separate equation is used to model the utilization of informal care (I), formal care at home (FH), and formal care in an institutional setting (FI). The dependent variable indicating the use of long-term care services can take the values 0, if the respondent receives no care, and 1, if he or she receives some type of care. The modelling for the use of each type of care is, thus, simply a discrete choice model. We opted for a probit specification. Model (Equation 15.5) specifies the use of informal care, formal care at home, and institutional care. It is given by using the same notation as before:

$$U_I^{t*} = g^t \gamma_I^1 + x^t \gamma_I^2 + y^t \gamma_I^3 + \alpha_I + u_I^t$$

$$U_{FH}^{t*} = g^t \gamma_{FH}^1 + x^t \gamma_{FH}^2 + y^t \gamma_{FH}^3 + \alpha_{FH} + u_{FH}^t$$

$$U_{FI}^{t*} = g^t \gamma_{FI}^1 + x^t \gamma_{FI}^2 + y^t \gamma_{FI}^3 + \alpha_{FI} + u_{FI}^t \qquad (15.5)$$

where U_I^{t*}, U_{FH}^{t*} and U_{FI}^{t*} are the latent continuous counterpart of the discrete variables U_I^t, U_{fh}^t and U_{FI}^t, and measure the underlying inclination for individuals to receive informal care, formal care at home and institutional care in period t. y^t is the set of the remaining independent variables described in the subsection 'Independent variables'. Individual effects α_I, α_{FH} and α_{FI} are assumed to be normally distributed, to have zero mean, and to be freely correlated. u_I^t, u_{FH}^t and u_{FI}^t are assumed to be independently and normally distributed with mean zero and unit variance. The individual effects are also assumed to be independent of u_I^t, u_{FH}^t and u_{FI}^t. It is important to point out that care alternatives are assumed to be correlated – unobserved determinants of care services being stochastically related. In Model 5, elderly individuals are allowed to opt for a combination of informal and formal services to more adequately meet their needs for care. Because of supply limitations, the needs of some elderly individuals may be unmet. This is represented in our model by N^* strictly greater than zero, and U_I^*, U_{FH}^*, U_{FI}^* smaller than zero.

Endogeneity of health status

The health status of respondents in wave t is characterized by the set of GoM g_k^t, for $k = 1, \ldots, 6$, representing the degree of involvement in specific health dimensions. As discussed above, health status of the elderly is a potentially endogenous variable. Health status affects the need for care, which, in turn, determines whether one is observed to receive some kind of care. The causality may also run in the opposite direction – receiving care may influence observed health status at a given point in time. Furthermore, unobserved individual factors may relate to observed health status, as well as to the need for and the choice of care arrangements. Either way, the GoM g^t in Equations 15.4 and 15.5 will be correlated with the unobservables, and direct estimation of this model would result in biased estimates of the parameters of interest.

In our model, GoM g^t are assumed to be correlated with individual effects α_N, α_I, α_{FH} and α_{FI}, and uncorrelated with u_N, u_I, u_{FH} and u_{FI}. A way to deal with this is to specify the correlation between g^t and the unobserved individual components directly, or to use a fixed effect approach[c]. In the fixed effect approach, the unobservables are allowed to be correlated with the included regressors, but are known to lead (in general) to a large number of nuisance parameters that have to be estimated along with the other parameters of the model. A way to deal with this, in the context of a qualitative choice model, is to use a conditional likelihood approach [2]. The fixed effects are eliminated from the specification by conditioning them on a sufficient statistic. The sum of the individual outcomes of the endogenous variable over the time span (for instance, for informal care, $\Sigma_t U_I^t$) is a sufficient statistic that is known to lead to consistent estimates in the logit model[d]. A drawback of this conditional likelihood approach is that, effectively, only observations for which a change in the endogenous variable has occurred are included in the analyses. In surveys with relatively short time spans, such as ours, this would mean that the majority of the observations need to be dropped from the analyses. Furthermore, as we will discuss below, a significant fraction of our initially selected respondents dies between the two waves. We will argue that this selection mechanism is endogenous in our model, and, therefore, needs to be explicitly modelled. As far as we know, a fixed effect estimator for the logit specification does not exist in the context of a qualitative sample selection model. As an alternative to the fixed effect approach, a random effect approach could be used. The correlation between the individual effects and the GoMs g^t is specified by augmenting the model with a separate model for g^t. However, estimation of an unrestricted model for N, U_I, U_{FH}, U_{FI} and g_k with $k = 1,...,6$ requires evaluation of the integrals of dimension 11, which will make the estimation extremely cumbersome. Moreover, other independent variables, such as income, network size, and the number of housing adaptations are potentially endogenous. This

will further complicate our random effects model and make it even less tractable. Another alternative for estimation of models with potentially endogenous variables has been suggested by Mundlak in 1978 [13]. In this approach, the correlation between individual effects of Equations 15.4 and 15.5 and the included regressors is specified directly. Assume that the individual effects are linearly related to a set of instruments z:

$$\alpha = z'\eta + \bar{\alpha}$$

where η is a set of parameters to be estimated and $\bar{\alpha}$ represents the residuals. Usually, z is taken to be the averages over time of the potentially endogenous variables. In our case, z would include the average GoM $\bar{g}^t$, and, possibly, averages over time of other potentially endogenous variables, such as income, network size, or housing adaptations. An advantage of this approach is that it is relatively simple to implement. A disadvantage is that the linear specification $z'\eta$ may be too restrictive to fully capture the correlation and that, when z includes time averages of the potentially endogenous variables, colinearity of z with x and g may obscure the estimation of the parameters of interest.

In the section 'Results', we will discuss estimates of our model, using the instrumenting procedure suggested by Mundlak [13]. Before that point, we will first discuss the consequences of mortality in the sample for our specification, present the full model, and report some estimation issues.

Correction for mortality between the two waves

A selection equation is added to our model of use of long-term care services to correct for attrition resulting from mortality between the two waves. A significant fraction (22.5%) of the initially selected respondents of our survey is indeed observed not to participate in the second wave. Seventy-nine percent of the 482 non-respondents for the second wave died in the 3-year time period. Mortality between the two waves is related to a range of demographic and socio-economic variables of wave I. The mortality equation is then given by:

$$M^* = x^1\zeta_M + u_M$$

using the same notation as before, and where M^* is the latent continuous counterpart of the discrete variable M and measures the underlying inclination for individuals to stay alive between the two periods. Individuals drop out of the panel (die, $M = 1$) if the latent index $M^* \geq 0$ and stay in the panel ($M = 0$) if the latent index $M^* < 0$.

u_M is assumed to have zero mean and a variance equal to two. As the focus of this paper is not on the determinants of mortality – we refer to Norton [14] for these issues – a reduced form equation is employed.

Full model for long-term care utilization

The complete model, in which we correct for attrition through mortality, combines information on the need for and the use of long-term care services from both waves of the data set. Using the instrumental procedure suggested by Mundlak [13], in which the correlation between individual effects and the included regressors is formulated explicitly, the complete model can be written as:

$$N^{t*} = g^t\beta_N^1 + x_N^t\beta_N^2 + z\eta_N + \overline{\alpha_N} + u_N^t$$

$$U_I^{t*} = g^t\gamma_I^1 + x^t\gamma_I^2 + y^t\gamma_I^3 + z\eta_{U,I} + \overline{\alpha_I} + u_I^t$$

$$U_{FH}^{t*} = g^t\gamma_{FH}^1 + x^t\gamma_{FH}^2 + y^t\gamma_{FH}^3 + z\eta_{U,FH} + \overline{\alpha_{FH}} + u_{FH}^t$$

$$U_{FI}^{t*} = g^t\gamma_{FI}^1 + x^t\gamma_{FI}^2 + y^t\gamma_{FI}^3 + z\eta_{U,FI} + \overline{\alpha_{FI}} + u_{FI}^t$$

$$M^* = x^1\zeta_M + u_M \tag{15.7}$$

with the same notation as before. z is a set of instruments including the averages over time of the GoM g_k^t, for $k = 1,\ldots,5$ of the monthly income, of the network size, and of the number of housing adaptations. Residuals u_N^t, u_I^t, u_{FH}^t and u_{FI}^t for $t = 1, 2$ are assumed to be independently distributed. All individual effects are assumed to be independent of u_N^t, u_I^t, u_{FH}^t and u_{FI}^t. The co-variances between the individual effects and u_M are crucial for the problem at hand, as, when all variances match the score zero, this implies that both the need for and the use of care are distributed independently from mortality, and that, hence, attrition resulting from mortality between wave I and II has no influence on the parameters of interest. It is important to note that the regressors and individual effects are, at present, assumed to be uncorrelated.

Standard likelihood methods are not appropriate for the estimation of Model 7 (Equation 15.7), as its likelihood function does not have any simple analytical form, as shown below. The individual effects are correlated across equations, and their presence, therefore, means that the whole set of equations should be jointly estimated. These individual effects are not observed and must be integrated out, introducing the presence of integrals of high dimension in the likelihood functions. The next subsection presents 'simulated maximum likelihood' methods that allow us to estimate Model 7 (Equation 15.7) by approximating integrals of high dimensions.

ESTIMATION PROCEDURE

As a first step, write u_M in the mortality equation into a part u_{M1} that is correlated with the unobserved individual components of the need and use equations and a part, u_{M2}, that is not. Both u_{M1} and u_{M2} are assumed to be independent of the noises u_N, u_I, u_{FH} and u_{FI}.

The sample likelihood function that needs to be optimized consists of the product of joint probabilities of observed needs for care and uses of care, as well as mortality. More specifically, we can write the likelihood contributions for deceased $M = 0$ and survivors $M = 1$ as:

$$\mathscr{L} = \int_{-\infty}^{+\infty} \cdots \int_{-\infty}^{+\infty} \left[\prod_{M=1} \prod_{N^t=1} f(N^t, M \mid \alpha_N, u_{M1}) \right.$$

$$\times \prod_{M=1} \prod_{N^t>1} f(N^t, U_I^t, U_{FH}^t, U_{FI}^t, M \mid \alpha_N, \alpha_I, \alpha_{FH}, \alpha_{FI}, u_{M1})$$

$$\times \prod_{M=0} \prod_{N^t=1} f(N^1, M \mid \alpha_N, u_{M1})$$

$$\left. \times \prod_{M=0} \prod_{N^t>1} f(N^1, U_I^1, U_{FH}^1, U_{FI}^1, M \mid \alpha_I, \alpha_{FH}, \alpha_{FI}, u_{M1}) \right]$$

$$\times \phi_{0,\Sigma_1}(\alpha_N, \alpha_I, \alpha_{FH}, \alpha_{FI}, u_{M1})\, d\alpha_N\, d\alpha_I\, d\alpha_{FH}\, d\alpha_{FI}\, du_{M1} \tag{15.8}$$

where ϕ_{0,Σ_1} is the multivariate normal density (zero mean and covariance matrix Σ_1) of the time constant unobserved individual effects and of u_{M1}. The unobservables α_N, α_I, α_{FH}, α_{FI} and u_{M1} need to be 'integrated out' of the likelihood, and the likelihood function needs to be optimized with respect to the remaining parameters. Conditional on these unobserved components, each individual contribution to the likelihood boils down to a simple product of univariate densities with unknown parameters β, δ, η and ζ. Using more concise notation, the generic problem for estimation of the model is to evaluate:

$$E(f(N^t, \ldots, M \mid \alpha, u_{M1}))$$

$$= \int_{-\infty}^{\infty} f(N^t, \ldots, M \mid \alpha, u_{M1})\phi_{0,\Sigma_1}(\alpha, u_{M1})\, d\alpha\, du_{M1}$$

where $\alpha = (\alpha_N, \alpha_I, \alpha_{FH}, \alpha_{FI})$. There is no explicit expression for this integral, and optimization of the likelihood function requires simulated maximum likelihood techniques. Simulated maximum likelihood methods [7,23] are based on an approximation of the actual likelihood function. The basic idea is to draw random variables from ϕ_{0,Σ_1} and use these to compute a sample mean of f, conditional on α and u_{M1}. The simulated maximum likelihood estimator of the parameters to be estimated, denoted by θ, is thus given by:

$$\theta_S = \text{Arg max}_\theta \sum_{r=1}^{R} \ln \frac{1}{S} \times \sum_{s=1}^{S} f(N_r^t, \ldots, M_r \mid \alpha_r^s, \omega_{1r}^s, \theta) \quad (15.9)$$

where R is the total number of observations. S accounts for the number of simulations and s indicates each simulation. The following steps should be taken in order to estimate Model 4 (Equation 15.4). First of all, expression for the distribution f conditional on u_{M1} and on the individual effects have to be derived. Second, the random variables u_{M1}, α_N, α_I, α_{FH} and α_{FI} have to be simulated. $S = (\alpha_N, \alpha_I, \alpha_{FH}, \alpha_{FI}, u_{M1})$ is assumed to be normally distributed with expectation zero and covariance matrix Σ_1. It is well-known that matrices can be written as the product $L * L' = \Sigma_1$, where L is an upper triangular matrix. In order to simulate S, we first simulate a matrix ε of standard normally distributed variables. It follows from standard statistical theory that the random variables (L_ε) are normally distributed with expectation zero and variance Σ_1. Coefficients of the matrix L are thus estimated and used to calculate the covariance between u_{M1} and the individual effects. Expression 9 is tractable using available computers. Antithetic acceleration [23] is an effective variance reduction method, and is used in the estimation procedure to reduce the computational time.

It should be added that all independent variables have been scaled by dividing them by the maximum of each variable, so that size of coefficients reflect the relative importance of these variables.

RESULTS

DETERMINANTS OF LONG-TERM CARE NEED AND UTILIZATION

Table 15.2(a) and (b) report parameter estimates for Model 7 (Equation 15.7).

It is important to emphasize that parameters associated with the potentially endogenous variables are not easy to interpret. One way to compute their marginal effects on the latent variables N^*, U_I^*, U_{FH}^* and U_{FI}^*, is given by the following expression:

$$\frac{\partial N^*}{\partial E} = \beta_{N,E} + \frac{\eta_{N,E}}{2}$$

$$\frac{\partial U^*}{\partial E} = \gamma_{U,E} + \frac{\eta_{U,E}}{2} \quad (15.10)$$

where E refers to the set of potentially endogenous variables, i.e. GoM g_k, for $K = 1, \ldots, 5$, monthly income, net-

work size and number of housing adaptations. The two terms composing the marginal effects in Equation 15.10 can be interpreted as a short- and a long-term effect, respectively. The parameters β and η are not reported in Table 15.2(a). Only the total marginal effects, namely $\beta + \eta/2$ of the endogenous variables, as well as their t-values, estimated using the delta method [8], are reported in Table 15.2(a).

Need for care

In the need equation, a positive sign indicates that high values of the included variables are associated with high needs for care. Not surprisingly, age and health disorders are found to be the major determinants of needs for care. After controlling for age and health status, females are found to have a lower need for care than males. Older individuals with higher GoM in pure type IV (serious arthritis), pure type I (chronic obstructive pulmonary diseases and cancer) and pure type V (cardiovascular diseases) face higher risks of needing assistance. Suffering from cognitive disorders or from chronic diseases related to pure type II also increases – but to a lesser extent – the probability of needing care. These diseases are generally not too serious and not typical for the elderly. Finally, individuals with high income tend to have lower needs for long-term care services.

Utilization of care services

Positive coefficients are here associated with greater utilization of care services. Remarkably, the emergence or aggravation of physical disabilities affects negatively the probability of receiving informal care. Pure types I (chronic obstructive pulmonary diseases and cancer), III (cognitively impaired) and at a lesser extent, IV (arthritis), are characterized by serious physical and cognitive limitations. High GoM in these health dimensions are significantly related to lower probabilities of receiving informal care. On the other hand, individuals with higher GoM in pure types IV (arthritis) and V (cardiovascular diseases) have greater uses of formal care, both at home and in an institutional setting. Individuals with higher GoM in pure type III (cognitive impairment) are also observed to have an increased probability of being institutionalized. We refer to the section 'Probabilities of use on long-term care services' for more details.

With respect to age, we find that, after controlling for health status, age is still associated with an increased probability of getting care services. It is noteworthy that the effect of age on use of formal care is stronger than on informal care. Possible explanations for this finding

Table 15.2

(a) Parameter estimates of Model 7 (controlled for region)[a]

Equations	Independent variables	Parameters	t-values
Need	Constant	−3.40	−5.78
	g_1	2.46	12.79
	g_2	0.79	0.79
	g_3	0.88	4.89
	g_4	2.57	5.25
	g_5	2.16	16.98
	Age	3.97	6.98
	Female	−0.55	−3.63
	Education	−0.29	−1.53
	Income	−0.90	−3.71
	l_N	1.05	26.87
Institutional care	Constant	−7.71	−4.30
	g_1	1.09	1.41
	g_2	−0.25	−0.32
	g_3	1.16	2.65
	g_4	1.51	2.67
	g_5	1.35	2.25
	Age	10.79	6.42
	Female	−1.12	−3.10
	Married	−1.88	−3.07
	Network size	−0.56	−0.65
	Degree of urbanization	1.59	0.96
	Education	0.62	1.44
	Income	−2.79	−3.55
	Home care maximum individual payments	3.91	2.95
	Institutional maximum individual payments	−5.79	−2.62
Informal care	Constant	−1.48	−1.65
	g_1	−0.85	−2.86
	g_2	−0.45	−1.51
	g_3	−0.59	−1.79
	g_4	−0.43	−1.87
	g_5	−0.22	−0.82
	Age	2.40	3.10
	Female	−0.34	−1.93
	Living alone	−0.63	−5.33
	Network size	−0.05	−0.12
	Education	−1.40	−4.66
	Income	0.68	1.03
	Degree of urbanization	−0.35	−0.27
	Housing adaptations	−0.24	−0.73
	Home care maximum individual payments	0.11	0.24
	Institutional maximum individual payments	−0.53	−0.78
Formal care at home	Constant	−6.62	−6.95
	g_1	0.51	1.62
	g_2	0.02	0.07
	g_3	−0.29	−0.90
	g_4	0.80	3.25
	g_5	0.53	1.95
	Age	5.03	6.05
	Female	0.35	1.82
	Living alone	0.67	5.50
	Network size	0.79	1.64
	Degree of urbanization	−0.14	−0.12
	Education	1.08	3.85
	Income	0.27	1.86
	Housing adaptations	0.79	1.64

Table 15.2 *(cont.)*

(a) Parameter estimates of Model 7 (controlled for region)[a]

Equations	Independent variables	Parameters	*t*-values
	Home care maximum individual payments	−0.91	−2.10
	Institutional maximum individual payments	1.51	2.61
Attrition	Constant	−6.49	−8.44
	Age	7.38	9.90
	Female	−0.87	−4.29
	Education	−0.37	−1.48
	Income	−0.61	−1.90

(b) Covariance matrix of Model 7; *t*-values in parentheses (calculated using the delta method)

$$
\begin{bmatrix}
1 & -0.16 & 0.20 & 0.29 & -0.39 \\
  & (-1.91) & (3.10) & (6.93) & (-11.52) \\
  & 1 & -0.18 & -0.08 & -0.36 \\
  & & (-1.73) & (-0.84) & (-3.31) \\
  & & 1 & -0.81 & -0.29 \\
  & & & (-10.73) & (-4.00) \\
  & & & 1 & -0.06 \\
  & & & & (-8.76) \\
  & & & & 1
\end{bmatrix}
$$

[a]Only the total effect of the endogenous variables is reported here (*t*-values calculated using the delta method).

include the fact that the oldest old needs more formal care, as he or she becomes more vulnerable. Not surprisingly, age is a very strong predictor for being in an institution.

After controlling for age differences, health status and living situation, women are found to have lower risks of being institutionalized than men. Women are also less likely to receive informal care. It is likely that women are more able to perform domestic tasks, and they, therefore, need less domestic assistance than men. Moreover, it is observed that elderly care recipients living alone have been found to receive considerably less informal assistance and more professional care than those sharing a household. Likewise, being married is significantly associated with a lower probability of being in an institution for the elderly. Married people are also more likely to have children, another source of information care, and this, in addition to the presence of a partner, may keep elderly people out of residential or nursing homes.

A positive effect of the network size on the probability of getting informal care would be expected, but is not observed. The social network is defined in our study by the children, family members, friends and neighbours with whom the elderly individual has regular contacts. A likely explanation is that most of the informal care is given within the household, namely by the co-residents of the elderly (for instance, the partner or resident siblings). The effect of network size on informal care is likely to

already be taken into account with the variable 'living alone'.

Residence in urban areas does not significantly affect the use of care services and, therefore, access to formal or informal care does not seem to be related to the degree of urbanization where elderly individuals live.

Significant effects are found for higher education levels and incomes. Higher education levels seem to increase the probability of getting formal care at home, at the expense of informal care. This could be related to the relative price of informal care, for two possible reasons. First, it is conceivable that educated people are more likely to have educated children, with a relatively high wage rate, and that, therefore, the opportunity cost to provide information care is higher for highly educated children. The second reason is related – educated children are likely to have less time available for caregiving, and may not live in proximity to their parents. In addition to issues related to the relative price of informal care, another possible explanation is that less educated elderly people may have less access to information about their options for formal care, and may not use the information they have as efficiently as more educated people.

Higher incomes positively influence the probability of getting formal care at home instead of in an institutional setting. People with higher financial resources may be willing to pay out-of-pocket for home help, supporting equipment and house adaptations, in order to remain at home as long as possible. Housing adaptations are significantly associated with a higher probability of getting formal care at home. Having housing adaptations, in combination with formal care, may help the elderly to remain at home as long as possible.

Finally, it can be seen that individual financial contributions have an additional effect on utilization of formal care after controlling for income levels. The results are in line with what one would expect *a priori*. Higher out-of-pocket costs for domestic assistance increase the probability of being in an institution and affect negatively the probability of getting home care. On the other hand, individuals with higher institutional charges are more likely to receive home care and less likely to live in an institution. The two products appear to be substitutes. As the individual charges are income-related, the relative price of public long-term care compared with private help is considerably higher for wealthier individuals. This is an additional incentive for people with higher incomes to purchase private help. For this, we may conclude that utilization of formal care seems price-sensitive, even when individual contributions are, as in the Netherlands, income-related. Consequently, price policies may be effective in controlling care service utilization.

Recently, regulations concerning out-of-pocket costs for formal care have been changed. We computed some simulations related to changes in formal individual charges. To compute these simulations, the contributions for each type of formal care are successively decreased and increased by 10%. The own-price elasticity of institutional care equals -2.15% for males and -2.55% for females, whereas the own-price elasticity of domestic formal care equals -0.08% for males and -0.07% for females. On the other hand, cross-price elasticities for institutional care equal 2.55% for males and 1.33% for men and women, respectively, while these are equal to 0.18% for men and 0.16% for women for formal care at home. These numbers are based on calculations for an individual of 85 years. It can be concluded that care use is inelastic, and that the price elasticities for domestic formal care are relatively small compared with the ones for institutional care. Therefore, use of institutional care is relatively more price-sensitive than utilization of formal care at home. Moreover, it can be concluded that changes in the prices of institutional care affect most the use of formal care, both at home and in an institutional setting.

Attrition

The parameters affecting mortality between waves I and II should be interpreted with caution, as the mortality equation is a reduced form specification – and, hence,

little can be concluded from the sign of the coefficients of the included variables. We find strong effects on mortality for age, gender, and, to a lesser extent, income and education level.

Covariance structure

With respect to the covariance structure, it is worth recalling that the covariance matrix Σ_1 of Model 4 (Equation 15.4) is given by the outer-product of the upper triangular matrix L. Σ_1 is a $5 * 5$ matrix, describing the covariance structure between u_{M1}, α_N, α_I, α_{FH} and α_{FI}. Matrix Σ_1 can easily be computed using $\Sigma_1 = LL'$, and the t-values can be computed using the delta method. Most of the covariances between u_{M1} and the individual effects are statistically significant, implying that mortality, need for care and use of care are stochastically related – and that, by consequence, the exclusion of deceased respondents in panel data analyses of use of care will lead to biased estimates. Consequently, attrition resulting from mortality must be taken into account in the estimation of models of use of long-term care services (see Table 15.2(b)).

PROBABILITIES OF USE OF LONG-TERM CARE SERVICES

To make the results of the previous subsections more insightful, one can calculate probabilities of getting care per age/gender groups. These probabilities are computed for all pure types, as well as for an individual with an 'average' health status (i.e. whose GoM in each health dimension equal the same averages frequencies). The results of these calculations are reported in Table 15.3(a)–(c).

First of all, age is a very strong predictor of institutionalization, as risks are multiplied by a factor of approximately 100 between the ages of 75 and 90. It can also be seen that the risks of institutionalization are low compared with those of getting formal care at home. Further, men enter old people's homes at lower ages than women. the probability of being institutionalized is significantly different from zero from the age of 75 for females and 70 for males. It is noteworthy that the risks of institutionalization of a male and a 5-years older female are quite similar for all health dimensions. Men face higher risks of being institutionalized than women – especially at younger ages. At age 75, the probability of men to be in an old people's home is at least five times higher than the one for women. This factor decreases to 2.5 when individuals are 90 years of age. A likely explanation for this finding is that men, in the case of death of the spouse, are not longer

Table 15.3

(a) Probabilities of institutional care (%)

	Female						Male					
	I	II	III	IV	V	Average health status	I	II	III	IV	V	Average health status
65	—	—	—	—	—	—	—	—	—	—	—	—
70	—	—	—	—	—	—	0.10	—	—	—	0.05	—
75	0.10	—	0.02	0.06	0.06	—	0.51	—	0.16	0.37	0.39	0.05
80	0.60	—	0.20	0.46	0.47	0.07	2.51	0.04	1.02	2.05	2.11	0.42
85	2.91	0.05	1.21	2.41	2.48	0.51	9.15	0.30	4.54	7.89	8.04	2.23
90	10.33	0.40	5.24	8.95	9.12	2.62	24.15	1.65	14.44	21.70	22.01	8.40

(b) Probabilities of informal care (%)

	I	II	III	IV	V	Average health status	I	II	III	IV	V	Average health status
65	7.22	25.27	11.98	16.64	37.90	24.73	9.84	31.62	15.69	21.19	44.45	30.34
70	9.35	30.61	15.01	20.37	43.33	29.35	12.49	36.75	19.28	25.47	50.20	35.40
75	11.91	35.68	18.51	24.56	48.88	34.35	15.60	42.14	23.35	30.16	55.58	40.73
80	14.93	41.02	22.48	29.17	54.45	39.62	19.19	47.67	27.84	35.20	61.04	46.23
85	18.42	46.53	26.89	34.15	59.94	45.10	23.24	53.25	32.72	40.52	66.29	51.81
90	22.38	52.11	31.70	39.42	65.24	50.67	27.72	58.76	37.92	46.52	72.23	57.35

(c) Probabilities of formal care at home (%)

	I	II	III	IV	V	Average health status	I	II	III	IV	V	Average health status
65	18.89	5.81	10.42	31.71	18.52	14.57	14.55	4.05	7.61	25.79	14.23	10.95
70	27.83	10.88	16.75	42.78	27.36	22.32	22.30	7.34	12.75	36.09	21.89	17.48
75	38.43	16.27	25.14	54.45	37.90	32.01	31.98	12.36	19.93	47.52	31.48	26.06
80	49.98	24.53	35.33	65.75	49.43	43.10	43.08	13.39	29.11	59.16	42.53	36.40
85	61.54	34.62	46.71	75.79	61.01	54.78	54.76	28.45	39.88	70.04	54.20	47.85
90	72.15	45.95	58.37	83.97	71.70	66.05	66.03	39.14	51.49	79.37	65.52	59.48

able to remain at home, mainly because of lack of house-keeping capabilities. Results also show that the probability of getting informal care is higher for males than for females. Men receive relatively more informal care at older ages than at younger ages. This finding may be explained by the higher needs of men for housekeeping assistance, possibly intensified by a generation effect – namely that the eldest old may have less experience with housekeeping tasks than the youngest elderly. Suffering from health disorders related to pure type I – i.e. physical disabilities, respiratory diseases, and cancer – most increase the probability of being institutionalized. Surprisingly, the probability of receiving informal care for pure type I is very low compared with other health dimensions – especially at younger ages. For a male with an average health status, the probability of receiving informal care at age 65 is three times higher than for a pure type I. This factor decreases to 2 above the age of 80. These numbers are even higher for females. On the other hand, pure type I is very likely to receive both types of formal care compared with other health dimensions. One may then conclude that the health disorders associated with pure type I require professional assistance. A similar effect of pure

type V – i.e. cardiovascular diseases – on the probability of getting informal care would be expected, but is not observed. A likely explanation is that health disorders associated with fifth health dimension are not responsible for severe physical disabilities, and individuals with high GoM in pure type V may be supported by informal assistance only. However, a look at the probabilities for formal care at home associated with this dimension shows that pure types V also face very high risks of getting formal care. Therefore, one may conclude that individuals with high GoM in the fifth dimension need a combination of informal and formal care to meet their care requirements. It is noteworthy that pure type II is very likely to receive informal care compared with other health dimensions. As a matter of fact, he or she receives relatively (very) little formal assistance. In consequence, it may be concluded that informal care is generally sufficient to support individuals with health disorders associated with health dimension II. Finally, pure type IV is found to demand on the average much formal and informal care.

Table 15.4 Probabilities of non-use of care by the elderly with needs for care (%)

	Male						Female					
	I	II	III	IV	V	Average health status	I	II	III	IV	V	Average health status
65	33.59	17.68	11.83	36.42	32.99	18.91	39.39	22.00	13.08	37.33	35.83	21.75
70	29.82	17.89	12.70	30.40	29.88	19.42	35.00	22.89	13.36	30.23	31.54	21.76
75	24.66	16.99	12.96	22.96	24.71	18.69	28.96	22.47	12.81	21.94	25.17	20.28
80	18.97	15.07	12.32	15.56	18.51	16.58	22.21	20.59	11.36	14.15	17.98	17.30
85	13.29	12.35	10.72	9.13	12.13	13.25	15.41	17.13	9.11	7.83	11.14	13.15
90	8.39	9.27	8.36	4.59	6.86	9.34	9.54	12.78	6.56	3.68	5.90	8.74

PROBABILITIES OF NON-USE OF CARE BY THE ELDERLY WITH NEEDS FOR CARE

One can also calculate the probabilities that individuals with a need for care receive neither informal nor formal services. There are several reasons why specific needs may not be met. First of all, elderly individuals may have a need for long-term care services, but still decide not to pursue or use care. This may be a result of perceived supply restrictions, but these individuals may also simply not know that they have access to care, or they may have already been rejected in the past and think that they still will not meet the eligibility threshold of the committee. Alternatively, they may be satisfied to live with their health problems without seeking care. Second, they may have expressed their demand for care, but have not received a positive recommendation from the state committees. Finally, individuals with a positive recommendation may have been put on a waiting list because of supply restrictions. For those individuals with a need for care, Table 15.4 shows the probabilities of not receiving any type of care at all – by health categories, age and gender.

First of all, it is worth recalling that about 20% of our respondents aged 65–85 that have needs do not receive any kinds of care services. In Table 15.4, about 22% of individuals aged 65, with an average health status, do not receive the care that they need. This percentage equals 13% at age 85. It can also be seen that, within each disease type, the oldest disabled have a higher probability of receiving some type of care than their younger counterparts. This could be partially a result of an age effect in the recommendation process of the state committees and to the actual selection process determined by the market. In other words, both the committee and institutions are predisposed to accepting the elder old – perhaps because care of these individuals is likely to have a shorter duration than for younger individuals, and, therefore, less impact both on costs and available capacity. Among the categories, at younger ages, individuals with arthritis (health dimension IV) are less likely to receive some type of care, but this pattern is reversed at older ages, where those with arthritis have more chance of obtaining care. In addition, we find that pure types V – individuals who suffer from cancer and/or respiratory diseases – are more likely to not receive care than others. Also, women are, in general, more likely to be denied care than are men, at all ages.

CONCLUSION

This paper proposes a characterization of the determinants of long-term care services utilization by the Dutch elderly. Major findings of these analyses may be summarized as follows. Emergence or aggravation of physical disabilities affects negatively the probability of receiving informal care. Individuals with higher GoM in pure types IV and V do have greater needs for formal care, both at home and in an institutional setting. Individuals with higher GoM in pure type III are also observed to have an increased probability of being institutionalized. Age is a major predictor of utilization of care services, especially of institutional care. After controlling for age differences, women are found to have lower risks of being institutionalized than men. Women are also less likely to receive informal care, and more likely to receive formal care at home. Significant effects are found for higher education levels and incomes. Higher education levels seem to increase the probability of getting formal care at the expense of informal care. Higher incomes positively influence the probability of getting formal care at home instead of in an institutional setting. Individual contributions have an additional effect on utilization of formal care after controlling for income levels. As a consequence, utilization of formal care seems to be price-sensitive, even when individual contributions are, as in the Netherlands, income-related.

ACKNOWLEDGEMENTS

The Longitudinal Ageing Study Amsterdam (LASA) kindly allowed us to use their data. The LASA study is mainly financed from a long-term grant from the Dutch Ministry of Health, Welfare and Sports. This paper has benefited substantially from the comments and suggestions of Edward C. Norton, Owen O'Donnell. Nol Merkies and two anonymous referees of this journal. We furthermore knowledge the valuable comments of the participants of the *Eighth European Workshop on Econometrics and Health Economics*.

NOTES

a. These individuals are given either a score 1 or 2, as it is not known which degree of impairment they actually experience. This is accounted for in the likelihood function of our model (see section 'Estimation procedure').

b. The Social and Cultural Agency (in Dutch: Sociaal en Cultureel Planbureau) kindly allowed us to use their operating procedure to calculate monthly maximum individual payments associated with different kinds of long-term care services [21].

c. This approach is only feasible in the context of a logit model.

d. An equivalent expression can be obtained by concentration of the likelihood with respect to the individual parameters.

REFERENCES

1. Beekman, A., Deeg, D., Braam, A., Smit, J. and van Tilburg, W. Consequences of depression in later life: associations of major and minor depression with disability, well-being, and service utilization. *Psychol. Med.* 1997; **27**: 1397–1409.
2. Chamberlain, G. Analysis of covariance with qualitative data. *Am. Economic Rev., Papers Proc.* 1980; **47**: 225–238.
3. Central Bureau of Statistics. Population Structure at 1 January 1999 Report (in Dutch), 1999.
4. Coughlin, T., McBride, T.D., Perozek, M. and Liu, K. Home care for the disabled elderly: predictors and expected costs. *Health Serv. Res.* 1992; **27**; 453–479.
5. Deeg, D.J.H. and Westendorp de Serière, M. Autonomy and well-being in the ageing population. In *Report from the Longitudinal Ageing Study Amsterdam 1992–1993*, Deeg, D.J.H. and Westendorp de Serière, M. (eds). VU University Press: Amsterdam, 1994.
6. Deeg, D.J.H., Beekman, A.T.F., Kriegsman, D.M.W. and Westendorp de Serière, M. Autonomy and well-being in the ageing population 2. In *Report from the Longitudinal Ageing Study Amsterdam 1992–1996*, Deeg, D.J.H., Beekman,

A.T.F., Kriegsman, D.M.W. and Westendorp de Serière, M. (eds). VU University Press: Amsterdam, 1998.
7. Gourieroux, C. and Monfort, A. *Simulation Based Econometric Methods.* Core Lecture Series. Oxford University Press: Oxford, 1994.
8. Greene, W.H. *Econometric Analysis.* Prentice Hall: Englewood Cliffs, NJ, 1993.
9. Grossman, M. *The Demand for Health: A Theoretical and Empirical Investigation.* National Bureau of Economic Research, vol. 39. University of Chicago: Chicago, 1972; 77–86.
10. Huijsman, R. A model for care facilities for the elderly (in Dutch), Thesis. Rijksuniversiteit Limbrug, 1990.
11. Manton, K.G. and Woodbury, M.A. A new procedure for analysis of medical classification. *Methods Inf. Med.* 1982; **21**: 210–220.
12. Manton, K.G., Woodbury, M.A., Stallard, E. and Corder, L.S. The use of grade of membership techniques to estimate regression relationships. *Sociol. Methodol.* 1992; **10**: 321–379.
13. Munklak, Y. On the pooling of time series and cross section data. *Econometrica* 1978; **46**: 69–85.
14. Norton, E. Long-term care. In *Handbook of Health Economics*, Culyer, A.J. and Newhouse, J.P. (eds). North Holland: Amsterdam, 2000; 21.
15. Pezzin, L., Kemper, P. and Reschovsky, J. Does publicly provided home care substitute for family care? *J. Human Res.* 1996; **XXXI**(3): 650–676.
16. Portrait, F., Lindeboom, M. and Deeg, D.J.H. Health and mortality of the elderly: the grade of membership method, classification and determination. *Health Economics* 1999; **8**: 441–457.
17. Portrait, F. Long-term care services for the Dutch elderly – an investigation into the process of utilization, Thesis. Vrije Universiteit, Amsterdam, Forthcoming (in press).
18. Robert, S. and House, J.H. SES differentials in health by age and alternative indicators of SES. *J. Ageing Health* 1996; **8**: 359–388.
19. Schrijvers, A. (ed.). *Health and Health Care in the Netherlands: A Critical Self-assessment by Dutch Experts in the Medical and Health Sciences.* De tijdstroom: Utrecht, Netherlands, 1997.
20. Sociaal en Cultureel Planbureau. *A Forecasting Model for the Health Care Services* (in Dutch). Sociaal en Centraal Planbureau: The Hague, Netherlands, 1999.
21. Stuurgroep Toekomstscenario's Gezondheidszorg. *The Elderly Population in 2005: Health and Care* (in Dutch). Stuurgroep Toekomstscenario's Gezondheidszorg: Houten, Netherlands, 1992.
22. Stern, S. Simulation-based estimation. *J. Economic Lit.* 1997; **XXXV**: 2006–2039.
23. Tilburg, T. Delineation of the social network and differences in network size. In *Living Arrangements and Social Networks of Older Adults in the Netherlands*, Knipscheer, C.P.M. (ed.). VU University Press: Amsterdam, 1995.
24. Wielink, G. *Elderly community resident's preference for care. A study of choices and determinants in hypothetical care – need situations*, Dissertation. Vrije Universiteit, Ridderprint, Ridderkerk, 1997.

16

HMO Selection and Medicare Costs: Bayesian MCMC Estimation of a Robust Panel Data Tobit Model with Survival

BARTON H. HAMILTON

Olin School of Business, Washington University in St. Louis, St. Louis, MO, USA

INTRODUCTION

Since the mid-1980s, an increasing proportion of the US Medicare population has chosen to enrol in health maintenance organizations (HMOs), with the fraction reaching 17% in 1997. HMOs have been promoted as a cost-containment measure, since most HMOs receive a fixed fee per patient (capitation). Capitation provides strong financial incentives to avoid unnecessary health care expenditures [1]. In addition, it is argued that HMO contracts align the incentives of physicians, hospitals and insurers, which should also help to restrain health care costs relative to those incurred by individuals in traditional fee for service (FFS) arrangements.

Despite the rapid growth in managed care in public health insurance programmes (Medicare and Medicaid) in the US, debate still exists as to whether HMOs constrain costs. A literature review by Miller and Luft [2] indicates that patients in HMOs generally had shorter lengths of stay, used fewer procedures and tests, and tended to receive less costly alternative interventions for conditions such as heart disease when compared to those in FFS. In a study of children covered by Medicaid, Goldman *et al.* [3] found that HMOs reduced expenditures relative to FFS. Finally, Baker [4] found that markets with higher HMO market share have lower expenditures. It is often claimed that these HMO cost savings simply reflect 'cream-skimming' on the part of HMOs, in which relatively healthy patients are enrolled into the managed care plan. For example, Morgan *et al.* [5] found that in the year prior to enrolment, the rate of use of inpatient services among future HMO members was only 66% of that for individuals remaining in FFS in southern Florida. Strumwasser *et al.* [6] found that employees switching to HMOs in a large firm tended to have lower health service utilization rates prior to the change. In addition, due to capitation, HMOs may have a strong financial incentive to disenrol high cost members from the plan [7].

This paper examines the role of selection in HMO enrolment between 1984 and 1991 for a random sample of 3876 Medicare recipients in the US aged 54+ in 1984 who were not initially HMO members. The panel nature of the data helps to identify the selection effect, since actual non-HMO health care expenditures are observed both pre- and post-enrolment for individuals who enrol in HMOs. Previous studies have generally relied on cross-sectional comparisons of HMO and non-HMO enrolees, which forces the analyst to make strong modelling assumptions with regard to what the health care expenditures of HMO enrolees would have been had they not in fact been in the HMO [3]. It is also difficult to assess selection effects using market level data, since the expenditures of individuals entering and leaving HMOs are not observed. The panel data approach presented here is used to quantify the selection effect by comparing the health care expenditures of prospective HMO members with other individuals in the sample prior to enrolment. The paper also examines the expenditures of individuals after they leave the HMO to determine whether high cost patients are disenroled.

A second issue, which arises when examining older (65+) individuals in a longitudinal setting, is that some individuals die over the course of the panel. Unobserved

Econometric Analysis of Health Data. Edited by Andrew M. Jones and Owen O'Donnell
© 2002 John Wiley & Sons Ltd. Previously published in *Health Economics*, Vol. 8; pp. 403–414 (1999). © John Wiley & Sons Ltd

(by the econometrician) characteristics affecting mortality are likely to be correlated with those that influence expenditure, since it is often claimed that health care expenditures are highest in the last year of life. Consequently, Medicare expenditures and mortality must be modelled jointly. In addition, the fact that many individuals have zero health care costs in a given year must be incorporated into the empirical model. One method is to model expenditures using a tobit framework, although other approaches have been taken in the literature. Finally, the longitudinal nature of the data allows the model to incorporate individual-specific differences in health care expenditures and mortality.

While classical methods for the estimation of the mixed tobit–probit model described above are available, such simultaneous equation limited dependent variable panel data problems are easily handled using Bayesian Markov Chain Monte Carlo (MCMC) simulation methods. The MCMC approach avoids high dimensional integration required by classical maximum likelihood methods. The Bayesian implementation of the model in this paper follows Chib's [8] analysis of the tobit model, and Chib and Greenberg's [9] simulation of the multivariate probit model. The model is also related to Cowles *et al.*'s [10] tobit model with non-random attrition. Because a preliminary examination of the data indicated the expenditure distribution was fat-tailed, the model differs from these previous approaches in that the disturbances are assumed to follow a multivariate *t* distribution rather than a normal one.

The results show that prior to enrolment, prospective HMO members had lower probabilities of positive health care expenditures. However, no evidence is found in this data set that HMOs disenrol high cost patients. Consequently, over the late 1980s and early 1990s, at least a portion of the difference in costs between HMO and non-HMO plans reflects cream-skimming effects rather than real cost-containment.

DATA AND INITIAL EVIDENCE

This paper analyses data from the 1982 New Beneficiary Survey (NBS), a random sample of newly eligible Social Security recipients in the US conducted by the Social Security Administration. These data were linked to administrative data on yearly Medicare expenditures covering the period 1984–1991 for each NBS sample member. These individuals tended to be between 65 and 70 years old, with a few aged 71+. The data set contains detailed information on demographics, health conditions, income, and assets of the sample members in 1982–1983. Demographics include age, years of education, gender and race.

Information on the number and type of health conditions, the number of days the individual had been ill in the previous year, and whether the individual had ever had a heart attack was also collected. Finally, asset information includes the net wealth of the sample member's household and whether he or she owns their house.

The individual level survey data is merged with administrative data from the Social Security Administration's Master Beneficiary Record and the Health Care Financing Administration's Medicare Automated Data Retrieval System of Medicare bills and enrolment. The administrative data provides information on the sample member's total Medicare charged expenditures (inpatient, outpatient, physician, home health, hospice and skilled nursing charges) for each year between 1984 and 1991. To cross-validate this data, a comparison of the number of hospital days with inpatient expenditures indicated that the correlation between the two variables was 0.883, suggesting the charge data accurately measures resource utilization. Finally, note that although Medicare may not recover all the charged expenditures, expenditures provide the best available measure of resource utilization by the individual.

The administrative data also lists the number of months of Medicare Part A and Part B coverage in each year, and whether the individual was enrolled in a HMO in each year. Medicare Part A covers inpatient hospital care, and some home health and nursing home services, while Part B covers outpatient, physician and hospice services. While Part B requires a small co-payment, virtually all sample members receive this coverage. Finally, the administrative data indicates the month and year of death, if mortality occurred between 1984 and 1991. The sample used here is limited to individuals who were not enrolled in a HMO in 1984, since pre-HMO enrolment health care expenditures are required to assess the selection effect. All expenditures are deflated to 1984 dollars using the Medical Care component for Urban Consumers in the Consumer Price Index.

Unfortunately, the health care expenditures of HMO members during their enrolment period is only sporadically reported. Consequently, the question of whether HMO expenditures are lower than non-HMO expenditures cannot be addressed directly. However, expenditures pre- and post-enrolment are reported accurately, as is mortality during the HMO enrolment (and non-enrolment) period.

After merging the survey and administrative databases, approximately 7% of the sample members had at least 1 year in which they reported zero months of Medicare Part A (and Part B) coverage. In many cases, these patients also reported positive Medicare expenditures for inpatient care, outpatient services, etc., in the same year, since Part A participation and Medicare expenditures are recovered from different administrative data files. Unfortunately, it was impossible to obtain HMO enrolment information for these individuals because Part A participation was not reported, so they were deleted from the sample. Little difference was found in the Medicare expenditures of the deleted group compared to those observations included in the sample, so their exclusion is unlikely to affect the results. After excluding the observations with missing Part A coverage information, the sample consists of 3876 individuals and 28 078 individual-year observations.

INITIAL EVIDENCE OF THE HMO SELECTION EFFECT

In order to investigate the magnitudes of pre- and post-enrolment selection effects, average monthly Medicare expenditures and mortality probabilities in each year from 1984 to 1991 are first examined. Let HMO_{it} equal 1 if individual i is enrolled in a HMO in year t, and 0 otherwise. Column (1) in Panel A of Table 16.1 shows that the average Medicare expenditures of non-HMO members is approximately $206 per month, with almost three-quarters of the individuals experiencing positive expenditure. While expenditure data is not reliably reported for HMO members, comparison of columns (1) and (2) shows that HMO enrolees are less likely to die in the current year, indicating that they are in better health. Column (3) of Panel A also provides evidence of non-random selection into HMOs. In the year prior to HMO enrolment,

the average expenditures of prospective HMO members was $100, about half of that shown in column (1). However, the probability of some positive expenditure was only slightly lower. Finally, in the year following disenrolment, the expenditure of former HMO members is higher than that of individuals not enrolled in the HMO. However, this might be somewhat misleading, since disenrolment occurs later in the panel when costs are likely to be higher due to advanced age and poorer health.

To provide additional information on the potential selection effect, Panel B of Table 16.1 summarizes the 1984 expenditures of individuals subsequently enrolling in HMOs versus those who do not. Recall that in the sample, no one is a member of a HMO in 1984. The first row of Panel B shows that in 1984 the average expenditures of individuals who subsequently enrol in a HMO is substantially less than the expenditures of individuals who do not, while the bottom row shows that the probability of positive expenditure is roughly the same. Consequently, it can be concluded from Table 16.1 that HMOs appear to be selecting low expenditure individuals for enrolment.

To examine whether the HMO selection effects shown in Panel B of Table 16.1 are reflected in the observed characteristics of sample members, Table 16.2 breaks down the demographic, health status and asset data as of the 1983–1984 baseline by prospective HMO status. Entries in Table 16.2 indicate little difference across prospective HMO status for the demographic and asset variables. However, it does appear to be the case that HMOs enrol individuals who are in better health, as indicated by the lower number of health problems, fewer days ill in 1983,

Table 16.1 Summary measures of Medicare expenditures and mortality

	Panel A: All individual-year observations			
	$HMO_{it} = 0$	$HMO_{it} = 1$	$HMO_{it} = 0$, $HMO_{it+1} = 1$	$HMO_{it-1} = 1$, $HMO_{it} = 0$
Variable	(1)	(2)	(3)	(4)
Average monthly expenditures (in year t)	206.1 (971.7)	—	100.2 (519.2)	304.9 (964.3)
Fraction of expenditures >0	0.73	—	0.65	0.74
Fraction died in year t	0.029	0.018	—	0.05
n	26 368	1710	274	120

	Panel B: 1984 data	
	Enrols in HMO in future year	Never in HMO in panel
	(1)	(2)
Average monthly expenditures (in 1984)	97.3 (504.5)	168.9 (822.6)
Fraction of expenditures >0	0.60	0.62
n	266	3610

SD in parentheses.

Table 16.2 Summary statistics, measured at baseline in 1983–1984

Variable	Enrols in HMO in future year (1)	Never in HMO in Panel (2)
Age	67.9 (2.2)*	68.2 (2.5)
Education (years)	11.3 (3.1)	11.2 (3.3)
Male	0.49	0.48
White	0.89	0.88
# Health problems	1.71 (1.48)**	1.96 (1.68)
Days ill in past year	5.60 (22.18)	6.56 (27.09)
Heart problem	0.35	0.38
Previous myocardial infarction	0.08***	0.11
Net worth/1000	100.4 (325.7)	99.6 (217.4)
Own home	9.76	0.78
n	266	3610

SD in parentheses.
*Difference between columns statistically significant at the 0.05 level.
**Difference between columns statistically significant at the 0.01 level.
***Difference between columns statistically significant at the 0.10 level.

and lower incidences of heart conditions and previous myocardial infarctions (heart attacks) as of 1984. These differences may account for some of the variation across HMO status observed in Table 16.1, and are controlled for in the model below.

A TOBIT MODEL OF MEDICARE EXPENDITURES WITH SURVIVAL

This section describes the econometric framework for jointly modelling individual health care expenditures and mortality. Joint estimation of these outcomes is important in this case since unobservables, such as health status, which increase mortality in any time period are also likely to increase Medicare expenditures. Consequently, attrition from the sample (through death) is likely to be correlated with expenditure [11]. The model is similar to Cowles et al.'s [10] framework for analysing compliance in the Lung Health Study in that it exploits the panel nature of the data by incorporating individual-specific, time-invariant random effects to account for correlations over time in an individual's expenditures and mortality probabilities.

To begin, let y_{1it} denote average monthly total Medicare health care expenditure for individual i, $i = 1, \ldots, n$ in year t, $t = 1, \ldots, T_i$. For all individuals, time period $t = 1$ refers to 1984. The notation T_i refers to the fact that some individuals die between 1984 and 1991. For those who survive over the course of the sample period, $T_i = 8$. Note

that y_{1i} is censored at zero for individuals with no health care expenditures in year t. The dichotomous variable y_{2it} indicates whether individual i died in year t.

As in any limited dependent variable problem, it is useful to write the model in terms of the latent dependent variables. Let y_{1it}^* denote the latent Medicare expenditures of individual i in year t, and specify the expenditure equation as

$$y_{1it}^* = \alpha_1 H_{1it} + x_{it}\beta_1 + b_{1i} + \varepsilon_{1it}, \quad (16.1a)$$

where H_{1it} is a vector of HMO enrolment indicators, described in greater detail below, α_1 is the corresponding coefficient vector describing the impact of HMO enrolment status on expenditures, and x_{it} is a vector of demographic, health status and asset variables thought to affect expenditures, with associated coefficient vectors β_1. b_{1i} is a individual-specific random intercept, which allows yearly Medicare expenditures to be correlated over time. Finally, ε_{1it} is period-specific error term. Latent Medicare expenditures map into observed expenditures according to:

$$y_{1it} = \begin{cases} y_{1it}^* & \text{if } y_{1it}^* > 0 \\ 0 & \text{if } y_{1it}^* \le 0 \end{cases}.$$

Equation 16.1a thus specifies a panel data tobit model with a random intercept.

Mortality is modelled using a probit framework. Let y_{2it}^* be the latent propensity of individual i to die in year t. The mortality equation may then be written as:

$$y_{2it}^* = \alpha_2 H_{2it} + x_{it}\beta_2 + b_{2i} + \varepsilon_{2it}. \quad (16.1b)$$

As above, H_{2it} is a vector of HMO enrolment indicators, and α_2 is the corresponding coefficient vector describing the impact of HMO enrolment on mortality. The vector x_{it} consists of demographic, health status, and asset variables with associated coefficient vector β_2. b_{2i} is an individual-specific random intercept and ε_{2it} is a period-specific error term. In the usual probit fashion, individuals are observed to die if the latent propensity is positive:

$$y_{2it} = I[y_{2it}^* > 0],$$

where $I[.] = 1$ if the expression in square brackets holds, and 0 otherwise. Equation 16.1b thus specifies a random intercept panel data probit model.

Since unobserved characteristics that affect Medicare expenditure may be correlated with those influencing mortality, the period-specific random error terms from Equations 16.1a and b are assumed to be jointly normally distributed with mean zero and variance

$$Var\begin{pmatrix}\varepsilon_{1it}\\\varepsilon_{2it}\end{pmatrix} = \Sigma = \begin{Bmatrix}\sigma_{11} & \sigma_{12}\\\sigma_{12} & 1\end{Bmatrix}. \tag{16.2}$$

Finally, to complete the model, distributional assumptions must be made for the individual-specific random intercepts. The random effects in Equations 16.1a and b are assumed to be jointly normally distributed, so that

$$\begin{Bmatrix}b_{1i}\\b_{2i}\end{Bmatrix} \sim N(0, D), \text{ where } D = \begin{Bmatrix}d_{11} & d_{12}\\d_{12} & d_{22}\end{Bmatrix}. \tag{16.3}$$

This specification allows further correlation between expenditures and mortality.

The parameters of the model to be estimated are β ($= [\alpha_1\beta_1\alpha_2\beta_2]$), Σ and D. The general form of the observed data likelihood is given by

$$L(\beta, \Sigma, D; y_1, y_2, x, H)$$

$$= \prod_{y_{1it}=0, y_{2it}=0} \Pr(y_{1it}^* \le 0, y_{2it}^* \le 0)$$

$$\times \prod_{y_{1it}=0, y_{2it}=1} \Pr(y_{1it}^* \le 0, y_{2it}^* > 0)$$

$$\times \prod_{y_{1it}>,0, y_{2it}=0} \Pr(y_{1it}^* = y_{1it}, y_{2it}^* \le 0)$$

$$\times \prod_{y_{1it}>0, y_{2it}=1} \Pr(y_{1it}^* = y_{1it}, y_{2it}^* > 0). \tag{16.4}$$

The first term on the right-hand side of this equation is the probability that individual i has zero Medicare expenditures in year t, and does not die that year; the second term is the probability that the individual has zero expenditures but dies in period t; the third term indicates that i has positive expenditures of y_{1it} and does not die; while the fourth term is the probability that the individual has expenditures of y_{1it} but dies in year t. Note that there is no simple classical estimation solution to this problem. Maximum likelihood estimation would require not only evaluation of the bivariate probabilities in the four terms of Equation 16.4, but also integration over the random individual-specific intercepts b_{1i} and b_{2i}.

Preliminary examination of the data suggested that the distribution of average monthly Medicare expenditures was heavy-tailed. Consequently, robust alternatives to the joint normality assumption on the period-specific error terms in Equations 16.1a and b and (1b) are considered. A simple alternative is to allow ε_{1it} and ε_{2it} to follow a multivariate t distribution with ν df. Lower

values of ν allow for heavier-tailed distributions of the type observed in the Medicare expenditure data. In the application below, $\nu = 5$ to allow for very heavy tails.

A minor complication in the construction of the model arises from the fact that health care expenditures y_{1it} are not observed during periods in which individual i is enrolled in a HMO, although mortality y_{2it} is. As a result, only the non-HMO observations are used to estimate the parameters of the expenditure equation. However, because death is observed for individuals enrolled in HMOs, all observations are used to estimate the mortality equation.

ESTIMATING THE IMPACT OF HMOS ON MEDICARE EXPENDITURES AND MORTALITY

To assess the selection effects associated with HMO enrolment and disenrolment, this paper follows a strategy similar to that of Heckman and Hotz [12] in their analysis of selection and cream-skimming effects in manpower training programmes. In particular, let H_{1it} consist of two variables: (1) PREHMO$_{it}$ which equals 1 if i enrols in a HMO in a subsequent period $t^* > t$; and (2) POSTHMO$_{it}$ = 1 if i had been enrolled in a HMO in a previous period $t^{**} < t$, but is not currently enrolled. Consider the interpretation of PREHMO$_{it}$. Because *future* HMO enrolment status cannot directly impact *current* health care expenditures, the coefficient on PREHMO$_{it}$ only reflects selection effects. For example, a negative coefficient on PREHMO$_{it}$ implies that HMOs enrol healthier patients, since prior to enrolment future enrolees had lower health care expenditures than other individuals. Similarly, if HMOs disenrol sicker, more costly patients, then one would expect a positive coefficient on POSTHMO$_{it}$ in the expenditure regression, since disenrolees would likely have greater expenditures than individuals never in a HMO.

For the mortality equation, H_{2it} includes indicators for HMO status, HMO$_{it}$, and disenrolment, POSTHMO$_{it}$. Note that PREHMO$_{it}$ is not included since it only equals 1 if the individual survives to enrol in a HMO. If HMOs cream-skim healthier individuals, then HMO members should have lower mortality probabilities, implying a negative coefficient on HMO$_{it}$ in the mortality equation. Of course, if HMOs provide lower quality care, perhaps by restricting access to health care resources, then HMO members might have a higher probability of death. Finally, if HMOs have an incentive to disenrol sicker, more costly patients, then a positive coefficient on POSTHMO$_{it}$ in the mortality equation might be expected, since these individuals may be more likely to die.

INTERPRETING THE CROSS-EQUATION CORRELATIONS

The model described in Equations 16.1–16.4 provides two useful insights into the relationship between health care expenditures and mortality. First, note that individuals with positive values of b_{2i} will tend to have higher probabilities of mortality at each period in the sample, which may be interpreted as being in poorer health throughout the panel. Positive values of d_{12} then indicate that these individuals also tend to have higher 'permanent' health care expenditures over the 1984–1991 period, i.e. a positive value of b_{1i}. Second, if individuals substantially increase their use of health care resources in the last year of life, then the covariance σ_{12} should be positive.

BAYESIAN MCMC SAMPLING FOR THE MODEL

The Bayesian MCMC implementation of the model described in the 'A Tobit Model of Medicare Expenditures with Survival' section closely follows Chib's [8] simulation of the tobit model and Chib and Greenberg's [9] analysis of the multivariate probit model. Much of the sampling algorithm is straightforward and will only be sketched here. Further information on the construction of MCMC samplers may be found in these papers, and in Carlin and Louis [13].

PRIOR SPECIFICATION

The first step in a Bayesian model is the formation of prior distributions for the parameters of the model, β, Σ, and D. Following standard practice, the prior on β is assumed to be multivariate Gaussian with $N(\beta_0, B_0)$. The free elements of the variance–covariance matrix, $\sigma = (\sigma_{11}, \sigma_{12})$, are assumed to follow a truncated normal prior distribution, $\sigma \sim TN(s_0, S_0)$. Truncation is required to assure that Σ is positive definite. Finally, the inverse of the random effect variance–covariance matrix, D^{-1}, is assumed to follow a Wishart distribution with parameters r_0 and R_0. For the estimates reported below, the parameters of these distributions are assigned subjectively to yield diffuse priors, although alternative priors generated from a training sample yielded similar results.

POSTERIOR SIMULATION ALGORITHM

The posterior density of the parameters, conditional upon the data, is

$$\pi(\beta, \sigma, D \,|\, y, x) \propto \pi(\beta, \sigma, D) f(y \,|\, \beta, \sigma, D, x), \qquad (16.5)$$

where the first term on the right-hand side of the equation is the prior density, and the second term is the data likelihood. The goal of the analysis is to learn about the joint posterior distribution of the parameters. For example, one may wish to know the mean value of the distribution of β and whether it is centred on zero. Although the left-hand side of Equation 16.5 is typically difficult to recover analytically, the posterior distribution of the parameters may be recovered by taking a large number of draws from it using Monte Carlo simulation methods. In addition, efficiency in the simulation process is often gained by drawing the current values of the parameters conditional upon their values from the previous iteration. After a 'burn-in' period of m iterations, this Markov chain should converge to a stationary distribution independent of the initial values of the parameters used in the simulation.

In Gibbs sampling, further simplifications can be gained by sequentially drawing values for subsets of the parameters (conditional upon the other parameters), rather than all the parameters at once, if the joint posterior distribution $\pi(\beta, \sigma, D \,|\, y, x)$ is very complex. To illustrate how this is carried out, consider the $(k + 1)$ iteration of the sampler. The sampler proceeds by drawing a value $\beta^{(k+1)}$ conditional upon the most recent values of the other parameters, $\sigma^{(k)}$ and $D^{(k)}$, from the full conditional distribution $\pi(\beta \,|\, \sigma^{(k)}, D^{(k)}, y, x)$. This draw is then followed by drawing $\sigma^{(k+1)}$ conditional upon $\beta^{(k+1)}$ and $D^{(k)}$ from $\pi(\sigma \,|\, \beta^{(k+1)}, D^{(k)}, y, x)$, and then by drawing $D^{(k+1)}$ conditional upon $\beta^{(k+1)}$ and $\sigma^{(k+1)}$ from $\pi(D \,|\, \beta^{(k+1)}, \sigma^{(k+1)}, y, x)$. These full conditional distributions take convenient functional forms such as the conditional normal distribution. This process is repeated a large number of times. At the end of the sampling process, analysis consists of examination of the n simulated values of (β, σ, D) obtained from the MCMC sampler, after excluding the first m values (the 'burn-in' phase).

A particular advantage of the Bayesian approach in limited dependent variable problems is that rather than maximizing the observed data likelihood, the MCMC sampler simplifies the problem by taking advantage of 'data augmentation' [14]. Evaluation of the data likelihood in Equation 16.4 is quite complicated, requiring high order numerical integration. However, if the underlying latent variables y_{1it}^{*} and y_{2it}^{*} were actually observed in the data, then Equations 16.1a and b would constitute a two equation Seemingly Unrelated Regression (SUR) model [15], which is easily estimated. The MCMC approach augments the parameter vector (β, σ, D) with the unobserved latent variables y_{1it}^{*} and y_{2it}^{*}, which will be generated using Equations 16.1a and b.

Note that y_{1it}^{*} is only observed if expenditures are positive. Consequently, in this case data augmentation only requires the construction of y_{1it}^* for observations where observed expenditures are zero (implying that $y_{1it}^* \leq 0$). These values are generated using Equation 16.1a by drawing ε_{1it} from a multivariate t distribution with mean zero and variance Σ under the constraint that the resulting y_{1it}^* must be less than or equal to zero. In the case of mortality, only the sign of y_{2it}^* is known, so values are generated using Equation 16.1b by drawing ε_{2it} from the multivariate t distribution with mean zero and variance Σ under the constraint that the resulting y_{2it}^* must be positive (negative) if $y_{2it} = 1$ ($= 0$). Then, conditional upon y_{1it}^* and y_{2it}^*, the remaining parameters (β, σ, D) can be simulated using the SUR model in Equations 16.1a and b, although further data augmentation is used to simulate D. Chib and Hamilton [16] provide a full discussion of this data augmentation step. Complete details of the simulation algorithm may be found in the Appendix.

POSTERIOR ANALYSIS

The model is fit to the Medicare data using 2500 MCMC iterations (due to the large sample size) with an initial burn-in of 500 iterations using default priors. The model was also estimated using priors constructed from a training sample of 373 observations not used in the analysis, and the results were virtually identical. To give an indication of the performance of the sampler, Figure 16.1 plots the autocorrelation functions for the 2500 simulated values of selected parameters, including the coefficients on PREHMO_{it} (α_{11}) and POSTHMO_{it} (α_{12}) in the expenditure equation, from the MCMC output for the analysis sample. If the sampler is performing well, any serial correlation in the simulated values of the par-

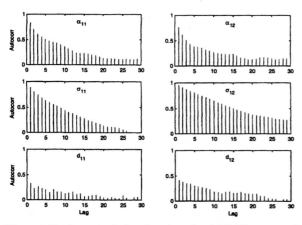

Figure 16.1. Autocorrelation functions for MCMC output of selected parameters

ameters should die out quickly. The plots show that the autocorrelations decline rapidly, indicating that the sampler is mixing well.

Because expenditures are so strongly skewed, models using both the level of expenditure (divided by 100 for scaling reasons) and a transformation of expenditure/100 as dependent variables in Equation 16.1a were estimated. While the natural logarithm is a commonly used transformation for right-skewed dependent variables, it cannot be used here because of the presence of individuals with zero expenditure. As an alternative, the transformation used in this paper takes the cube root of expenditures/100. The cube root transformation is often used in statistics when the dependent variable is right-skewed and takes on non-negative values including zero. In addition to the multivariate t models with $\nu = 5$ df reported in the paper, I also attempted to estimate the model assuming normally distributed disturbances. However, it was impossible to fit the normal model when using the level of expenditure as the dependent variable because of the large number of outlying observations, which caused the estimates of Σ to continually bump up against the positive definiteness constraint. Consequently, distributions allowing for heavier tails are required for this data.

Table 16.3 reports the posterior means and SDs of the 2500 values for each of the parameters in the model. The left two columns present the results using the cube root of expenditures in Equation 16.1a, while the right two columns report the results when the level of expenditure is used as the dependent variable. Note that the coefficient estimates in the expenditure regressions refer to changes in latent expenditures, which incorporates both the effect on the probability of positive expenditure, and the change in expenditures conditional on positive expenditure.

The estimates are generally similar when using the level of expenditure or its cube root transformation. For the expenditure equations in the first and third columns, the negative coefficient estimates on PREHMO in the second row indicate that prior to enrolment, prospective HMO members had lower health care expenditures. This finding is stronger using expenditure levels, perhaps reflecting the presence of influential outliers. This provides evidence of cream-skimming on the HMOs part, and the result is similar to Morgan et al.'s [5] finding that future HMO members were less likely to have used inpatient services in the year prior to enrolment compared to those remaining in FFS.

Table 16.3 also shows that individuals disenroled from HMOs had lower health care expenditures, as indicated by the negative mean value of the coefficient on POSTHMO. This surprising result is at odds with some of the previous literature [5,7], which finds that disenrolees have higher expenditures. Some of the difference

Table 16.3 Posterior estimates for training and analysis samples

Variables	Cube root transformation		Levels	
	Expenditure/100	Mortality	Expenditure/100	Mortality
HMO	—	−0.643 (0.240)	—	−0.228 (0.224)
PREHMO	−0.149 (0.098)	—	−0.311 (0.126)	—
POSTHMO	−0.258 (0.102)	0.035 (0.287)	−0.401 (0.158)	0.064 (0.532)
Age	0.032 (0.010)	0.111 (0.015)	0.058 (0.013)	0.121 (0.024)
Education	0.021 (0.011)	−0.029 (0.015)	0.030 (0.011)	−0.047 (0.016)
Male	−0.037 (0.061)	1.022 (0.143)	−0.026 (0.063)	1.205 (0.091)
White	0.107 (0.078)	0.071 (0.184)	0.288 (0.116)	−0.077 (0.146)
# Health conditions	0.094 (0.019)	0.099 (0.029)	0.160 (0.025)	0.029 (0.036)
Days ill	0.001 (0.001)	0.007 (0.002)	0.002 (0.001)	0.008 (0.002)
Heart condition	−0.006 (0.066)	0.133 (0.092)	0.153 (0.084)	0.207 (0.084)
Previous myocardial infarction	−0.011 (0.099)	0.561 (0.149)	0.052 (0.122)	0.796 (0.150)
Net income/100	0.000 (0.001)	−0.001 (0.0002)	0.000 (0.001)	−0.001 (0.0002)
Owns home	−0.070 (0.098)	−0.372 (0.143)	−0.098 (0.089)	−0.386 (0.160)
Time	0.026 (0.012)	0.134 (0.058)	0.041 (0.021)	0.250 (0.086)
Time^2	0.021 (0.009)	−0.046 (0.068)	0.043 (0.023)	−0.258 (0.098)
Constant	−2.424 (0.686)	−12.589 (1.079)	−5.008 (0.887)	−13.717 (1.719)
σ_{11}	0.289 (0.003)		2.260 (0.037)	
σ_{12}		0.276 (0.006)	0.237 (0.024)	
d_{11}	0.747 (0.028)		1.839 (0.061)	
d_{12}		0.227 (0.033)	0.076 (0.053)	
d_{22}		3.214 (0.100)		3.304 (0.108)
n		28 078		28 078

Dependent variables are average monthly expenditure/100 or its cube root, and mortality.
Table presents posterior means with SD in parentheses.

may be due to the fact that previous studies have focussed on expenditures within 3–12 months after disenrolment, whereas the findings from this paper examine expenditures from disenrolment until the end of 1991. To investigate this possibility, the model was re-estimated after changing POSTHMO to be equal to one only for the first year after discharge, and zero thereafter. The estimate for this specification of POSTHMO in the (cube root) expenditure equation was 0.026, with a SD of 0.075, indicating that the result in the literature reflects short-term effects.

Turning to the mortality estimates in the second and fourth columns, HMO members have a lower probability of mortality. Thus, the evidence does not indicate that HMOs increase the mortality risks of their members, perhaps through restricted access to health care resources, as some have argued. Moreover, former HMO members do not have substantially higher mortality probabilities.

The remainder of the coefficients behave as expected. Individuals with more health problems have higher health expenditures, while the presence of a heart condition or a previous myocardial infarction (heart attack) increases the probability of mortality over the panel. Of notable interest are the estimates for σ_{12} and d_{12}. The positive estimate for σ_{12} indicates that period-specific

shocks, which increase mortality probabilities, are also associated with higher levels of expenditure. Thus, Medicare costs are higher in the last year of life. The positive estimate of d_{12} indicates that individuals who were more likely to die earlier in the panel also tended to have higher expenditures in each year.

A TWO-PART MODEL OF EXPENDITURE

To further investigate the relationship between HMO selection and Medicare expenditures, a two-part model of health care expenditures was estimated specifying separate equations for the probability of positive expenditure by individual i in year t, and the (cube root of) total expenditure of the individual in the given year if it was positive. Let y_{11it} be a 0–1 indicator of positive health care expenditure for individual i in year t, and let y_{11it}^* denote its associated latent variable. Let y_{12it} be the level of expenditure if expenditure is positive (i.e. when $y_{11it} = 1$), and y_{12it}^* be the associated latent variable. Equation 16.1a now becomes

$$y_{11it}^* = \alpha_{11}H_{1it} + x_{it}\beta_{11} + b_{11i} + \varepsilon_{11it}, \qquad (16.1a.1)$$

and

$$y^*_{12it} = \alpha_{12}H_{1it} + x_{it}\beta_{12} + b_{12i} + \varepsilon_{12it}. \qquad (16.1a.2)$$

The error terms and random intercepts follow multivariate t and normal distributions, respectively, with mean zero and variances

$$Var\begin{pmatrix}\varepsilon_{11}\\ \varepsilon_{12}\\ \varepsilon_2\end{pmatrix} = \Sigma = \begin{pmatrix}1 & \sigma_{12} & \sigma_{13}\\ \sigma_{12} & \sigma_{22} & \sigma_{23}\\ \sigma_{13} & \sigma_{23} & 1\end{pmatrix},$$

$$Var\begin{pmatrix}b_{11}\\ b_{12}\\ b_2\end{pmatrix} = D = \begin{pmatrix}d_{11} & d_{12} & d_{13}\\ d_{12} & d_{22} & d_{23}\\ d_{13} & d_{23} & d_{33}\end{pmatrix}.$$

Equations 16.1a.1, 16.1a.2 and 16.1b now form the model to be estimated. This model differs from many two-part models discussed in the literature by allowing for non-zero correlation between unobservables affecting the probability of positive expenditure and those influencing the level of expenditure if it is positive (i.e. σ_{12} is not restricted to equal 0).

Simulation of the two-part model is similar to that for the two equation model presented above. Table 16.4 shows that the differences between prospective HMO enrolees and those who do not enrol in a HMO reflects differences in the probability of positive expenditure, rather than differences in expenditure itself. HMOs thus appear to select individuals who are substantially less likely to have a history of high utilization. Similarly, disenrolees have a much lower probability of positive expenditure, but no difference in expenditure if it is positive. With regard to the remaining independent variables, in most cases the sign of the coefficient estimates are the same across the probability and level of expenditure equations. The notable exception to this pattern occurs in the case of gender, where males have a lower probability of positive expenditure than do females. However, conditional upon utilization, males have significantly higher expenditures.

The positive estimates of σ_{13} and σ_{23} indicate that both the probability and level of expenditure increase in periods when mortality is more likely. The estimate of σ_{12} implies a correlation coefficient of approximately 0.95, so that unobservables affecting the probability and amount of expenditure are highly correlated. Finally, as in Table 16.3, the covariance matrix of the random effects indicates a positive correlation between unobserved 'permanent' individual-specific factors affecting mortality and expenditures. The cross-equation correlations thus reflect both the period-specific relationships between unobservables and permanent effects.

CONCLUSIONS

This paper develops a Bayesian panel data tobit model of Medicare expenditures for recent US retirees, which is implemented using MCMC simulation methods. The results indicate the importance of accounting for survival over the panel, since unobservables which lead to higher mortality probabilities are positively correlated with those implying higher health care expenditure. The model is also novel in that a multivariate t-link is used in place of normality to allow for the heavy-tailed distributions often found in health care expenditure data. The findings indicate cream-skimming on the part of HMOs, since patients with a lower probability of positive expenditure tend to enrol in HMOs. Surprisingly, it does not appear that HMOs disenrol sicker, higher cost patients, and mortality rates are not higher among HMO members.

The findings of this study suggest that Medicare may have difficulty in achieving cost savings through the use of HMOs, given current reimbursement methodologies. Morgan et al. [5] note that the capitated rate paid to Medicare HMOs is 95% of the average cost of FFS care. If HMOs have lower expenditures due in part to selection, then this methodology rewards HMOs for cream-skimming rather than cost reduction, as is desired by Medicare. Clearly, further research is important for understanding the impact of managed care on Medicare. Because of data limitations, the sample only covers the 1984–1991 period, while substantial increases in the HMO enrolment occurred in the early 1990s. It would be useful to know whether the selection of low expenditure patients into HMOs continued during this expansionary period. More importantly, the data is limited in that expenditures are not reliably reported during the period of HMO enrolment. As a result, HMO and non-HMO costs cannot be directly compared. The availability of data on health care expenditures during HMO enrolment would certainly be of great value in assessing whether HMOs constrain costs, net of selection effects. With the appropriate data, the statistical framework developed in this paper could easily be adapted to address these issues.

ACKNOWLEDGEMENTS

I would like to thank Sid Chib, Vivian Ho, Dana Goldman, Rab Manning, two referees and participants at the Seventh European Workshop on Econometrics and Health Economics in Helsinki for many helpful comments, and Terry Lum for bringing the data set to my attention.

Table 16.4 Posterior estimates for two-part model of expenditure

	Pr(expenditure > 0)	Cube root of expenditure/100	Mortality
HMO	—	—	−0.530 (0.147)
PREHMO	−0.345 (0.091)	0.033 (0.046)	—
POSTHMO	−0.522 (0.129)	0.002 (0.067)	0.116 (0.265)
Age	0.061 (0.012)	0.037 (0.004)	0.105 (0.017)
Education	0.054 (0.010)	0.010 (0.007)	−0.032 (0.016)
Male	−0.178 (0.056)	0.129 (0.052)	0.994 (0.078)
White	0.390 (0.073)	0.019 (0.036)	−0.146 (0.120)
# Health conditions	0.183 (0.022)	0.061 (0.009)	0.080 (0.042)
Days ill	0.001 (0.001)	0.002 (0.0005)	0.006 (0.001)
Heart condition	0.312 (0.057)	0.037 (0.047)	0.088 (0.093)
Previous myocardial infarction	−0.008 (0.089)	0.018 (0.043)	0.504 (0.117)
Net income/1000	0.0004 (0.0001)	−0.0001 (0.00005)	−0.0004 (0.0004)
Owns home	0.008 (0.060)	−0.152 (0.034)	−0.434 (0.098)
Time	0.035 (0.020)	0.003 (0.007)	0.095 (0.045)
Time^2	0.148 (0.023)	0.013 (0.008)	−0.069 (0.060)
Constant	−4.905 (0.821)	−2.252 (0.301)	−11.440 (1.136)
σ_{12}	0.418 (0.009)		
σ_{13}	0.448 (0.013)		
σ_{22}		0.190 (0.003)	
σ_{23}		0.204 (0.008)	
d_{11}	1.908 (0.058)		
d_{12}	0.335 (0.020)		
d_{13}	0.069 (0.044)		
d_{22}		0.413 (0.012)	
d_{23}		0.149 (0.022)	
d_{33}			2.182 (0.069)

Dependent variables are indicator of positive expenditure, cube root of expenditure/100|expenditure > 0, mortality.
Table presents posterior means with SDs in parentheses. Estimates based on sample of 28 078 observations.

APPENDIX: DETAILS OF THE MCMC SIMULATION ALGORITHM

This simulation algorithm is very similar to that in Chib and Hamilton [16]. The main complication in the sampling of the model is that restrictions must be imposed on Σ, namely that the $Var(\varepsilon_{2it}) = 1$. Consequently, the Metropolis–Hastings algorithm must be used to sample σ. In addition, to allow the errors to follow a multivariate t distribution, suppose that the error terms in Equations 16.1a and 16.1b are now specified as

$$\begin{pmatrix} \varepsilon_{1it} \\ \varepsilon_{2it} \end{pmatrix} \sim N\left(\begin{pmatrix} 0 \\ 0 \end{pmatrix}, \lambda_{it}^{-1}\Sigma \right),$$

where the independently distributed random variable λ_{it} follows a gamma $(v/2, v/2)$ distribution. In this case, it can be shown that the error terms follow a multivariate t distribution with v df [14].

Let y_{it}^* denote (y_{1it}^*, y_{2it}^*). The $(k + 1)$ iteration of the simulation algorithm involves the following steps:

1. Sample $\{y_{it}^*\}^{(k+1)}$ from $\{y_{it}^*\} \mid \{y_{1i}, y_{2i}\}$, $\{b_i\}^{(k)}$, $\beta^{(k)}$, $\Sigma^{(k)}$, $\{\lambda_{it}\}^{(k)}$ (data augmentation).
2. Sample $\sigma^{(k+1)}$ from $\sigma \mid \{y_{it}^*\}^{(k+1)}$, $\{b_i\}^{(k)}$, $\beta^{(k)}$, $\{\lambda_{it}\}^{(k)}$ using the Metropolis–Hastings algorithm.
3. Sample $\beta^{(k+1)}$ from $\beta \mid \{y_{it}^*\}^{(k+1)}$, $\{b_i\}^{(k)}$, $\Sigma^{(k+1)}$, $\{\lambda_t^i\}^{(k)}$.
4. Sample $\{\lambda_{it}\}^{(k+1)}$ from $\{\lambda_{it}\} \mid \{y_{it}^*\}^{(k+1)}$, $\{b_1\}^{(k)}$, $\Sigma^{(k+1)}$.
5. Sample $\{b_i\}^{(k+1)}$ from $\{b_i\} \mid \{y_{it}^*\}^{(k+1)}$, $D^{(k)}$, $\beta^{(k+1)}$, $\Sigma^{(k+1)}$, $\{\lambda_{it}\}^{(k+1)}$ (data augmentation).
6. Sample $D^{(k+1)}$ from $D \mid \{b_i\}^{(k+1)}$.
7. Repeat steps (1)–(6) using the most recent values of the conditioning variables.

The algorithm indicates that once data augmentation for the dependent variable is performed in Step (1), the remainder of the simulation steps condition on the latent dependent variable y_{it}^*. Note that in Step (1), y_{1it}^* is drawn from a normal distribution truncated to the interval $(-\inf, 0)$ if $y_{1i} = 0$ (recall that $y_{1i} = y_{1i}^*$ if $y_{1i} > 0$). Similarly, y_{2i}^* is drawn from a normal distribution truncated to the interval $(-\infty, 0)$ if $y_{2i} = 0$, and from the interval $(0, \infty)$ if $y_{2i} = 1$ [17].

REFERENCES

1. Phelps, C. *Health Economics*, 2nd edn. New York: Harper Collins, 1997.
2. Miller, R. and Luft, H. Managed care plan performance since 1980: a literature analysis. *Journal of the American Medical Association* 1994; **271**: 1512–1519.
3. Goldman, D., Leibowitz, A. and Buchanan, J. Cost-containment and adverse selection in Medicaid HMOs. *Journal of the American Statistical Association* 1998; **93**: 54–62.
4. Baker, L. The effect of HMOs on fee-for-service health care expenditures: evidence from Medicare. *Journal of Health Economics* 1997; **16**: 453–481.
5. Morgan, R., Virnig, B., DeVito, C. and Persily, N. The Medicare–HMO revolving door – the healthy go in and the sick go out. *The New England Journal of Medicine* 1997; **337**: 169–175.
6. Strumwasser, I. *et al.* The triple option choice: self-selection bias in traditional coverage, HMOs and PPOs. *Inquiry* 1989; **26**: 432–441.
7. Riley, G., Ingber, M. and Tudor, C. Disenrollment of Medicare beneficiaries from HMOs. *Health Affairs* 1997; **16**: 77–92.
8. Chib, S. Bayes inference in the Tobit Censored Regression Model. *Journal of Econometrics* 1992; **51**: 79–99.
9. Chib, S. and Greenberg, E. Analysis of multivariate probit models. *Biometrika* 1998; **85**: 347–361.
10. Cowles, M., Carlin, B. and Connett, J. Bayesian tobit modeling of longitudinal ordinal clinical trial compliance data with nonignorable missingness. *Journal of the American Statistical Association* 1996; **91**: 86–98.
11. Little, R. and Rubin, D. *Statistical analysis with missing data*. New York: John Wiley, 1987.
12. Heckman, J. and Hotz, J. Choosing among alternative nonexperimental methods for estimating the impact of social programs: the case of manpower training. *Journal of the American Statistical Association* 1989; **84**: 862–874.
13. Carlin, B. and Louis, T. *Bayes and empirical Bayes methods for data analysis*. London: Chapman & Hall, 1996.
14. Tanner, M. and Wong, W. The calculation of posterior distributions by data augmentation (with discussion). *Journal of the American Statistical Association* 1987; **82**: 528–550.
15. Zellner, A. An efficient method of estimating seemingly unrelated regressions and tests for aggregation bias. *Journal of the American Statistical Association* 1962; **57**: 348–368.
16. Chib, S. and Hamilton, B. Bayesian analysis of cross-section and clustered data selection models. Mimeo, Olin School of Business, Washington University, 1999.
17. Albert, J. and Chib, S. Bayesian analysis of binary and polychotomous response data. *Journal of the American Statistical Association* 1993; **88**: 669–679.

Index